Muscular Exercise and the Lung

Proceedings of a symposium held at the
University of Wisconsin-Madison
1976
with support from the Syntex Laboratories, Inc.
and Boehringer Ingleheim Ltd.

MUSCULAR
EXERCISE
and the
LUNG

Edited by

Jerome A. Dempsey

Charles E. Reed

The University of Wisconsin Press

Published 1977

The University of Wisconsin Press
Box 1379, Madison, Wisconsin   53701

The University of Wisconsin Press, Ltd.
70 Great Russell Street, London

First Printing

Printed in the United States of America

For LC CIP information see the colophon

ISBN 0-299-07220-7

Contents

Preface

Historically, substantial precedence exists for the use of exercise stress to elucidate problems of human pulmonary physiology. In the early 1900's August Krogh and J. S. Haldane incorporated exercise testing as an integral part of their fundamental studies into human pulmonary gas exchange and high altitude adaptation. The respectability of "exercise physiology"--at both a basic and applied level of study--is probably attributable to the extensive work of David B. Dill and his colleagues at the Harvard Fatigue Laboratory in the 1920's and 1930's. This broad field of exercise physiology gradually encompassed adaptative mechanisms in all organ systems, with particular emphasis in recent years on muscle biochemistry and clinical cardiology; and in the mid-50's the ever expanding interest in this field in North America was expressed in the formation of the present day American College of Sports Medicine.

The work presented in this symposium proceedings represents an extension and a tribute to the contributions of Erling Asmussen of Copenhagen's August Krogh Institute. Professor Asmussen's work has spanned more than three decades in this area of human pulmonary adaptations to muscular work. While he is best known for his studies of the problem of human exercise hyperpnea, he and his colleague, Marius Nielsen, also conducted landmark investigations into such problems as pulmonary gas exchange, dead space and lung-volume subdivisions and high altitude acclimatization in exercising man. On the occasion of the publication of these proceedings, we are pleased to recognize the contributions of Professor Asmussen which have truly provided much of the essential impetus for present-day studies of muscular exercise and the lung.

This symposium presents research findings in four basic areas of pulmonary physiology, with specific emphasis on their application to man at work in both health and disease. The first section on mechanics of the lung and chest wall emphasizes newer work on the control of respiratory muscle function and the neural control of breathing. The dilemma of mechanisms of exercise hyperpnea is discussed and debated with adequate representation from the various schools of thought. As expected this perplexing question remains controversial; although the reported findings and lively, lengthy discussions clearly provide a basis for new, meaningful interpretations of the traditional concepts of "neural" and "humoral" mediation of exercise hyperpnea. The control of airway calibre is covered in two sessions; the first dealing with basic questions of neural, chemical, pharmacologic and mechanical control of the airways; and the second attempting to apply the basic mechanisms to the clinical dilemma of exercise-induced bronchospasm. The final section deals with the broad question of control of pulmonary gas exchange during exercise and highlights the application of newer techniques to problems of ventilation:perfusion distribution, regulation of pulmonary capillary blood flow and alveolar:capillary diffusion.

We are indebted to Ms. Naomi Wells who almost single-handedly conducted the arrangements for this symposium and the preparation of the proceedings. We also gratefully recognize the interest and financial support provided by the Syntex Laboratories, Inc. (Palo Alto, California) and Boehringer Ingleheim Ltd. (Elmsford, New York).

We wish to acknowledge the contributions of several individuals at the University of Wisconsin: to graduate students, fellows and colleagues; Charles Irvin, Dale Pelligrino, Martin Mastenbrook, Brent Kooistra, Robert Bush, Timothy Musch, Peter Hanson, Burt Olson, Monique Wanner and William Reddan who assisted in the conduct of the meetings and the transcription of the discussion sessions; to Ms. Edith Heggland for the conference center arrangements; to Candace Anderson and Judith Mayfield for secretarial assistance; and to Ms. Elizabeth Reddan for direction of the social program.

We are also indebted to Dr. John Rankin for his opening remarks which set the stage for the conference and discussions and to Dr. Alfred Fishman for his eloquent summary and interpretations of the conclusions.

Jerome A. Dempsey
Charles E. Reed

Part I
Respiratory Muscles and Breathing Mechanics

1

Respiratory Muscles
& Breathing Mechanics: Introduction

Michael D. Goldman

The goal of studies in respiratory mechanics is the description and analysis of the mechanisms by which the elements of the respiratory system produce the result we call breathing, or pulmonary ventilation. Since the respiratory system includes skeletal muscles, the neural organization of the activity of these muscles represents an important aspect of the mechanisms by which ventilation is produced and controlled. It is only natural then that recent advances in the understanding of respiratory muscles and breathing mechanics have come from the joint efforts of neurophysiologists and respiratory physiologists in this area of investigation. This and the following four chapters bring together the disciplines of neurophysiology, respiratory physiology, biomedical engineering, and clinical chest medicine in an attempt to integrate current knowledge of the organization of the active breathing mechanisms into a useful "package" which may be applied by those studying other aspects of respiration as well as mechanics and control. Our aim is to direct other investigators toward the major issues in the neuromuscular control of breathing (some of which are admittedly unresolved as yet), using ventilation during exercise as a framework for analysis.

Studies of neural (or neuromuscular) respiratory events and those of mechanical events do not provide sufficient basis when viewed separately for an integrated understanding of the functional organization of breathing. These two approaches compliment each other however, and the effectiveness of studies measuring both kinds of events in providing useful insights into the behavior of respiratory muscles is exciting. Indeed the combination of neural and mechanical studies is a common theme in the following chapters.

The most persistently recurring theme in the following four chapters, however, is the fractionation of neural and mechanical events into their component parts. This is done not simply to classify and codify observed phenomena, but rather to gain insight into the way respiratory muscles work. Its usefulness is justified below.

The major role of the respiratory muscles is to develop the pressure changes necessary to produce adequate pulmonary ventilation. From time to time they may be called upon to develop forces in assisting postural movements, to aid in the expulsion of the contents of abdominal viscera, and to control phonation. Thus there

3

is a dichotomy between respiratory acts and non-respiratory acts
(although some might argue that phonation should be considered a
respiratory act). And it is tempting to label the non-respiratory
acts as "voluntary" and the respiratory acts as "automatic." However, volitional control over breathing is everyday knowledge; and
it is clear that the motor act of breathing at the level of the
spinal motor neuron serves two masters — metabolism and volition.
There is reasonably good evidence now (14,15) for believing that
the neural pathways providing voluntary and metabolic control are
largely separate anatomically. In this and the succeeding four
chapters we are concerned with the organization of breathing to
serve the needs of metabolism. However, we can make use of non-
respiratory acts and volitional factors by designing our studies
and structuring our analyses so as to produce known directional
changes in the nature of the neural input to the respiratory muscles
or the mechanical load placed upon them when comparing different
metabolic states.

   We assiduously avoid use of the phrase "central respiratory
drive," for its meaning depends entirely upon one's functional definition of "center." Some investigators view the "respiratory center" as a bulbopontine pacemaker, while others view the spinal
motor neuron as the central integrator of all input to the respiratory muscles. And the emerging importance of segmental and extra
segmental reflex effects on breathing is now becoming increasingly
clear, as is outlined in Chapter 5.

   It should be noted here that while we recognize the importance
of the laryngeal muscles in regulating respiratory airflow (3,4,10),
we largely neglect this important group of respiratory muscles in
the following chapters. That they are important respiratory muscles
and not simply "accessories" is clear to anyone who observes their
remarkable phasic displacements during ordinary breathing. However,
they are not directly accessible for either neural or mechanical
studies in man; and we concentrate our attention instead on the
remaining three major groups of respiratory muscles, namely: the
diaphragm, the rib cage musculature (intercostals and accessories),
and the abdominal musculature.

   Electromyographic studies of the diaphragm suggest that this
muscle contracts uniformly (5). In contrast, studies of the intercostals and thoracic accessories reveal highly non-uniform activation (7,16,17). However, mechanical studies of the effects of contraction of the rib cage muscles cannot distinguish these nonuniformities; and except where specifically stated to the contrary,
inferences drawn from mechanical measurements will be confined to
describing the behavior of the rib cage musculature as a unit.
Similarly, although differences in the behavior of the abdominal
external oblique and rectus have been reported (6,8,9) little is
known of the activation of the other layers of abdominal muscles
(internal oblique and transversus). And again, mechanical measurements permit conclusions only regarding the entire group of abdominal muscles as a unit.

   The conceptual framework for relating neural and mechanical
events in muscle is the length-tension diagram. The three-

dimensional analog of the muscle length-tension diagram is the volume-pressure (V-P) diagram which is the major analytical tool of respiratory mechanics. These diagrams are discussed in detail in Chapter 2. Here we develop the rationale for partitioning the mechanical events represented in such diagrams into their component parts.

The thoracic cavity is bounded by the rib cage and the diaphragm. The rib cage may be viewed as representing the "walls" of the thoracic cavity, and the diaphragm its "floor." Clearly the volume of the thoracic cavity can be increased by outward movement of its walls, or downward movement of its floor, or some combination of both. Since the volume of intestinal gas is normally very small, the abdominal contents behave essentially as a liquid, and downward movements of the diaphragm are associated with outward movements of the abdominal wall. Thus movements of the body surface (rib cage and abdomen) will reflect changes in thoracic volume.

Konno and Mead (13) measured changes in the anteroposterior (A-P) diameters of the rib cage and abdomen in a number of different locations. They found that a large part of the anterior surface of the rib cage moved as a unit as did a significant portion of the anterior abdominal wall. They next investigated whether recordings of A-P diameter change at a single site on each of the two parts — rib cage and abdomen — could be summoned to measure the change in lung volume during spontaneous breathing, and found that they could be to a useful approximation (±10%). Calibration of the rib cage and abdominal A-P diameter signals was accomplished by having subjects perform "isovolume maneuvers." In this maneuver, the subject fixes lung volume by closure of the upper airway and then voluntarily changes abdominothoracic configuration by alternately contracting his abdominal muscles while simultaneously expanding his rib cage and then relaxing the abdominal muscles while depressing the rib cage. That lung volume changes could then be assessed with reasonable accuracy from A-P diameter changes at a single site on each of the rib cage and abdomen was only slightly more remarkable than the wide variety of abdominothoracic shapes that could be maintained voluntarily at a single lung volume.

Mead and coworkers (11,12,13) described the configuration of thorax and abdomen at different lung volumes with all the respiratory muscles relaxed voluntarily, and showed that during spontaneous breathing at rest, the relaxed abdominothoracic configuration is maintained. In agreement with earlier workers (1,2) they found that the abdomen and thorax were distorted from their relaxed configuration by muscle activity during breathing at increased levels of ventilation. It is thus clear that a given change in lung volume can be produced by different combinations of rib cage and abdominal displacements. Displacements of these structures depend not only on muscle activity within each structure but also upon activity of muscles in other parts of the abdominothoracic wall; and any attempt to describe systematically the patterns of respiratory muscle activity and the results of such activity during breathing must therefore take into account the separate volume displacements of rib cage and abdominal walls.

Having established our priorities, we may now proceed to develop the "ground rules" by which we shall evaluate different experimental approaches and review the recent evidence describing the neuromuscular organization of breathing at rest and during exercise. That is the business of Chapters 2, 3, and 5. Chapter 4 presents a systematic approach to the modelling of the respiratory system, integrating recent advances in the analysis of respiratory muscle function from the "physiological engineering" point of view.

REFERENCES

1.   Agostoni, E. and P. Mognoni. J. Appl. Physiol. 21: 1827-1832, 1966.

2.   Agostoni, E. and G. Torri. Respiration Physiol. 3: 318-322, 1967.

3.   Bartlett, D., Jr. and J. E. Remmers. J. Physiol. 247: 22-23P, 1975.

4.   Bartlett, D., Jr. and J. E. Remmers. Respir. Physiol. 18: 194-204, 1973.

5.   Boyd, W.H. and J.V. Basmajian. Am. J. Physiol. 204(5): 943-948, 1963.

6.   Campbell, E.J.M. J. Physiol. 117: 222-233, 1952.

7.   Campbell, E.J.M. J. Anat. (Lond.) 89: 378-386, 1955.

8.   Campbell, E.J.M. and J.H. Green. J. Physiol. 120: 409-418, 1953.

9.   Campbell, E.J.M. and J.H. Green. J. Physiol. 122: 282-290, 1953.

10. Gautier, H., J.E. Remmers and D. Bartlett, Jr. Respir. Physiol. 18: 205-221, 1973.

11. Grimby, G., J. Bunn and J. Mead. J. Appl. Physiol. 24: 159-166, 1968.

12. Grimby, G., M. Goldman and J. Mead. Scand. J. Resp. Dis. (Suppl.) 77: 407, 1971.

13. Konno, K. and J. Mead. J. Appl. Physiol. 22: 407-422, 1967.

14. Newson Davis, J. In: The Respiratory Muscles: Mechanics and Neural Control, edited by E.J.M. Campbell. Saunders: Philadelphia, 1970.

15. Plum, F. In: Breathing: Hering-Breuer Centenary Symposium, edited by R. Porter. Churchill: London, 1970.

16. Sears, T.A. and J. Newson Davis. Ann. N.Y. Acad. Sci. 155: 183-190, 1968.

17. Taylor, A. J. Physiol. 151: 390-402, 1960.

2

Respiratory Muscles: The Generator

Michael D. Goldman

The results of respiratory muscle contraction depend upon the nature of the neural input to the muscles, the effectiveness of the muscles in converting this neural drive into mechanical output, and the mechanical properties of the respiratory system itself (including the passive properties of the chest wall as well as those of the lung). The last-mentioned properties have been more extensively studied, but understanding the functional organization of the active breathing mechanism demands an integrated approach which includes analysis of neural and neuromuscular events as well. This chapter presents an account of the analysis we have developed based upon the study of two aspects of respiratory muscle function, namely, the electrical events associated with muscle contraction.

Neural and Neuromuscular Studies

Electromyographic (EMG) measurements tell us which muscles are active and something about the gradation of such activity. Since a single cell creates the anatomical continuity between the body of a spinal motor neuron and the motor end-plate of a muscle fiber, it is not unreasonable to presume that the intensity of EMG activity in a muscle bears a direct relationship to the excitatory state of the motor neuron innervating the muscle. However, the spinal motor neuron represents the final common pathway which integrates a variety of central and reflex neural inputs, and it is a common error to infer that an increased EMG in a respiratory muscle means an increase in "the output of the respiratory center." Such an inference is justified only when it is known that all cortical and reflex influences have remained constant.

Another limitation of EMG measurements is the practical problem of sampling. Because of the anatomical separation of the intercostal muscles, both in different interspaces and into internal and external layers within a single interspace, it is not possible to infer generalized intercostal activity from measurement at a single site. Indeed, the available evidence (6,24,25) indicates that the pattern of muscle activation during respiratory efforts is highly nonuniform among the different interspaces. Within a given interspace, the internal layer shows activity generally during expiration, and the external layer during inspiration, but phase overlap may occur. And because it is technically difficult to obtain a "pure" single layer recording, the mixed layer recordings obtained in

7

common practice present difficulties in interpretation. The same
considerations apply to the abdominal muscles, where three distinct
layers can be identified anatomically. In contrast, limited evidence describing diaphragm activity (4) suggests the EMG activity
is spatially relatively uniform throughout the muscle. The relatively straightforward interpretation of diaphragm EMG measurements
accounts for its usefulness in neuromuscular studies.

In many instances it is useful to know simply whether or not
a muscle is active; and nothing suits this purpose better than the
EMG. No quantitation is necessary, and the interpretation is either
"on" or "off". The most important limitation of even such a direct
approach is that the electrical activity of a muscle tells us nothing about the mechanical effects of such activity, however. Ultimately we want to know how the respiratory muscles produce breathing,
that is to say, how they produce changes in lung volume appropriate
to metabolism. The first step in acquiring that knowledge is to
define the effect of muscle electrical activity in producing tension. The second step is to relate muscle tension (or its three-
dimensional equivalent, pressure) to the pressure necessary to produce volume displacements of the respiratory system. In the remainder of this section we consider the first step.

The framework for the analysis of electrical and mechanical
studies is the muscle length-tension diagram, illustrated schematically in Figure 2.1a

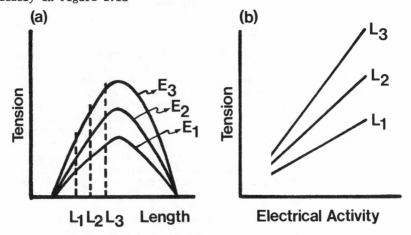

Fig. 2.1 Schematic representation of muscle length-tension diagram
(a) and the relationship between muscle electrical activity and
tension (b). Each curve in (a) represents measurements made during
isometric contraction at a fixed submaximal electrical stimulation
(E_3 E_2 E_1). The maximal stimulus beyond which no further increases
in tension develop is not represented. Each line in (b) represents
the relationship obtained from the family of curves in (a) along a
vertical iso-length line (L_3 L_2 L_1). See text for discussion.

If a muscle is made to contract isometrically with a fixed electrical stimulus, the resulting tension will increase with muscle length
up to a maximum at some optimal length. At any given length, the
tension developed will be greater, the greater the electrical stimulus (up to some maximal stimulus level, not illustrated). Moreover,
the same tension may be developed at different stimulus levels if
length is permitted to change. Thus it is clear that in order to
define the muscle tension resulting from a given amount of muscle
electrical activity, it is necessary to know the length-tension
curve for the muscle and the particular length at which the electrical activity was measured.

Accurate measurements of respiratory muscle length are not
available. The common assumption has been made that all inspiratory
muscles shorten during inspiration and vice-versa for expiratory
muscles. This has led to the notion that lung volume is an adequate
index of respiratory muscle length. However, as outlined in Chapter
1, many recent reports have convincingly demonstrated that thoraco-
abdominal configuration and respiratory muscle geometrics can change
markedly at a given lung volume during both static and dynamic respiratory efforts (2,3,16,17,18). Thus, reports of respiratory
muscle pressure-volume relationships in which lung volume is used as
a direct index of muscle length (21) must be viewed with considerable reserve.

This author and his associates have followed a different
approach (11,13,15). Stimulated by the observation that the abdominal contents behave essentially as a liquid (9) and are thus
virtually incompressible, we reasoned that to a first approximation
the volume displaced by movement of the diaphragm should be closely
similar to that displaced by the abdominal wall. We predicted then
that change in diaphragmatic length should be more directly reflected
in abdominal displacements than in change of lung volume per se. We
demonstrated that this was the case in upright human subjects using
an analysis suggested by Figure 2.1b. During an isometric contraction, there is a unique relationship between electrical activity of
a muscle and the resultant tension, which is different for different
muscle lengths. We instructed subjects to produce such a relationship for the diaphragm by gradually increasing the strength of a
voluntary diaphragmatic contraction while at the same time keeping
the glottis closed and the rib cage and abdomen fixed. Thus, since
no displacements were permitted of lung, rib cage, or abdomen, we
reasoned that such a diaphragmatic contraction was as nearly isometric as possible. We plotted transdiaphragmatic pressure (Pdi)
as an index of tension in the muscle against the intensity of the
diaphragmatic EMG and obtained relationships similar to those in
Figure 2.1b. We found that at a given lung volume we could obtain
very different EMG-Pdi relationships depending on abdominal wall
displacement. Conversely, with the abdominal wall fixed we could
obtain virtually identical EMG-Pdi relationships at different lung
volumes (15). This suggested to us that the diaphragm could be
maintained at a virtually constant length at different lung volumes,
if the thoracoabdominal configuration was properly adjusted by
appropriate activity of rib cage and abdominal muscles; and led to

the somewhat surprising conclusion that inspiratory airflow could
occur with a nearly isometric contraction of the diaphragm. This
prediction was easily tested, again with reference to Figure 2.1b,
since the EMG-Pdi relationships obtained during an isometric contraction (at a given lung volume and thoracoabdominal configuration)
represent the maximum Pdi that can be obtained at a given EMG intensity. If the muscle is allowed to shorten, then the Pdi developed
at that EMG level (measured as the respiratory system passes through
the same lung volume and thoracoabdominal configuration at which the
static, isometric relationship was obtained) must be less than the
isometric Pdi due to the velocity of shortening. Conversely, if
the same Pdi is developed dynamically during inspiratory airflow as
the static isometric contraction produced at a given EMG level,
then we can conclude that the diaphragm contracted isometrically
during inspiratory airflow. We found that the dynamic Pdi indeed
fell in the static EMG-Pdi relationship if outward displacement of
the abdominal wall was prevented during inspiratory airflow. This
maneuver required simultaneous contraction of the abdominal muscles
(antagonistically) during inspiration. Conversely, if outward
abdominal displacements occurred during inspiratory airflow, the
dynamic Pdi was substantially less than the static Pdi, and the
decrement was quantitatively related to the velocity of abdominal
displacement (11,15).

    Thus, for one respiratory muscle, we have established tentative
volume-pressure (analog: length-tension) curves and pressure-flow
(analog: force-velocity) curves using quantitative measurements of
diaphragm electrical activity and mechanical output. Once having
defined these relationships (but only after having done so), we
can infer changes in the output of neural control mechanisms from
measurements of mechanical changes. Thus, with reference to Figure 2.1 again, if we observe an increase or decrease in Pdi at
constant diaphragm geometry, we can infer corresponding increases
or decreases in diaphragm electrical activity. Conversely, if
increases or decreases in Pdi are associated with appropriate
increases or decreases in diaphragmatic length, we can conclude that
diaphragmatic activation has remained constant.

    We have much less extensive information on the rib cage and
abdominal musculature, but in the following section we describe a
comparable approach based upon mechanical measurements alone.

Mechanical Studies

    In the preceding section we showed that it is necessary to have
quantitative measurements of electrical activity as well as mechanical output in order to develop the length-tension relationship for
contracting muscle. We were able to accomplish this for the diaphragm because our sample of diaphragm EMG activity is believed to be
representative of a uniform activity throughout the muscle. The
evidence for this belief is limited to the finding of simultaneous
equal changes in EMG activity in two or more locations in humans and
animals (4,12). We have no such assurance of uniform activity
throughout the rib cage or abdominal musculature. Indeed, as noted
earlier for the intercostals, there is good evidence that activity
is highly nonuniform. Because of this sampling problem, we are

limited to interpreting intercostal and abdominal EMG's as indicating that the muscles are either "on" or "off" and some rough notion
of "great" or "small" activity. But even these limited statements
are of assistance in permitting inferences of respiratory muscle
behavior during spontaneous breathing, along the lines developed
below.
    In Figure 2.1a we represented the active component of the
length-tension diagram of a contracting muscle. But it is well
known that if a relaxed muscle is not stimulated but is stretched
sufficiently, it will develop tension due to lengthening of passive
elastic elements. This is represented schematically in Figure 2.2a
for the purpose of comparison with the volume-pressure diagram shown
in Figure 2.2b.

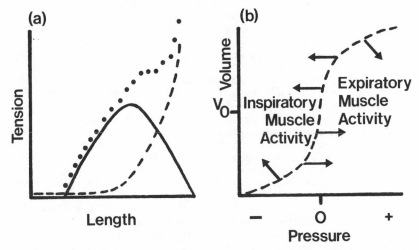

Fig. 2.2 Schematic representation of length-tension curves (a) and
the three-dimensional equivalent (b). In (a), active (continuous
line), passive (dashed), and total (dotted) curves are represented
for one level of muscle activity. The dotted curve is the sum of
dashed and continuous curves. In (b), only the passive curve is represented. The three-dimensional equivalent of length is plotted
on the vertical axis and that of tension on the horizontal. In a
structure with both inspiratory and expiratory muscles, the passive
curve above V0 represents the stretching of passive expiratory muscles, while below V0, it represents stretching of passive inspiratory muscles. In (a) any total tension greater than the passive tension at a given length implies active contraction of the muscle.
In (b) any pressure greater in the positive direction than the
passive pressure at a given volume implies active contraction of
expiratory muscles, and any pressure greater in the negative direction,   activity of inspiratory muscles.

    If the respiratory volume-pressure (V-P) curve is obtained with

all the respiratory muscles relaxed (i.e., passive), then any departure from the passive curve implies activity of some respiratory
muscles(s), and the difference between the active pressure and the
passive pressure at a given volume is a quantitative measure of the
mechanical result of the muscle activity. This was the approach
used by Rohrer (23) and Rahn et al. (22), and later modified by
Campbell (7). The Campbell V-P diagram represented the overall
volume displacements of the respiratory system (i.e., lung volume
changes) on the vertical axis and transthoracic pressure on the
horizontal. This representation was useful to show the inspiratory
and expiratory muscle pressures developed during spontaneous breathing by comparing the dynamic transthoracic pressure developed during
breathing with the static pressure measured during relaxation at the
same lung volume. But as we have already pointed out in the preceding section, lung volume is not an adequate index of respiratory
muscle length, and thus the interpretations one might make from the
Campbell diagram are limited to assessment of net inspiratory or
expiratory muscle activity and some rough notion of gradation. Moreover, as pointed out by others (1,20) the contributions of the
abdominal muscles are not represented at all, nor are those of the
diaphragm which produce changes in abdominal pressure, when only
transthoracic pressure is recorded.

     Konno and Mead (19) partitioned the overall respiratory V-P
curve between the rib cage (rib cage volume vs. transthoracic pressure) and abdomen-diaphragm (abdominal volume vs. transabdominal
pressure). This partitioning made it possible to infer net mechanical activity of muscles operating on these separate parts, and in
particular the activity of the abdominals during inspiration as well
as expiration, could be assessed. However, the specific contributions of the diaphragm, apart from other inspiratory muscles, were
not readily identifiable until after the development of the concept
of mechanical interaction between the diaphragm and rib cage (14)
and the further partitioning of the pressure applied to the rib cage
between the diaphragm on the one hand (rib cage volume vs. transdiaphragmatic pressure) and the intercostals/accessories on the
other (rib cage volume vs. transabdominal pressure).

     Using these V-P diagrams, the contributions of the diaphragm,
the abdominals as a unit, and the intercostals/accessories as a
unit were all represented separately; and the authors concluded that
during quiet breathing, the rib cage as well as the abdomen were both
essentially passive structures and the diaphragm alone performed all
of the mechanical work of breathing (14). Moreover, since the volume
displacements of the separate parts of the chest wall are directly
related to the geometry of the respiratory muscles within each part,
these partitioned V-P diagrams permit inferences as to the neuromuscular organization of breathing. Based on these concepts, an
analysis was developed of the action and coordination of respiratory muscles during breathing at rest and as ventilation increased
progressively during exercise (10) as summarized below.

     In normal subjects, separate passive volume-pressure curves are
obtained for the rib cage, abdomen, and diaphragm. The "passivity"
of such V-P curves is inferred from the consistency of measurements

in trained "relaxers" (14), and is supported by absence of EMG activity from a variety of locations over the thorax and abdomen. Measurements during spontaneous breathing at rest show that the rib cage and abdomen are both moved along their passive V-P curves by the action of the diaphragm. In contrast, the diaphragm departs substantially from its passive curve during inspiration, and rejoins it during the latter portion of expiration. These results are interpreted to indicate that the diaphragm does the whole job during quiet breathing at rest. While the rib cage and abdomen remain passive, the diaphragm develops the entire pressure necessary to produce the volume displacements of the lung and chest wall.

It should be noted here that Taylor's (25) work provides convincing evidence of contraction of internal intercostal muscles in a limited area in the parasternal region during quiet inspiration and in another restricted area anterolaterally during quiet expiration. These observations are not inconsistent with the notion that the diaphragm alone develops the total muscular pressure necessary to produce the inspiratory displacements of the respiratory system during quiet breathing. The absence of EMG in all but these very restricted areas supports our interpretation that the rib cage is essentially a passive structure during quiet breathing in man. Our volume-pressure measurements are not sufficiently sensitive to permit us to infer the intercostal activity to respiratory pressure changes are trivial. Indeed, Taylor noted that "under conditions of quiet breathing, the intercostals contributed little to the effort of respiration" (25). However, when viewed from the perspective of neural control mechanisms, the importance of such activity should not be underestimated. Taylor suggested that the parasternal activity during inspiration is likely to oppose the tendency of the diaphragm to pull the sternum inward. This suggestion is supported by the observations of Bryan and coworkers (26), who showed decreased inspiratory rib cage volume displacements during REM sleep associated with decreased intercostal activity.

As ventilation increases above resting levels, EMG activity of intercostals and abdominal muscles increases (8,25). The volume-pressure diagrams of rib cage and abdomen reflect such activity even at low (50-100W) levels of exercise (10). The departures of abdominal tracings from the passive curve suggest phasic contraction of abdominal muscles beginning in the latter portion of expiration and decreasing during inspiration; while the rib cage tracings indicate activity of inspiratory intercostals/accessories which diminishes during expiration. At moderate exercise levels (100-150W), the rib cage and abdominal V-P tracings indicate that the activity of the rib cage and abdominal musculature is coordinated and timed so as to permit these muscles to take over completely the movement of the chest wall, thereby allowing the diaphragm to expend the pressure it develops entirely on the lung. With further increases in exercise and ventilation, the finely coordinated activity of diaphragm, intercostals, accessories, and abdominals appears to be maintained, each major muscle group increasing its mechanical output together with the others.

It is of interest that the increased abdominal displacements observed during exercise are all in the expiratory direction (10,16, 17). This results in the diaphragm having a greater length (i.e., a more favorable "mechanical advantage") with which to initiate the subsequent inspiration. Furthermore, diaphragmatic length at end-inspiration appears to be no shorter at high levels of ventilation during exercise than during quiet breathing. Thus the rib cage and abdominal muscles, in addition to their contribution to active expiration, appear to permit the diaphragm to operate within a mechanically favorable length range during inspiration as well.

Finally, we may compare this coordinated behavior with the respiratory muscle behavior during encapneic voluntary hyperpnea. In the latter condition, we find a relatively greater participation of rib cage and abdominal musculature at any given ventilation, associated with increased abdominothoracic distortion (5). The volitional element then appears to be associated with a preferential increase in activity of muscles other than the diaphragm. Indeed, during such voluntary hyperpnea at levels which lead to exhaustion of the respiratory muscles within five to ten minutes, we find that just prior to exhaustion there appears to be a great increase in expiratory muscle activity, as if to spare the diaphragm and other inspiratory muscles. The limited usefulness of such expiratory activity is analyzed in Chapter 3.

It must be emphasized that while the conclusions drawn herein are entirely plausible and supported by mechanical measurements, they remain to be confirmed by detailed electromyographic studies. Nevertheless, it is hoped that they will provide a useful framework for the analysis of respiratory muscle behavior until more definitive studies are performed.

Summary
    The complimentary nature of measurements of electrical and mechanical events in muscle is reviewed and the advantages of simultaneous measurements employing both approaches are considered for analyzing the neuromuscular organization of breathing. The muscle length-tension diagram is examined as the basis for studying the relationship between electrical and mechanical measurements in contracting muscle. Results of experiments in upright human subjects during voluntary contraction of the diaphragm are reviewed. These experiments show that diaphragmatic length is reflected most directly in abdominal displacements rather than in change of lung volume per se. Accordingly, the separate volume-pressure diagrams of rib cage and abdomen are developed as three-dimensional analogues of the muscle length-tension diagram. Analysis of the volume-pressure tracings partitioned between the rib cage and abdomen is based on a comparison of pressures developed during spontaneous breathing with those developed by the passive muscular structures during voluntary relaxation of the respiratory muscles. Results in upright man during exercise are reviewed, showing that while the diaphragm performs all of the mechanical work of breathing at rest, activity of rib cage and abdominal musculature increases progressively during exercise, and appears to be coordinated to assist and optimize diaphragmatic function.

REFERENCES

1. Agostoni, E. J. Appl. Physiol. 16(6): 1055-1059, 1961.
2. Agostoni, E. and P. Mognoni. J. Appl. Physiol. 21: 1827-1832, 1966.
3. Agostoni, E. and G. Torri. Respir. Physiol. 3: 318-322, 1967.
4. Boyd, W.H. and J.V. Basmajian. Am. J. Physiol. 204(5): 943-948, 1963.
5. Bradley, M. and M.D. Goldman. Unpublished observations.
6. Campbell, E.J.M. J. Anat. (Lond.) 89: 378-386, 1955.
7. Campbell, E.J.M. The Respiratory Muscles and the Mechanics of Breathing. Chicago: The Yearbook Publishers, Inc., 1958.
8. Campbell, E.J.M. and J.H. Green. J. Physiol. 127: 423-426, 1955.
9. Duomarco, J. and R. Rimini. La Presion Intraabdominal en el Hombre. Buenos Aires, 1947.
10. Goldman, M. In: Loaded Breathing, edited by L.D. Pengelly, A.S. Rebuck and E.J.M. Campbell. Longman Canada Limited, 1974, pp. 50-63.
11. Goldman, M. Bull. Physio-path. Resp. 11(2): 98-101P, 1975.
12. Goldman, M.D., E.N. Bruce, L. Loh, and J. Mead. Fed. Proc. 34(3): 371, 1975.
13. Goldman, M., A. Grassino, J. Mead and T. Sears. Fed. Proc. 31(2): 321, 1972.
14. Goldman, M. and J. Mead. J. Appl. Physiol. 35: 197-204, 1973.
15. Grassino, A. In: Loaded Breathing, edited by L.D. Pengelly, A.S. Rebuck, and E.J.M. Campbell. Longman Canada Limited, 1974, pp. 64-72.
16. Grimby, G., J. Bunn, and J. Mead. J. Appl. Physiol. 24: 159-165, 1968.
17. Grimby, G., M. Goldman, and J. Mead. Scand. J. Resp. Dis. (Suppl.) 77: 407, 1971.
18. Konno, K. and J. Mead. J. Appl. Physiol. 22(3): 407-422, 1967.
19. Konno, K. and J. Mead. J. Appl. Physiol. 24(4): 544-548, 1968.
20. Milic-Emili, J. and J.M. Tyler. J. Appl. Physiol. 18(3): 497-504, 1963.
21. Pengelly, L.D., A. Alderson, and J. Milic-Emili. J. Apply. Physiol. 30(6): 797-805, 1971.
22. Rahn, H., A.B. Otis, L.E. Chadwick, and W.O. Fenn. Amer. J. Physiol. 146: 161-178, 1946.
23. Rohrer, F. Arch, f.d. Ges. Physiol. 165: 419, 1916.
24. Sears, T.A. and J. Newson Davis. Ann. N.Y. Acad. Sci. 155: 183-190, 1968.
25. Taylor, A. J. Physiol. 151: 390-402, 1960.
26. Tusiewicz, K., H. Moldofsky, and A.C. Bryan. Fred. Proc. 35(30: 396, 1976.

3

Pulmonary Mechanics:
The Load

Gunnar Grimby

The increased ventilation during exercise requires that the respiratory muscles produce larger negative pleural pressures during inspiration and positive pressures during expiration. In contrast to inspiration, during expiration there is a maximum pleural pressure at a certain lung volume beyond which airflow does not increase further (1, 11). If pleural pressure exceeds that pressure, ventilation can be termed inefficient (11) as there will be an increased work of breathing without an increase in ventilation.

The extent to which pressure, volume and flow "reserves" are used at various ventilatory levels can be estimated by comparing the pressure-volume and flow-volume curves during spontaneous breathing with those measured during maximum forced inspiration and expiration (MIFV and MEFV). At rest only a minor fraction of the potential volume and flow changes are used, and even at heavy exercise the MIFV and MEFV curves are not usually reached in sedentary young men. With increasing age the MEFV curve becomes more curvilinear (10) and the flow-volume curve during heavy exercise may reach the MEFV curve. In patients with chronic airways obstruction the MEFV curve may be reached already at rest or during moderate exercise (5,12), see Figure 3.1. Such patients are faced with several problems in increasing their ventilation during exercise. They must either increase their inspiratory flow to be able to use a proportionately larger time for expiration, or increase their expiratory flow, which implies that they must increase their end-tidal volume. In the first instance, the flow resistive inspiratory work will increase, and in the latter the elastic inspiratory work will increase. Thus, in both situations to solve the problem of a limitation of the expiratory flow, a greater stress will be placed on the inspiratory muscles. The choice is often, as shown in Figure 3.1, that the end-tidal volume increases during exercise in the patients with airways obstruction (5, 12). The patient then takes advantage of the higher elastic recoil and lower airway resistance in the flow-limiting segments which occur at higher lung volumes (10). Besides the increase in the elastic inspiratory work, an extra amount of work will also be added due to "deformation" of the chest wall. As demonstrated by Mead et al. (9) and Goldman et al. (2) in normal subjects, the abdominal muscle activity acts to maintain the diaphragm in a relatively curved position and, thus, working within its most favorable range. For that purpose, an extra amount of work by the rib cage muscles has to be accepted when they

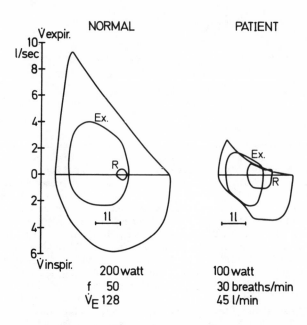

Fig. 3.1. Maximal expiratory and inspiratory flow-volume curves
together with the flow volume curves during breathing at rest (R)
and during exercise (Ex.) in a normal subject (left panel) and a
patient (right panel) with obstructive lung disease (FEV$_1$=1.4 1,
corresponding to 38% of predicted normal value (5).

cause a deviation of the chest wall from its relaxation characteristics. In patients with airway obstruction the larger than normal
increase in tidal volume in an inspiratory direction during exercise
will be achieved by an increase of the rib-cage volume at end-
expiration. However, the diaphragm moves in an expiratory direction
and is, thus, maintained under optimal working conditions for the
subsequent inspiration (3).

It has already been mentioned that at forced expirations at
most lung volumes, a critical pleural pressure is reached at which
a maximum expiratory flow is achieved. As is shown by the isovolume
pressure-flow curves from the paper by Olafsson and Hyatt (11, Fig.
3.2), increases in pressures above the "maximum effective pleural
(transpulmonary) pressure" (Peffmax) do not give a further increase
in flow, because they result in dynamic compression of large airways.

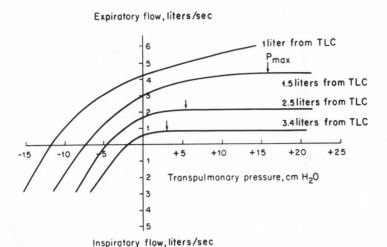

Fig. 3.2. Isovolume pressures - flow curves for a normal subject.
Volume at which each curve was measured is given in liters from
total lung capacity (TLC). Arrows indicate "maximum effective
transpulmonary pressures" (Peffmax).

The question then arises do normal subjects and patients with
lung diseases exceed these pressures. In normals (< 45 yrs),
Olafsson and Hyatt (11) found that the transpulmonary pressure did
not exceed Peffmax even at exhaustive exercise. Thus, it was
suggested that the mechanical properties of the lung do not limit
ventilation during exhaustive exercise in normal sedentary subjects.
Very well-trained men will attain higher ventilation volumes at maximal exercise. In a study of 8 athletes in the age group 19-34
years, with maximal oxygen uptakes of 3.7-5.2 ℓ/min and ventilations
of 128-195 ℓ/min at maximal exercise, it was found that all subjects
reached their MEFV at their highest work load on a bicycle ergometer
(4). In fact, the majority of athletes used most of their "flow
reserve" in achieving their high tidal volumes (Fig. 3.3). They
reached only slightly higher transpulmonary pressures (7-38 cm H_2O)
than normals in spite of higher ventilation and did not exceed their
Peffmax. At fairly heavy, but still submaximal exercise, the pressures were only around or slightly above atmospheric pressure.
Thus, even at very high exercise ventilations, the expiratory pressures in these men were controlled in an "economical" way.
    In patients with obstructive lung disease, somewhat varying
results have been reported. Potter et al. (12) found transpulmonary
pressures in excess of Peffmax indicating that ventilation became
mechanically inefficient. Peffmax values were also lower than in
normal subjects. Grimby and Stiksa (5) showed that these patients

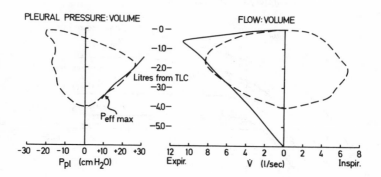

Fig. 3.3. Simultaneous pressure-volume and flow-volume curves for
a tidal breath at near "maximal" exercise in a well-trained young
man with a ventilation of 129 ℓ/min at an oxygen uptake 4.03 ℓ/min.
Respiratory frequency 30 breaths/min. Data from ref. 4. The maximum expiratory flow-volume curve is shown by the continuous line
and the curve during tidal breathing by the interrupted line. On
the pressure-volume curve the continuous line shows the Peffmax-
volume curve and the interrupted curve is the tidal change in
pleural pressure.

reached their MEFV curves at a lower than normal maximal heart rate.
These results demonstrated clearly that the patients were limited
by their ventilatory function. However, the question is how often
inefficient ventilation, as defined above, occurs in patients with
airway obstruction. Leaver and Pride (8) reported that their
patients usually avoided pressures in excess of Peffmax (Fig. 3.4)
and concluded that obstructive patients were able to adjust their
respiratory muscle force properly during heavy exercise. We do not
know why some patients have lost this ability or to what extent in-
struction and training in breathing can help them.
     The work done on the lung during one breath corresponds to the
area encircled by the pulmonary pressure-volume loop (the Campbell
Diagram). In normals there is a relationship between the pulmonary
work of breathing and the ventilation (6). However, the total work
of breathing is not only determined by the pressure-volume loop for
the lung, but also from any amount of work added by the work to dis-
tort the thoraco-abdominal shape from the relaxed configuration.
To estimate this part of the actual work of breathing, the separate
rib cage and abdominal pressure volume loops must be known (2),
assuming that the chest wall is made up of these two parts (7).
At rest, Goldman et al. (2) showed that the two techniques gave
comparable values for the work of breathing. However, the Campbell
Diagram does not give deviating results, but as ventilation increases,
the estimates developed from the rib cage and abdominal tracings

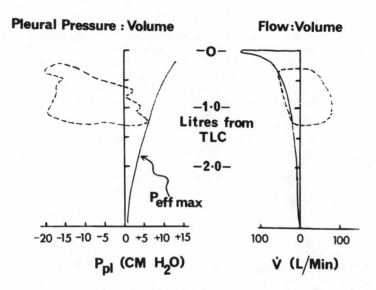

Fig. 3.4. Simultaneous pressure-volume and flow-volume curves for a tidal breath during exercise in a patient with severe airflow obstruction. From ref. 8. For further explanation, see text Fig. 3.3.

revealed greater mechanical work than that estimated from the Campbell Diagram. The differences between methods were as great as 25% in normal subjects at heavy exercise. This is consistent with distortion of the chest wall from the relaxed thoraco-abdominal configuration at higher levels of exercise (9). Such a distortion can be expected to be still more pronounced in patients with airways obstruction (3) (see above). Furthermore, in patients, there may be distortions within the rib cage. The rib cage, then, will no longer behave as if it had only one degree of freedom (7). This problem of distortion, both within the rib cage and between abdomen and rib cage, may also contribute to an "inappropriateness of length-tension relationships", thereby leading to sensations of breathlessness.

These measurements of the total work of breathing have clearly demonstrated that the total work of the respiratory muscles during moderate and heavy exercise is larger than that produced only by the lungs. Thus, analysis of only the pressure-volume relationship for the lung does not demonstrate the total load placed on the generator during increased ventilation at exercise.

Summary

From recordings of the flow-volume and pressure-volume repre-
sentations for the lung, it does not appear that the mechanical
properties of the lung limit ventilation during exhaustive exercise
in normals. The transpulmonary pressures do not exceed those required to produce maximal expiratory flows and ventilation therefore
remains "efficient", also in well-trained subjects, who reach high
ventilations. Patients with airways obstruction reach their maximal expiratory flow-volume curves already at rest or at low work
loads; some of them may even exceed their maximum effective pressures. Besides the work on the lung, deviation of the chest wall
from its relaxed configuration adds an extra amount to the total
work of breathing during moderate and heavy exercise.

REFERENCES

1. Fry, D.L. and R.E. Hyatt. Amer. J. Med., 29:672-689, 1960.
2. Goldman, M., G. Grimby and J. Mead. J. Appl. Physiol., In
    Press, 1976.
3. Grimby, G., B. Elgefors and H. Oxhöj. Scand. J. Resp. Dis.,
    54:45-52, 1973.
4. Grimby, G., B. Saltin and L. Wilhelmsen. Bull. Physio-path.
    Resp., 7:157-168, 1971.
5. Grimby, G. and J. Stiksa. Scand. J. Clin. Lab. Invest., 25:
    303-313, 1970.
6. Holmgren, A., P. Herzog and H. Åström. Scand. J. Clin. Lab.
    Invest. 31:165-174, 1973.
7. Konno, K. and J. Mead. J. Appl. Physiol. 22:407-422, 1967.
8. Leaver, D.G. and N.B. Pride. Scand. J. Resp. Dis. Suppl 77:
    23-27, 1971.
9. Mead, J., M. Goldman and G. Grimby. Scand. J. Resp. Dis.
    Suppl 77:8-13, 1971.
10. Mead, J., J.M. Turner, P.T. Macklem and J.B. Little. J. Appl.
    Physiol. 22:95-108, 1967.
11. Olafsson, S. and R.E. Hyatt. J. Clin. Invest. 48:564-573,
    1969.
12. Potter, W.A., S. Olafsson and R.E. Hyatt. J. Clin. Invest.
    50:910-919, 1971.

DISCUSSION

Goldman: When patients with COPD exercised and exceeded their effective maximal pressure you mentioned that ventilation became inefficient. By "inefficiency" did you mean only that extra pressures
were developing or were you implying that regional distribution of
air flow was inefficient?

Grimby: We don't know what happens to the flow distribution, only
that the COPD patient during exercise can develop flow limiting pressures. In health we have two strong expiratory muscles, but thank-
fully, we do not need that much force during expiration in heavy
exercise.

Dempsey: What is the major distortion that occurs in the coupling
of the rib cage and the abdomen during exercise, or during rebreathing at high ventilatory volume, that causes the work of
breathing to be so much higher when you measure it your way, i.e.,
combining abdominal and rib cage work components, than when you
measure it via the Campbell Diagram.

Grimby: Both rib cage and abdomen are distorted during heavy exercise.

Goldman: I think that both Dr. Grimby and I would agree that it is
the elastic cost of this distortion of rib cage and abdomen that
accounts for the difference between the Campbell Diagram and the
work measured from the separate rib cage and abdominal volume-
pressure tracings. In other words, the Campbell Diagram cannot
tell whether you are breathing normally in a relaxed fashion or with
a squeezed-in belly.

Grimby: In the patients with airway obstruction in whom I showed
the motion: motion diagram for the rib cage and abdomen, one would
assume that there is quite an increase in the distortional work of
the rib cage. The rib cage may then depart from one degree of freedom and it will move differently in different parts. But we do not
know anything about the size of that increased work of breathing.
We can just assume that it is larger than in normals.

McFadden: Are the changes in lung volume that you are reporting
with exercise in the chronic obstructive patients, actively determined by the muscles of the chest wall and abdomen or passively
determined by mechanical properties of lung, per se, i.e. premature
airway closure.

Grimby: I have no definite reasons to believe that they are passively caused by changes in the properties of the lung. In these
patients we measured flow-volume loops immediately after exercise
and they were identical with those just before exercise. We also
followed the diameters of the rib cage and abdomen with the
magnetometers. That was our way to assure that there were no

major change in the total lung capacity so that we could superim-
pose the flow-volume curves on each other.

McFadden: So the residual volumes, for instance, or total lung
capacities before and after exercise in the people with chronic
obstructive lung disease did not change?

Grimby: We assume that these volumes did not change significantly
as far as we could record from the shape of the chest wall; and we
selected people who didn't show exercise induced airway obstruction
for these experiments.

4

Modeling the Respiratory System: Essentials

F. S. Grodins & S. M. Yamashiro

Modeling in General (6). Let me begin by suggesting that all of us in science are modelers in one form or another, implicitly or explicitly, for modeling is an essential component of science. Thus, someone has defined the goal of science as the compression of the maximum number of observations into the minimum number of conceptual principles. This is a good definition because it emphasizes the essential duality of science, i.e., it is neither a collection of facts alone (like a telephone directory) nor a set of conceptual schemes alone (like philosophy) but an inter-dependent combination of both.

It is most appropriate for us to illustrate this definition by a model which we will call a block diagram of the "Science Servo-System" (Fig. 4.1). Its objective as noted above is to compress the maximum number of observations into the minimum number of conceptual principles. To do this it makes hopefully reliable and valid observations on the real word and feeds them through a poorly understood process of bold and inspired abstraction to produce a conceptual scheme. This scheme is simply a set of propositions which help us to think about some aspect of the real world. Depending partly upon our own pre-tentiousness and partly upon currently popular jargon, we could equally well call it an hypothesis, theory, law, or model. To decide whether it really does provide a useful summary of real world behavior, we must feed its propositions into an "Infallible Deducer" in order to obtain logically consistent and directly observable implications which can then be compared with nature. Thus we have a closed loop servo-system designed to minimize the error between the testable implications of our conceptual scheme and real world observations by appropriate modification of the scheme itself. In engineering terminology, this model represents a non-linear adaptive control system, a clear characteristic of its human operator!

We now turn to another problem. Our scheme or model is useless until it is expressed in some form or language which can be communicated to others and processed by our "Deducer." Such expressions may assume a variety of forms as shown in Figure 4.2. Symbolic models may be verbal, pictorial, mathematical, or special purpose computer programs. Physical models may represent

25

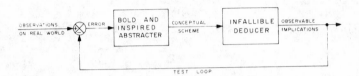

Fig. 4.1 The Science Servosystem

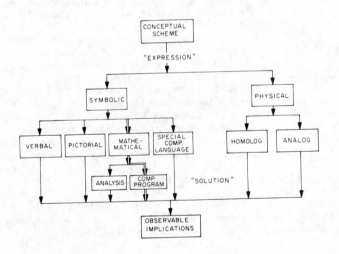

Fig. 4.2 Expression and Solution

structure (homologs), function (analogues), or both. Although useful models may appear in any of these forms, the most highly developed and powerful mode of expression is the mathematical one. This compact, unambiguous, and emotionless language provides rigorous operational rules for manipulation of its symbols, and it is thus able to keep track of complex dynamic causal chains which the human mind cannot trace in any other way. Thus, we are hard pressed to think fruitfully about three interacting variables simultaneously, let alone 100 or more! Moreover, the usefulness of mathematical models has been increased immeasureably in recent years by the development of computer technology which can solve intractable equations numerically at incredible speeds.

Although Figure 4.2 displays a number of forms in which our models can be expressed, it says nothing about their content. This question is addressed in Figure 4.3. If we assume no internal structure but simply express our raw observations directly in one form or another, we have an empirical or descriptive model. This is the least abstract and least general type of model content. If we assume some internal structure and express this rather than our observations, we have a theoretical or explanatory model. Such models may be analytical, i.e., involve the invention of new unit processes, or synthetic, i.e., involve selection and arrangement of conventional unit processes or empirical descriptions into new configurations, or both.

Models of the Respiratory System. Now that we know what models are and how they can be expressed and solved, let us look at some examples of models of the respiratory system. Figure 4.4 is an overall block diagram of the respiratory control system, which, depending on one's point of view, could be called either orienting or disorienting! It does serve to identify the major functional components and their connectivities, and thus allows one to fit detailed models of the various blocks (e.g. respiratory mechanics, cycle control, gas exchange and transport) as well as overall models of the respiratory chemostat into their proper context. In what follows we shall briefly describe two kinds of respiratory models. The first is concerned with optimal control of the respiratory cycle and is closely related to the pump and muscle mechanics we have been discussing this morning. The second is concerned with the chemical control of pulmonary ventilation and will serve to briefly introduce the main issue of this afternoon's session on the hyperpnea of exercise.

Optimal Control of the Respiratory Cycle. Pulmonary ventilation is a cyclic process in which average minute volume is the product of respiratory frequency and tidal volume. Since the same minute volume may be achieved by a variety of such frequency-tidal volume combinations, it is natural to ask what

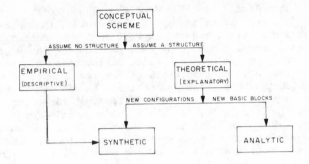

Fig. 4.3 Content of Models

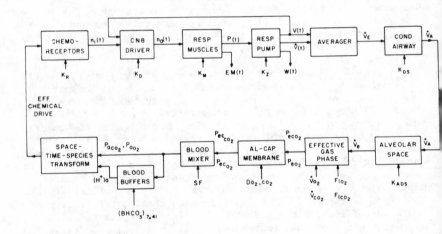

Fig. 4.4 Overall Block Diagram of Respiratory
Control System

criteria determine the particular choice the system makes. Rohrer (13) was the first to advance the hypothesis that the magnitude of mechanical respiratory work is important in the regulation of respiratory frequency. To explore this notion, Rohrer needed a model of the pump mechanics. He assumed the very simple two element mechanical structure shown in Figure 4.5. This mechanical model can also be represented by the electrical analog of Figure 4.6. The equation of motion of this simple first order linear system is:

$$R_{rs} \dot{V} + \frac{1}{C_{rs}} V = P_m. \tag{1}$$

To calculate the work, Rohrer simplified his problem by assuming passive expiration, $\dot{V}$ = constant during inspiration, and $T_I = T_E$. Under these conditions it is easily shown that work per inspiration, W_i, is

$$W_i = \left(\frac{1}{2fC_{rs}} + 2R_{rs} \right) (\dot{V}_A + fV_D)^2. \tag{2}$$

By differentiating (2) with respect to f and setting the result equal to zero, we obtain the optimal frequency for minimal inspiratory work as shown below:

$$f_{opt} = \frac{\sqrt{1 + 32R_{rs} C_{rs} \dot{V}_A/V_D} - 1}{16R_{rs} C_{rs}}. \tag{3}$$

Rohrer noted that resting human breathing rate could be closely predicted by equation (3).

Otis, Fenn and Rahn (10) modified Rohrer's basic model by adding a non-linear resistance, R'_{rs}, and also assumed a sinusoidal air flow pattern. The work rate equation then became:

$$\dot{W} = \left(\frac{1}{2fC_{rs}} + \frac{\pi^2}{4} R_{rs} \right) (\dot{V}_A + fV_D)^2 + \frac{2\pi^2}{3} R'_{rs} (\dot{V}_A + fV_D)^3 \tag{4}$$

and the optimum frequency predicted by setting $d\dot{W}/df$ equal to zero again was close to normal human respiratory rates at rest. If R'_{rs} is omitted from Otis' model but the sinusoidal airflow assumption retained, the optimum frequency is given by

$$f_{opt} = \frac{\sqrt{1 + 4\pi^2 R_{rs} C_{rs} \dot{V}_A/V_D} - 1}{2\pi^2 R_{rs} C_{rs}}. \tag{5}$$

Mead (8) found that equation (5) did not adequately describe frequency changes in moderate to severe exercise in man. Using the same linear, two element model and assuming sinusoidal air flow, Mead explored an alternative criterion which he described

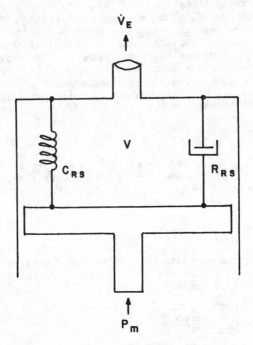

Fig. 4.5 Two Element Mechanical Model

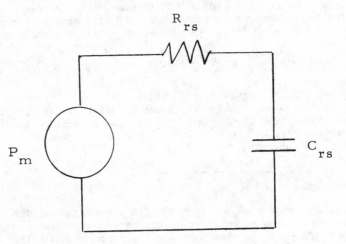

Fig. 4.6 Electrical Analog of Fig. 4.5

as "minimum average force of the respiratory muscles." He developed the following expression for average pressure:

$$\bar{P} = \frac{V_T \sqrt{(2\pi fRC)^2 + 1}}{C} \, . \tag{6}$$

Differentiating (6) with respect to f and equating the derivative to zero yielded the optimal frequency:

$$f_{opt} = \left(\frac{\dot{V}_A}{V_D}\right)^{1/3} (2\pi RC)^{-2/3} \tag{7}$$

Mead concluded that equation (7) predicted frequency behavior in guinea pigs at rest, and in man both at rest and during exercise better than did equation (5), which was based on the minimum work criterion.

In his analysis, Mead equated minimal average force to peak to peak force amplitude, and this presents some problems in interpretation. For the first order linear model used by Mead, the average pressure over one cycle is not in general given by equation (6) (which is pressure amplitude) but rather by:

$$\bar{P}_{2\pi} = \frac{1}{2C} \, (\dot{V}_A/f + V_D) \tag{8}$$

which clearly has no optimal frequency, i.e., $\bar{P}$ decreases monotonically with increasing f. If we take our average over inspiration only, we get:

$$\bar{P}_I = \left(\frac{1}{2C} + 2Rf\right)(\dot{V}_A/f + V_D) \tag{9}$$

and this does yield an equation for f_{opt} which, however, differs from (6):

$$f_{opt} = \sqrt{\frac{1}{4RC} \times \frac{\dot{V}_A}{V_D}} \, . \tag{10}$$

As pointed out by Ruttimann and Yamamoto (14), the problem arises from equating average pressure with pressure amplitude because this ignores the constant term, $(1/C) V_T/2$, corresponding to lung mid-position, which appears in the driving pressure function:

$$P(t) = (V_T/2)\left[\left(\frac{1}{C}\right) + 2\pi fR \sin(2\pi ft) - \left(\frac{1}{C}\right)\cos(2\pi ft)\right] . \tag{11}$$

This means that (6) and (7) contain the implied constraint that chest mid-position stays constant and independent of f and V_T; this in turn implies that any increase in V_T, ΔV_T, is accompanied by a decrease in FRC of $1/2 \, \Delta V_T$.

A qualitative departure from traditional optimization formulations was made by Yamashiro and Grodins in 1971 (16). In all of the studies described above, a particular air flow pattern was always assumed (e.g. constant or sinusoidal) in order to determine an optimal frequency. The latter then became a familiar problem in ordinary calculus, i.e., to determine a minimum point on a function curve. Yamashiro asked instead whether airflow pattern itself could be chosen to minimize work for any given $\dot{V}_A$ and V_D. Note that this complicates the mathematics, for the problem is converted from a familiar one in ordinary differential calculus into a problem in the calculus of variations. Instead of finding a single point on a function, we must now find an entire function which will minimize a given functional (i.e. a function of the function sought). This kind of problem lies at the heart of modern control theory (2,11).

Using the same linear, two element model employed by Rohrer, Otis, and Mead, Yamashiro predicted optimal flow patterns for minimum work with either passive or active expiration. Figure 4.7 shows the pattern for passive expiration, comprising a rectangular inspiratory and exponential expiratory flow. Figure 4.8 shows the pattern predicted for active expiration, and now both phases are rectangular. The rectangular pattern resembles human flow records obtained during exercise but not of those at rest which are nearly sinusoidal. It is of interest that Mead's pressure criterion (3) does not predict an optimal flow pattern for the linear two element model, as shown by Ruttimann and Yamamoto (14).

In a subsequent study, Yamashiro and Grodins (17) examined the idea of including FRC as an optimization variable rather than a fixed constraint. They used a two element model similar to those already described but with the non-linear compliance characteristic shown in Figure 4.9 which was based on the data of Rahn et al. (12). Residual volume was assumed constant so that any change in FRC could be expressed in terms of ERV changes. It was shown that the optimum ERV for minimum elastic work per breath was:

$$\text{ERV}_{opt} = V_r - \frac{V_T}{(1 + a)} \tag{12}$$

where V_r is relaxation volume, V_T is tidal volume, and a is the ratio of inspiratory to expiratory compliance, C_I/C_E. Frequency was optimized for minimum total inspiratory work rate, assuming a rectangular inspiratory flow pattern, an optimum ERV, and also that inspiratory viscous work for volumes below V_r was provided by the elastic energy stored during expiration. Under these conditions, total inspiratory work rate becomes:

$$\dot{W}_I = 2R\left(\frac{a}{1 + a}\right)f^2 V_T^2 + \frac{1}{2C_I}\left(\frac{a}{(1 + a)^2}\right)f V_T^2 \tag{13}$$

and the optimal frequency is given by:

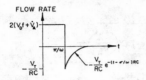

Fig. 4.7 Optimal Flow Pattern for Passive Expiration

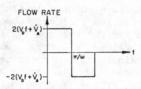

Fig. 4.8 Optimal Flow Pattern for Active Expiration

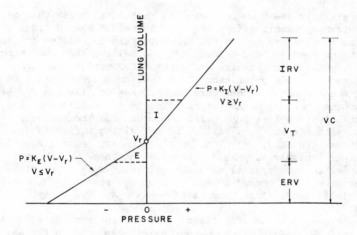

Fig. 4.9 Non-linear Compliance Characteristic

$$f_{opt} = \frac{\sqrt{1 + 32\left(\frac{1+a}{a}\right)RC_I\left(\frac{\dot{V}_A}{V_D}\right)} - 1}{16\left(\frac{1+a}{a}\right)RC_I}.$$

(14)

Figure 4.10 compares the frequency predicted by equation (14) for two different time constants with experimental data reported by Silverman et al. (15), and optimization of both flow pattern and ERV clearly improves the fit at higher levels of ventilation. The ERV predictions of equation (12) are compared with the observations of Asmussen and Christensen (1) in Figure 4.11. The experimental data were obtained in a human subject exercising on a bicycle ergometer. Again the fit becomes better as ventilation increases. Figure 4.12 shows that the theory also predicts a shift in lung mid-position (i.e., ERV + $(1/2)V_T$) with tidal volume (which, we recall, would invalidate equation (7)), and if the resting data are excluded, Figure 4.11 shows such a shift during exercise.

What all this seems to be saying is that it is worth the cost of the expiratory muscle effort required to reduce ERV in order to minimize inspiratory work rate. Perhaps this is related to the concepts of Mead (9) and Goldman (4) who believe that breathing may be organized to optimize diaphragmatic function, and that respiratory muscles other than the diaphragm operate mainly to assist the diaphragm rather than to increase ventilation per se. This becomes more important at high levels of ventilation, and it is certainly true that pump performance becomes increasingly optimal with respect to a variety of optimizing variables (e.g. f, flow pattern, ERV, T_I/T_E) as ventilation increases (18). It is not particularly surprising that some of these variables do not appear to have optimal values to minimize work rates at rest, for here the total energy consumption of the respiratory muscles is trivially small (less than 1% of total $\dot{V}_{O_2}$) (7).

This brings us to some challenges for the future. First it is clear that the models of the mechanical system used so far have been very simple ones. We have not even distinguished between the lungs and the chest wall, let alone recognizing that the former has multiple parallel units and the latter has at least two (i.e., rib cage and abdomen). The general importance of "unlumping" rib cage and abdomen, and their separate roles in accurately estimating the work of breathing have both been emphasized by the previous speakers (Goldman; Grimby). We can expect that future optimization models will take this into account. Finally let us point out that optimization studies of the sort we have described only ask whether certain variables appear to be chosen to meet some particular performance criterion; they do not provide any particular physiological control

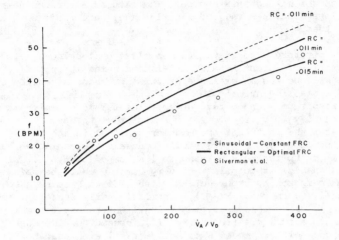

Fig. 4.10 Comparison of Predicted Optimal
Frequencies with Data of Silverman et al (11)

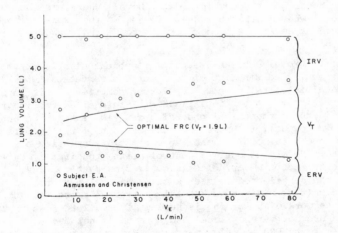

Fig. 4.11 Comparison of Predicted Optimal
ERV (or FRC) with Data of Asmussen and
Christensen (12)

mechanism for making this choice. The latter is the business of
people like John Remmers, and clearly, they have their work cut
out for them.

The Respiratory Chemostat. Let me close by looking briefly at
a completely different kind of model, and using it to define what
I think will be the major issue of this afternoon's session on
the hyperpnea of exercise. Figure 4.13 is a simplified version of
Gray's respiratory chemostat, a very fruitful model which is now
almost exactly 30 years old (5). Among other things, it
illustrates the fact that one modeler's signal is another
modeler's noise, since it carefully conceals everything we have
talked about so far this morning in its lumped controller block!
But this enables it to point out very clearly what the main
problem is in the hyperpnea of exercise. If we breathe a CO_2
mixture (i.e., increase F_{ICO_2}), ventilation will increase, as
will P_{aCO_2}, since this is a proportional control system which will
always have a steady state error. If, instead, we increase $\dot{V}_{CO_2}$,
the response of this model will be identical with that to CO_2
inhalation, i.e. both $\dot{V}_A$ and P_{aCO2} will increase along the same
CO_2 response curve. The catch is that when $\dot{V}_{CO2}$ increases during
exercise, $\dot{V}_A$ rises as expected but P_{aCO2} stays at its resting
level. This means that some signal proportional to $\dot{V}_{CO_2}$ must
drive the controller during exercise. It is the physiological
nature of this signal which is the central issue in exercise
hyperpnea, an issue which is at least 88 years old (3). Is it
neural, humoral, or a combination of both? Where are the
receptors, what do they receive, and how do they work? These are
the kinds of questions I look forward to having answered this
afternoon.

Summary. Models are an essential component of science which is
an interacting combination of real world observations and
conceptual interpretations. The latter comprise models in one
form or another. A particularly useful form of expression for
models is the mathematical one which can take maximum advantage
of modern computer technology. Many aspects of the respiratory
system have been modeled, and two particular varieties are
reviewed. Models of optimal control of the respiratory cycle
ask whether certain variables (e.g. f, flow pattern, ERV,
T_I/T_E) can be selected to meet some mechanical performance
criterion (e.g. minimum work, minimum average pressure, etc.).
Since the work of breathing is negligibly small at rest, optimal
choices are not very critical and apparently not made, at least
with regard to ERV and flow pattern. However, when ventilation
increases during exercise, optimization of many of these variables
is achieved asymptotically as high levels of exercise are
reached. A simple model of the respiratory chemostat clearly
identifies the major issue of the enigma of exercise hyperpnea:
What is the physiological signal mechanism which makes $\dot{V}_E$
proportional to $\dot{V}_{CO_2}$ in exercise?

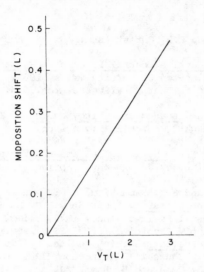

Fig. 4.12 Predicted Lung
Mid-position Shift With
Tidal Volume

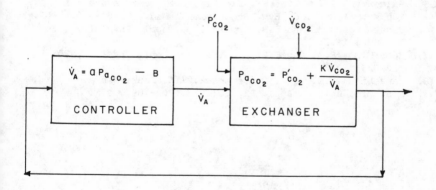

Fig. 4.13 The Respiratory Chemostat

REFERENCES

1. Asmussen, E. and E.H. Christensen. Skand. Arch. Physiol., 82:
    201-211, 1939.
2. Bellman, R. Adaptive Control Processes: A Guided Tour.
    Princeton: Princeton University Press, 1961.
3. Geppert, J. and N. Zuntz. Pflügers Arch. f.d. ges. Physiol.,
    42:189, 1888.
4. Goldman, M. In: Loaded Breathing, edited by L.D. Pengelly
    et al. Edinburgh: Churchill Livingston, 1974, p. 50-63.
5. Gray, J.S. Science, 103:739-744, 1946.
6. Grodins, F.S. In: Physiological and Behavioral Temperature
    Regulation, edited by J.D. Hardy. Springfield: Thomas, 1970,
    p. 722-726.
7. Grodins, F.S. and S.M. Yamashiro. In: Annual Review of Bio-
    physics and Bioengineering, edited by L.J. Mullins et al.
    Palo Alto: Annual Reviews, Inc., 1973, Vol. 2, p. 115-130.
8. Mead, J. J. Appl. Physiol., 15:325-336, 1960.
9. Mead, J. In: Loaded Breathing, edited by L.D. Pengelly et
    al. Edinburgh: Churchill Livingston, 1974, p. 35-49.
10. Otis, A.B., W.O. Fenn and H. Rahn. J. Appl. Physiol., 2:592-
    607, 1950.
11. Pontryagin, L.S., V.G. Boltyanskii, R.V. Gamkrelidze and
    E.F. Mischchenki. The Mathematical Theory of Optimal Pro-
    cesses. New York: Wiley, 1962.
12. Rahn, H., A.B. Otis, L.E. Chadwick and W.O. Fenn. Am. J.
    Physiol., 146:161-178, 1946.
13. Rohrer, F. In: Handbuch der Normalen und Pathogischen
    Physiologie, edited by A. Bethe et al. Berlin: Springer,
    1925, p. 70-127.
14. Ruttimann, U.E. and W.S. Yamamoto. Annals Biomed. Eng.,
    1:160-181, 1972.
15. Silverman, L., G. Lee, T. Plotkin, I.A. Sawyers and A.R.
    Yancey. Arch. Ind. Hyg. Occupational Med., 3:461-478, 1951.
16. Yamashiro, S.M. and F.S. Grodins. J. Appl. Physiol., 30:
    597-602, 1971.
17. Yamashiro, S.M. and F.S. Grodins. J. Appl. Physiol., 35:
    522-525, 1973.
18. Yamashiro, S.M., J.A. Daubenspeck, T.N. Lauritsen and
    F.S. Grodins. J. Appl. Physiol., 38:702-709, 1975.

DISCUSSION

Goldman: I am not at all upset by the fact that the resting data does not appear to be consistent with optimized variables because my point of view is that at rest the respiratory mechanical problem is a trivial one. In normal people we have so much reserve so that we could be far off from our optimum pattern and it wouldn't cost us much in terms of ventilatory work or force. It may be different for patients--would you agree with that?

Grodins: Yes. The cost of ventilation in a resting person is extremely small--maybe 2% of the metabolic rate or less, so that it really doesn't matter very much whether you are optimized or not. One would expect that optimization criteria would become more important as one increased the ventilatory load, as during exercise, or in obstructive lung disease.

5

Neural Control Mechanisms

J. E. Remmers & D. Bartlett, Jr.

In mammalian breathing, a host of skeletal muscles participate in producing a continuous series of respiratory movements of immediate, life sustaining importance to the organism. These movements are executed automatically and, in the limit, involuntarily; volitional control impinges on the respiratory control system to mold and shape the act for non-respiratory purposes. Ultimately, however, breathing is autonomous, and voluntary control is constrained by the so-called automatic mechanism.

Traditionally, regulation by this automatic mechanism has been evaluated in a stimulus-response framework. The nervous system is treated as a "black box" controller with an input (chemical stimulus) and a motor output (minute volume). The components of the "black box" are now the subject of considerable investigation, and the aim of this review is to examine the behavior of this neural machinery under condition of its most natural stress, the metabolic load produced by muscular exercise. The strategy is to fractionate the motor output in search of changes uniquely associated with the exercise state and, thereby, gain insight into fundamental neural adjustments associated with the state.

The neural machinery responsible for breathing

Exactly how we should view the central neural mechanism underlying breathing has received considerable debate. For the purposes of this article we shall contrast two extreme views: control by respiratory center(s) and control by sensory-motor comparison. Both explain a substantial portion of our present knowledge and elements of both would seem to be required ultimately to develop a fully valid view of neural respiratory control.

Control of "respiratory centers". This view holds that breathing resembles deglutition, vomiting and other stereotyped functions that can reasonably be attributed to the action of centers. A center consists of functionally linked set of neurons, which generates a stereotyped movement when triggered by the proper sensory input (13). The act originates in a localized set of neurons, capable of generating the appropriate central neuronal activity, which then preempts the final common pathway to produce a pre-programmed discharge pattern in the periphery. Present evidence from anesthetized animals leaves little doubt that, under these admittedly abnormal circumstances, inspiration is an act that neatly fits the center concept.

Inspiration is triggered by afferent feedback utilizing the
time integral of lung volume as the important variable (9,22).
Once triggered, a pre-set pattern of excitation evolves in the
neurons of the tractus solitarius and retroambigualis nuclei (15,
26). Short latency excitatory projections descend over anatomically established pathways to convey a central respiratory drive
to phrenic motoneurons resulting in efferent traffic to the principal respiratory muscle (30). Consequently, the activity of the
diaphragm, the principal pressure generator, closely parallels
the central excitatory phenomenon. Central inspiratory excitation
continues to increase autonomously until it is terminated when inhibitory feedback from pulmonary stretch receptors reaches the
time-dependent threshold curve set by an inspiratory off switch
(7). The respiratory pattern is, therefore, determined by the
interaction of vagally mediated reflexes and the central inspiratory activity which dictates the rate of increase of phrenic
efferent discharge (40).

Breathing as a sensory-motor act. A contrasting view of the
respiratory control machinery derives from the observation that
under normal circumstances breathing is a highly plastic act where-
by a variety of muscles are coordinated to execute both respiratory
and non-respiratory movements. Under many circumstances breathing
resembles other movements not governed by discrete centers, eg.
postural actions, travel movements and manipulation. The out-
standing feature of the nervous system in executing such acts is
that several levels of the nervous system participate in the process of matching sensory information and motor commands. Since
continuous comparison of demand and achievement at all levels of
the nervous system from cortical to spinal level is the essential
feature of such behavior, the idea of an autonomous medullary
command center seems simplistic. Experiments in the unanesthetized state involving mechanical loading and unloading of the
respiratory system support this view. Sudden changes in upper
airway resistance evoke short latency compensatory responses in
diverse respiratory muscles apparently consisting of coordinated
"tracking" of what seems to be a desired time-course of lung
volume (4). Similarly, mechanical loading during vocalization
in humans evokes transient inhibition followed by a facilitating
response (31). Segmental, medullary or cortical responses may be
involved in these short latency, automatic responses. Of particular interest is the likelihood that the spinal neurons play an
important integrative role, inasmuch as they are impinged on by
mechanoreceptor afferents, by phasic command signals and by tonic
descending influences (14). The last play directly on the motoneuron and modulate the inflow of sensory information as well (25).
During muscular exercise, for instance, one must combine respiratory and postural actions, inasmuch as the same muscle group often
are involved in both. In this case, respiratory and postural demands project onto the spinal motoneurons, both α and γ, and the
segmental feedback provided by the muscle spindle allows fulfill-

ment of both demands. Similarly, during volitional movements,
such as speech, cortical influences project onto the respiratory
motoneuron and the muscle spindle plays a role in integration of
respiratory and non-respiratory demands (31).

Nowhere is the divergence between the two views presented
above more apparent than in regard to the level of integration.
The "center" theory holds that dominant integration occurs at the
respiratory centers, with their output being transmitted straight
to the periphery. The sensory-motor comparison view, on the other
hand, places particular emphasis on spinal integration. However,
integration of respiratory and non-respiratory functions probably
occurs at both levels. Multi-level integration is suggested by
observations that intercostal muscle spindle afferents initiate
segmental and brain stem arcs which influence the intensity of
motoneuron output as well as the rhythm of breathing (38,41).

Another reconciliation of the two views is illustrated by the
control of relative activation of the diaphragm and the inspiratory intercostals. Under anesthesia and during sleep the diaphragm
is the dominant inspiratory muscle (35). However, during muscular
exercise inspiratory activity is prominent in the rib cage musculature. The likely explanation is that anesthesia depresses intercostal motoneurons and their gamma loop activation system. In
fact, the consequent loss of rib cage motion represents a major
factor in the lessened ventilatory response to hypercapnia under
anesthesia (44). Also, in the awake animal the larynx contributes
importantly to the regulation of airflow. The posterior cricoary-
tenoid, the primary laryngeal abductor, receives phasic respiratory
activation (5,28). This muscle controls upper airway resistance
and, together with post-inspiratory contraction of the diaphragm,
regulates expiratory airflow and duration (4,16).

Respiratory motor output during exercise

This raises the question of the nature of the respiratory
motor output during muscular exercise. Does exercise alter the
relative activation of inspiratory muscles, or does it simply increase the respiratory motor output? Almost nothing is known
about the factors controlling the relative activation of different
inspiratory muscles, and experiments we have recently carried out
relate to the question. We reason that changes in the central
neural state might be associated with changes in the behavior of
respiratory neurons and muscles. For instance, one can envision
a spectrum of CNS states of arousal extending from sleep to muscular exercise. Changes in degree of arousal along this spectrum
will be associated with differences in the mode of execution of
the respiratory act. For instance, sleep is known to be associated
with selective depression in intercostal motoneuron activity which
progresses with deeper sleep until activity is completely eliminated during REM sleep (35).

Our specific hypothesis is that exercise has effects opposite
to sleep on the respiratory motor output, i.e., that it engenders
a shift in the balance of activation of the various respiratory

motoneurons toward intercostal and other "accessory" motor units
acting on the rib cage. The ideal approach would be to compare
quantitatively respiratory muscle action potentials in various
states when comparable levels of ventilatory output were achieved.
However, such EMG studies are technically difficult in humans and,
therefore, we used an indirect method, that of examining rib cage
and abdominal movement. Abdominal motion reflects movement of the
diaphragm, whereas rib cage motion is the complex result of the
action of the diaphragm as well as contraction of rib cage inspiratory muscles (17).

Our approach is to compare the relative motion of the two
components of the chest wall when the same tidal volume is generated by each of two respiratory stimuli: hypercapnia and muscular exercise. Four subjects were studied in the supine posture.
They were made hypercapnic by rebreathing into an oxygen filled
spirometer. Exercise was performed either with calf or forearm
musculature. Ventilation was recorded spirometrically, while rib
cage and abdominal anterio-posterior (A-P) dimensions were recorded by the method of Konno and Mead (23) using Hookian springs
connected to force transducers. Data for isovolume calibration
maneuvers and for tidal excursions were analyzed by a digital
computer. Isovolume regressions were fitted using a cubic expression, and tidal volumes were estimated as the sum of rib cage
and abdominal excursions. This calculated tidal volume differed
from the spirometrically measured tidal volume by less than 10%
during either hypercapnia or muscular exercise, as shown in Figure
5.1, and in most instances the method provided accuracy to the 5%
level.

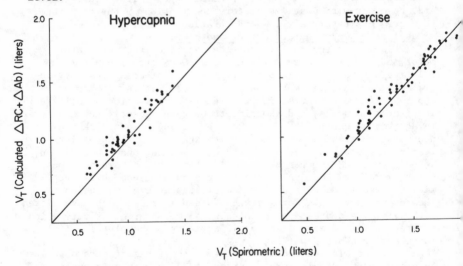

Fig. 5.1. Validation of volume estimation from A-P dimensions.
Abscissa: spirometrically measured V_T; ordinate: calculated V_T.
Each point represents one breath.

Illustrative records are shown in Figure 5.2, where rebreathing
and exercise conditions can be compared at roughly comparable
levels of tidal volume and minute volume. In the pre-stimulated
portions of both records, tidal volume was achieved primarily
through abdominal movement, an observation which agrees with the
results of Konno and Mead (23) for the supine posture.

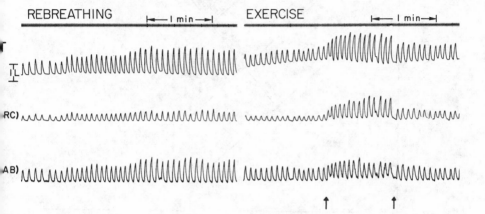

Fig. 5.2. A typical polygraph tracing of V_T and volume excursions
of rib cage and abdomen, $L_{(RC)}$ and $L_{(Ab)}$ respectively. The latter
two signals have been adjusted in gain to be of equal significance
with regard to volume. Note that during leg exercise (period between vertical arrows) the increase in tidal volume was produced
primarily by an increase in rib cage excursion.

During CO_2 stimulated hyperpnea, the excursion of both compartments increased, but the relative contribution of each remained
unchanged. In other words, hypercapnia increases the respiratory
motor output without altering the relative activation of respiratory muscles. By contrast, exercise substantially increased rib
cage excursion, so that the relative contribution of both compartments shifted in favor of the rib cage. A plot of tidal excursion of each compartment for individual breaths in a typical
experiment is shown in Figure 5.3. During hypercapnia, the abdominal
movement accounted for 70% of the tidal volume, whereas for exercise induced hyperpnea the relative contribution of each compartment was equal. This finding, that exercise increased the importance of the rib cage movement, was apparent in all four subjects.

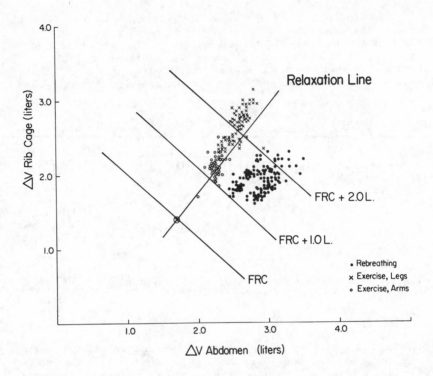

Fig. 5.3. Results of a typical experiment on one subject showing rib cage and abdominal volume excursions above FRC for individual breaths observed during hypercapnia (rebreathing) and
muscular exercise of arms or leg. Relaxation line indicates
the passive configuration of the chest wall. Note that rebreathing produced points lying to the right of this line whereas
exercise resulted in points lying on or to the left of this line.

        The relationship between end-inspiratory volumes of the rib
cage and abdomen, and the relaxed configuration of the chest wall
is also shown in Figure 5.3. The relaxation line describes the configuration of the passive chest wall and has a slope approximating
45°, indicating that equal volume changes of each compartment occur
when the relaxed respiratory system changes volume. For CO_2 stimulated breathing, abdominal movements predominated so that the end-
inspiratory points lay to the right of the passive configuration
line. This means that during inspiration the rib cage is pulled

inward from its relaxed position at any given lung volume, presumably by the negative intrapleural pressure resulting from diaphragmatic contraction. Under these circumstances, then the chest
wall is distorted during inspiration, and some of the force developed by diaphragm contraction is expended inefficiently doing
work on the rib cage.

During exercise, end-inspiratory points scatter upward along
the passive configuration line since the volume excursions of the
rib cage and abdomen are nearly equal. This finding indicates
that breathing is executed more efficiently during exercise because the rib cage inspiratory muscles are activated sufficiently
to avoid distortion of the chest wall. In other words, the evidence confirms our initial speculation that muscular exercise may
be associated with a shift in the relative activity of different
respiratory muscles, and as a result, the overall motor act is
executed more efficiently.

What changes underlie this shift in the balance of rib cage
versus diaphragmatic motion? The work of Goldman and Mead (17,
see also Goldman in this volume) indicates that, in the upright
posture, contraction of the diaphragm and increase in abdominal
pressure account in large measure for the motion of the rib cage.
Although there are indications that this interpretation cannot be
transposed to the supine posture, the importance of tidal swings
in abdominal pressure (P_{Ab}) must be considered when interpreting
these results. Of particular concern is the possibility that during
supine leg exercise abdominal compliance may change owing to contraction of abdominal muscles. This would increase the respiratory
fluctuations in P_{Ab} and according to the theory of Goldman and
Mead, lessen abdominal excursion and augment rib cage movement.
That this is not a tenable explanation of our results is demonstrated, on the one hand, by the finding that arm exercise produced the
same mode of breathing as leg exercise (Fig. 5.3) and, on the other
hand, by direct measurements of gastric pressure. Figure 5.4 shows a
pressure-volume relationship of the abdomen at the beginning and
end of inspiration for one subject during hypercapnia and muscular
exercise. The end-inspiration and end-expiration points for the
two conditions occupy a single continuous compliance curve, and
the inspiratory fluctuations in abdominal pressure were similar in
both situations. These findings manifest a similar abdominal compliance during hypercapnic and exercise induced hyperpnea and, accordingly, we conclude that the greater rib cage motion during exercise resulted not from altered action of the diaphragm or abdominal
muscles, but from greater activation of rib cage inspiratory muscles.
The principal lesson from these experiments is that the respiratory
motor output cannot always be characterized by measuring tidal volume or inspiratory flow rates. A corollary is that the exercise
stimulus qualitatively changes the motor output by altering the
sequence of recruitment of respiratory muscles. Using the respiratory motor output as a gauge of the respiratory stimulus, we
suggest that whatever factors underlie the hyperpnea of exercise,
they differ fundamentally from those operating in hypercapnia.

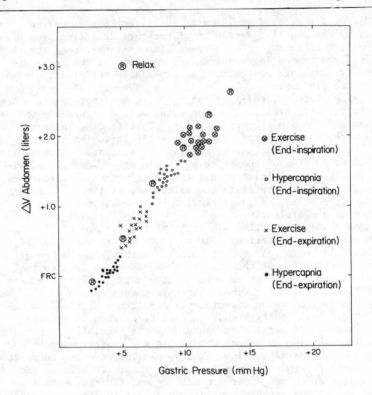

Fig. 5.4. Relationship between abdominal volume (above FRC) and gastric pressure in a single experiment. ℝ represents static value observed with relaxation against a closed airway. Points observed during hypercapnia and leg exercise fall along a common regression.

Respiratory sensation and reflexes

We shall conclude with a discussion of respiratory reflexes and sensations as they may apply to muscular exercise. Respiratory sensations fall into two categories, conceptually. One is the continuous feedback which constitutes the sensory matrix on which breathing, like other complex motor acts, is based. The results reported by Bakers and Tenney (2) manifest a rich sensory input from respiratory receptors which allows appreciation of pressure, volume and total ventilation with roughly the same accuracy as in other motor acts. The other type of sensation is noxious, so called dyspnea or breathlessness. Here, the sensation links the automatic and volitional control systems and con-

stitutes the means by which the automatic mechanism constrains
volition. When volitional inhibition approaches its limits, unpleasant sensations overcome volitional control and release the
automatic mechanism. Although this categorization of sensation
may be artificial, there is no reason to assume that all respiratory sensations carry the same implication for the brain, particularly during muscular exercise.

The pioneering work of Campbell and coworkers on detection
of added mechanical loads (6,8), led to an intuitive concept which
fits subsequent notions regarding sensory-motor comparison in the
respiratory system. This theory attempted to provide a unitary
explanation for both types of respiratory sensation. Their theory
of "length tension (in)appropriateness" was developed to account
for the observation that perception of an added elastic load, for
instance, does not depend on the consequent reduction in inspired
volume or the greater pressure generated. Rather, a load is
detected whenever pressure generated is excessive in relation to
the volume inspired. Reducing this concept to respiratory muscles
and their receptors led them to postulate that the factor of
unique significance in load detection was the force developed
by the muscle in relation to its length. In other words, awareness of a mechanically hindered breath stems from sensing
length-tension inappropriateness.

The list of possible sources of respiratory sensations is
staggering, and the relative importance of each is unknown at
the present time. Airway receptors, both intra-thoracic and extra-
thoracic, are plentiful. Intra-thoracic pulmonary stretch receptors, located primarily in the large airways, relate instantaneous
lung volume (27). Whereas they play a dominant role in determining
the pattern of breathing in animals, their role in human respiration
at rest is questionable. During exercise, however, they may importantly determine the timing of respiratory phase switching.
The extra-thoracic trachea is also the locus of abundant stretch
receptors (3). These provide information of the relation of upper
airway resistance to airflow and may be important in feedback regulation of laryngeal resistance and in "tracking" behavior. Afferent impulses from both types of airway receptors travel up the
vagus nerve and since its fibers have been shown to project to the
cortex (32), it is reasonable to presume that they provide a basis
for conscious perception of lung volume. Of interest in this regard is the finding that elastic loading is detected more readily
when applied at the mouth than when the thorax alone is loaded.
Increases of respiratory elastance of 50% are not detected when
applied by a head-out body plethysmograph (42). This load is
easily detected when applied at the mouth (8). Presumably, activation of extra-thoracic airway receptors (oral, pharyngeal or
tracheal) account for this difference.

Nonetheless, the airway sensory input is probably not of
great importance in the awareness of mechanical loading since they
sense volume, not pressure. Evidence from load detection studies
using oral anesthesia, blocking the vagus and glossopharyngeal

nerves, and in patients with cervical cord lesions, suggests that
the rib cage is an important sensory source relating to the mechanical loads (19,29). Originally, costo-vertebral joint receptors
were favored as the responsible receptor based on the common im-
pression that muscle spindle afferents did not project to the
cortex (29). However, we now have abundant evidence in cats and
primates that the sensorimotor cortex receives afferent projections from these receptors (1,24,33,36,45).

Intercostal muscle is richly endowed with muscle spindles,
which, in the phraseology of Granit, are "the only endorgans
reflecting both demand and execution" (18). The salient feature
of this receptor complex is co-activation of gamma and alpha
efferent fibers. "Demand" for movement transmitted to the spinal
level causes activation of both types of motoneurons, those
innervating extrafusal (alpha) as well as the parallel intrafusal
(gamma) fibers. The latter activate spindle afferent discharge
unless appropriate shortening of the extrafusal fibers occurs.
Accordingly, gamma activation signals "demand" and overall receptor length measures "execution"; receptor discharge reflects the
difference between the two. In the framework of the length-
tension relationship, the muscle spindle would seem to constitute
a key receptor; its output is an error signal indicating the
extent to which actual motion parallels desired motion. This
type of signal is, in essence, what Campbell and coworkers presumed to provide the awareness of a mechanically hindered breath.
Similarly, the inferences of Bakers and Tenney regarding the
sensory modality used in estimating respiratory movements and
efforts are consistent with a muscle spindle signal (2).

What is known about the reflex actions of intercostal muscle spindle afferents? The primary endings (fast adapting)
exert powerful facilitatory actions segmentally and similar effects
have been documented now for the secondary endings (43). This
class of reflex provides a load compensating servo loop of considerable importance in anesthetized cats (11) and awake humans
(31) providing the principal means for spinal integration of
postural and respiratory movements. At the next level in neural-
respiratory machinery a surprising twist occurs: afferents from
the secondary endings of inspiratory intercostal muscle spindles
exert inhibitory actions on inspiratory activity (41).

The discovery of this neural circuitry was disconcerting in
that it stands at odds with a strong bias about motor control,
namely: the nervous system relies on negative-feedback, "load-
compensating" reflexes in motor execution. This reflex is apparently load "de-compensating", and its function remained
obscure until recently, when studies on infants elucidated a
possible role. Chest wall distortion owing to rib cage collapse
is a problem of major mechanical significance in this setting,
particularly with loss of intercostal tone during REM sleep.
Knill et al. have demonstrated that rib cage distortion, whether
a spontaneous occurrence during inspiration or experimentally

induced, foreshortens inspiration by means of this reflex (20,21).
The inspiratory terminating actions of intercostal spindle afferents may constitute an efficiency promoting reflex enabling the
infant to terminate mechanically disadvantageous breaths. The
secondary ending would appear to constitute an ideal "distortion"
receptor owing to its strategic placement; the receptor receives
the inspiratory drive which projects onto phrenic motoneurons.
If the activation of inspiratory intercostal alpha motoneurons is
deficient relative to the phrenic activity, the rib cage will be
distorted, the muscle spindle will either lengthen or fail to
shorten as expected, and the inappropriate behavior of the rib
cage will be reflected in the resultant error signal.

Another set of reflexes derived from intercostal mechanoreceptors provides connections with phrenic motoneurons via
laryngeal and abdominal motoneurons (39). These extra-segmental
loops manifest intimate integration of the various respiratory
muscles and suggest that the higher nervous system supervises
breathing using these reflexes to coordinate complimentary motions.
Noteworthy is the projection of intercostal spindle afferents to
a region of cerebellar cortex, which modulates these reflexes and
also exerts direct control of inspiratory activity (10,12).

Finally, one can anticipate that the secondary endings of
intercostal afferents project to the sensorimotor cortex; such
connections, demonstrated in monkeys for other motor systems,
probably mediate a cortical load-compensating reflex (45). It
also seems likely that this ascending information can be consciously appreciated.

Our own view is that intercostal muscle spindles may signal
mechanical loading as "performance-demand" mismatching. Based on
the suggestion that these receptors sense rib cage distortion, we
speculate that load detection may be equivalent to detection of
distortion.

That mechanical loading and lung disease exert reflex effects
on breathing during exercise is apparent in the studies of
Phillipson et al. using exercising dogs with experimental pneu-
monitis (37). This condition results in an exaggerated exercise
hyperpnea, tachypnea and decreased exercise tolerance. The
hyperpnea depends upon the integrity of the vagus nerves and
presumably results from abnormal stimulation of pulmonary afferents. Pulmonary stretch receptors could sense the decrease in
lung compliance and promote tachypnea but, presumably, not hyperventilation. Another possibility is that J-receptors were activated, and Paintal has speculated that these receptors, responding to increases in pulmonary vascular pressure, engender sensations of breathlessness during exercise (34). In any case, the
abnormal tachypnia persisted after vagal blockade suggesting
the participation of a chest wall reflex. The inspiratory terminating reflex derived from intercostal muscle spindles could
be expected to produce such an action.

Summary
    Current understanding of the motor control of breathing is
reviewed. Two concepts of the neural machinery are contrasted:
one emphasizing autonomous control by respiratory centers, and one
holding that execution depends upon sensory-motor comparisons
throughout the nervous system. Results of experiments on supine
humans, comparing rib cage and abdominal movements, show that
muscular exercise causes equal movements of both components of
the chest wall, whereas CO_2 causes predominantly abdominal movements. This disparity suggests that chemical and exercise
stimuli influence the neural control system differently, the
latter causing relatively greater recruitment of the rib cage
inspiratory musculature. The neurophysiologic basis for awareness
of respiratory movements is considered. The possible role of the
intercostal muscle spindle in sensing chest wall distortion leads
to the proposition that sensing of length-tension inappropriateness may be equivalent to sensing rib cage distortion.

REFERENCES

1.   Albe-Fessard, D. and J. Liebeskind. Expl. Brain Res. 1:127-146,
      1966.
2.   Bakers, J.H.C.M. and S.M. Tenney. Resp. Physiol. 10:85-92, 1970.
3.   Bartlett, D.Jr., P. Jeffery, G. Sant'Ambrogio and J.C.M. Wise.
      J. Physiol. (In press) 1976.
4.   Bartlett, D.Jr. and J.E. Remmers. J. Physiol. 247:22-23P, 1975.
5.   Bartlett, D.Jr., J.E. Remmers and H. Gautier. Respir. Physiol.
      18:194-204, 1973.
6.   Bennet, E.D., M.I.V. Jayson, D. Rubenstein and E.J.M. Campbell.
      Clin. Sci. 23:155-162, 1962.
7.   Bradley, W.G., C. vonEuler, I. Marttila, B. Roos. Biol. Cyber-
      netics, 1-12, 1975.
8.   Campbell, E.J.M., S. Freedman, P.S. Smith and M.E. Taylor.
      Clin. Sci 20:223-231, 1961.
9.   Camporesi, E. and G. Sant'Ambrogio. Pflugers Arch. 324:311-318,
      1971.
10.   Coffey, G., R.B. Godwin-Austen, B.B. MacGillivray and T.A. Sears.
      J. Physiol. 201:96-97P, 1969.
11.   Corda, M., G. Eklund and C. vonEuler. Acta. Physiol. Scand.
      63:391-400, 1965.
12.   Decima, E.E. and C. von Euler. Acta. Physiol. Scand. 76:148-
      158, 1969b.
13.   Doty, R.W. In: Simpler Networks and Behavior, edited by J.C.
      Fentress. Sinauer Associates: Sunderland, Mass., 1976.
14.   Euler, C. von. In: Loaded Breathing, edited by E.J.M. Camp-
      bell, L.D. Pengelly and A.S. Rebuck. Churchill Livingston:
      Edinburgh.
15.   Euler, C. von, J.N. Hayward, I. Marttila and R.J. Wyman.
      Brain Res. 61:1-22, 1973.
16.   Gautier, H., J.E. Remmers and D. Bartlett, Jr. Respir. Physiol.
      18:205-221, 1973.

17. Goldman, M. and J. Mead. J. Appl. Physiol. 35:197-204, 1973.
18. Granit, R. Brain 95:649-660, 1972.
19. Guz, A., M.I.M.Noble, J.G. Widdicombe, D. Trenchard, W.W. Mushin, A.R. Makey. Clin. Sci 30:161-170, 1966.
20. Knill, R., W. Andrews, A. Bryan and M. Bryan. J. Appl. Physiol. 40:357-361, 1976.
21. Knill, R. and A. Bryan. J. Appl. Physiol. 40:352-356, 1976.
22. Knox, C.K. J. Neurophysiol. 34:284-295, 1973.
23. Konno, K. and J. Mead. J.Appl. Physiol. 22:402.
24. Landgren, S. and H. Silfvenius. J. Physiol. 200:353-372, 1969.
25. Lundberg, A. Physiology of Spinal Neurones 12:197, 1964.
26. Merrill, E.G. Brain Res. 24:11-28, 1970.
27. Miserocchi, G., J. Mortola and G. Sant'Ambrogio. J. Physiol. 235:775-782, 1973.
28. Murakami, Y. and J.A. Kirchner. The Laryngoscope 82:454-467, 1972.
29. Newsom-Davis, J. Clin Sci. 33:249-260, 1967.
30. Newsom-Davis, J. In: The Respiratory Muscles edited by E.J.M. Campbell. Saunders: Philadelphia, 1970.
31. Newsom-Davis, J. and T.A. Sears. J. Physiol. 209:711-738, 1970.
32. O'Brien, J.H., A. Pimpaneau and D. Albe-Fessard. Electroenceph. and Clin. Neurophysiol. 31:7-20, 1971.
33. Oscarsson, O. and I. Rosen. J. Physiol. 182:164-184, 1966.
34. Paintal, A.S. Physiol. Rev. 53:159-222, 1973.
35. Parmeggiani, P.L. and L. Sabattini. Electroenceph. Clin. Neurophysiol. 33:1-13, 1972.
36. Phillips, C.G., T.P.S. Powell and M. Wiesendanger. J. Physiol. 217:419-446, 1971.
37. Phillipson, E.A., E. Murphy, L.F. Kozar and R.K. Schultze. J. Appl. Physiol. 39:76-85, 1975.
38. Remmers, J.E. Respir. Physiol. 10:358-383, 1970.
39. Remmers J.E. J. Physiol. (London) 233:45-62, 1973.
40. Remmers, J.E. Chest (In press), 1976.
41. Remmers, J.E. and I. Marttila. Respir. Physiol. 24:31-41, 1975.
42. Remmers, J.E., J.F. O'Donnell, S.H. Loring and D. Bartlett, Jr. Physiologist 13:291, 1970.
43. Sears, T.A. In: Respiratory Centers and Afferent Influences edited by B. Duron, I.N.S.E.R.M., in press.
44. Tusiewicy, K., A.C. Bryan and A.B. Froese. Personal communication.
45. Wiesendanger, M. J. Physiol. 228:203-219, 1973.

DISCUSSION

Goldman: I should point out that Dr. Remmers' supine exercise data
are not inconsistent with our data on upright exercise. We are not
quite certain of the mechanical interaction between diaphragm and
rib cage in the supine posture, but we have limited data in the
prone posture and it is the same as upright position data. Dr.
Remmers, you talk about a drive (to breathe) being reflected in
inspiratory mean flow rate that is accomplished on a reflex basis.
Overall drive increases with either exercise level or CO_2, and
there is an increased activation of expiratory muscles. Gene Bruce
has suggested to me that this activation might be purely on a vagal
reflex basis which abolishes expiratory braking without involving
the respiratory center. Is that the way you see things? Is it
primarily dependent on vagal afferents?

Remmers: That has been the traditional view but the notion is that
as one has an increase in the stimulus to breathe one might have
an increase in inspiratory flow rate and go to higher tidal volume.
That higher tidal volume during expiration, triggers an increase in
vagal reflexes. Vagal stimuli or pulmonary stretch receptor stimuli
during expiration do, in fact, turn on the dilator muscle of the
larynx, so that would act to decrease upper airway resistance.
They also turn on the abdominal muscle and turn off the antagonistic
action of the diaphragm which would assist active expiration. One
would expect then, on these bases, faster expiration and, in the
anesthetized animal, the duration of expiration is now fixed.
Similarly, in our unanesthetized animal, who is vagotomized below
the recurrent laryngeal nerve so we were able to preserve the innervation of the larynx, we have found that in general the duration
of expiration now fits. So I place a lot of importance on the
volume feedback during expiration in allowing the shortening of
expiration and really don't know if I would talk about expiratory
drive in the same way. The nice feature about drive during inspiration is that the center or the mechanism seems to be relatively
immune to vagal and other reflex inputs during inspiration. Once
triggered, it goes along a pre-programmed course evolving its
neural excitation until it is shut off. But you do not have continuous modulation of the activity. Whereas during expiration you
have moment-to-moment modulation.

Swanson: Could you speculate on how voluntary ventilation fits
into your scheme?

Remmers: Certainly. You have ill defined cortical mechanisms and
we really don't know a lot about them. But they are extremely important in controlling respiratory muscles and may be important in
mediating the ventilatory response to exercise. A lot of credence
should be given to the notions of Newsom, Davis and Sears that the
cortical descending influence summates with the segmental reflexes
and with other descending influences from the cerebellum or from
brain stem neurons at the respiratory motor neuron pool. This

respiratory motor neuron and other associated neurons can be viewed as integrating mechanisms which allow all of these combinations and influences to be combined and come up with an output which satisfy a variety of needs. It satisfies the ventilatory need for posture, for breathing, for speaking and for other kinds of movements.

Discussion

Dempsey: John, I am worried about your idea of "brakes" on expiration. Does this just happen in cats and in vagal animals or is there any evidence in man that there is this sort of a volume mediated brake on expiration.

Remmers: In man the diaphragm doesn't stop at the end of inspiration, i.e., you have antagonistic contractions of the inspiratory muscles. This is a brake in man. The larynx is actively moving in man, and may act as a brake. Other evidence for a brake is that the duration of expiration is longer than the spontaneous collapse time for a paralyzed intubated human respiratory system. So I believe the brakes are working, but quantitatively how important they are in man, I don't know.

Goldman: I agree that the diaphragm certainly does contract during expiration, that is, it's inspiratory discharge continues on into the first part of expiration. That's in resting breathing, but as we stimulate ventilation in exercise this discharge becomes less and less of a factor.

Filley: Dr. Grodins, I really appreciate your emphasis on mid-position of the lung. Have I got the message right, that the concept of the FRC is particularly appropriate for the static phase of quiet expiration when the balance of forces between the lung and chest are important. Whereas, during exercise the very dynamic circumstance seems to arise in which the position of greatest importance with respect to how the lung is functioning, is determined by what is going on in both chest and diaphragm. So, firstly, is mid-position defined as the volume of the lung halfway between inspiration and expiration?

Grodins: Yes.

Filley: Secondly, you say that Dr. Mead's analysis was only valid if that mid-position was maintained constant.

Grodins: Yes, the point is that when Dr. Mead derived the equation for his analysis, he equated minimum average pressure with minimum pressure amplitude. In those equations, setting those two quantities equal is only valid under a special condition, which is the constancy of the mid-position of the lung.

Filley: This concept has been neglected because it is hard to know exactly where mid-position is during walking on a treadmill. But the literature shows that mid-position isn't too far from constant because when you breathe in during exercise you breathe out an increased amount, i.e., inspiratory and expiratory reserve volumes both increase at the same time. So I would think that Mead's model for minimum work would apply; correct?

57

Goldman: The fact is that of course inspiratory reserve and expiratory reserve do both decrease simultaneously in exercise. If they would decrease by equal amounts, then the mid-position would be the same. In Dr. Grodins' data taken at rest and at the highest exercise load mid-position was unchanged; but in the rest of the data the mid-position did change because of different relative changes in inspiratory and expiratory reserve. Data obtained by Gunnar Grimby and I have shown that same thing. Mid-position does in fact change.

Grodins: If you plot Asmussen's exercise data with mid-position vs. ventilation, ERV and IRV changes are not equal and mid-position does rise.

Gee: You are using mid-lung volumes as a volume weighted average of the lung volume and that is obviously reasonable. However, when we consider respiratory work, one also gets into time factors and the power exerted during ventilation. Therefore, I am wondering whether averaging around a volume, mid-lung capacity, is necessarily the same average as opposed to a time weighted average. This problem occurs repeatedly in the definition of alveolar gas. I suspect it occurs in this problem depending upon the exact time course of inspiration and expiration. Is there any data to elucidate this?

Goldman: I would agree that perhaps tension-time would be a better index of chemical energy utilization by muscle, but experimentally we are a long way from getting there and we have to, at this point, content ourselves with rough approximations, such as pressure and volume.

Eldridge: John, you implied that once an inspiration starts it is fully programmed, and that the end of expiration is a function of vagal feedback. I know that you are aware this only applies when there are no interventions during the inspiration. If you put in a stimulus from the carotid body or a peripheral receptor, you can easily change the size of the breath immediately during that inspiration. This has been shown by several investigators (Black and Torrance, Resp. Physiol., 13:221, 1971; Eldridge, J. Physiol., (Lond.), 222:297-318, 319-333, 1972). I recently have found that if you stimulate the carotid body or nerve during expiration, you can actually make that specific expiration deeper (Eldridge, Resp. Physiol., 26:395, 1976). This happens with vagi intact or not.

Remmers: I wouldn't be too surprised about expiration. It seems to me that you are providing the kind of feedback that Dr. Grodins was alluding to before. This is a model that was developed because it applies primarily to vagal feedback and volume feedback, i.e., inspiration is relatively unperturbed by changes in the volume feedback during inspiration. The phrenic ramp continued along the same time course. I think that you are only pointing out that certainly excitatory chemical stimuli will alter that ramp in mid-inspiration. We are dealing with an approximation in my book.

Farber: John Remmers has brought up the possibility that muscles
of the abdomen and chest wall may have altered effects upon breathing when they are concomitantly used as muscles for exercise. Does
anyone on the panel have evidence that differing demands upon respiratory muscles with different kinds of exercise will modify
breathing pattern or optimization of breathing pattern?

Goldman: The data that Dr. Grimby showed suggested that there were
two major differences between exercise and re-breathing. First,
there was greater overall distortion during exercise. Secondly,
with exercise on a bicycle ergometer, contractions of the abdominal
masculature are required as you life the legs so that there are
postural demands on respiratory muscles with exercise which must
be satisfied. This led us to the point of view that those postural demands might determine the relationship between breathing
phase and leg movement. Dr. Loring in our laboratory looked at
treadmill exercise. His notion was that there might be a locking
of respiratory frequency with the leg movement frequency due to
the "slosh of the guts", i.e., accelerative pressures. We found
in treadmill exercise that when we took measurements of esophageal
and gastric pressures and of the separate volumes of the rib cage
and abdomen in people who chose to lock breathing with stride
frequency, there was a clear phasic relationship between the rapid
accelerative pressure change due to "slosh of the guts" and tidal
volume. I think that these are factors that have not been taken
into consideration in modeling, i.e., the locking of breathing to
leg movement frequency; and I agree that they should be.

Filley: This is the first time I have ever heard at a formal
meeting something which is very true, i.e., the "slosh of the
guts". This is an amusing phrase but it really does happen when
you first jump on the treadmill. I am quite convinced that the
very first breath of exercise does not have to be neurogenic, in
as much as many things can happen when your guts slosh. Namely,
get a little bit of air in the lungs and you start things.

Goldman: Those of us who have more guts are more aware of it.

Bake: Dr. Remmers, I think that you mentioned during sleep you
often saw paradoxical motion of rib cage and abdomen.

Remmers: This is work of Bryan and co-workers in Toronto. Certainly there is a departure from the relaxation characteristics
and an extreme paradoxical motion of the rib cage.

Bake: Would you know how frequent it is and the quantitative
importance in terms of volume?

Remmers: It occurs in REM sleep when you have a virtual atony of
the rib cage masculature and all I can say is that you can see
paradoxical motion. I am not sure how common it is. These same
workers have pointed out the importance of this kind of loss of

rib cage tone on the CO_2 response particularly under anesthesia.
They find that some portion of the depression of ventilatory response to CO_2 which occurs in light anesthesia can be attributed
just to loss of intercostal tone and the attending paradoxical
motion of the rib cage. If you look at the abdominal motion during
CO_2 response it is not much changed by anesthesia.

Godfrey: I was one of the experimentors who worked on the CARP,
i.e., the continuous apneic respiratory physiologist with Moran
Campbell (Campbell, E.J.M., et al. Clin. Sci., 36:323-328, 1969).
While the concept of length:tension inappropriateness as the cause
of respiratory sensation is very interesting, I don't think that
you need anything below the neck, or in fact, below the cortex to
produce the sensation of dyspnea. When we paralyzed Moran Campbell,
while conscious, he had no sensation while he relaxed and was left
alone. Only if he tried to make any respiratory effort did he then
feel uncomfortable and experience unpleasant sensations. As his
intrafusal and electrafusal fibers were knocked out during paralysis
the sensation could be attributed purely to cortical influences.

Remmers: This theory of dyspnea was a very general one and I'm not
sure that we ought to apply it that generally. The authors wanted
to go from ordinary respiratory sensations, to sensations in detecting the mechanically hindered breath, all the way over to dyspnea;
and my focus is that it is a very viable explanation for detecting
the mechanically hindered breath and normal respiratory sensations.
I'm not sure where dyspnea fits into that category, and it was that
part of Moran Campbell's generalization that bothered me. I think
it is too sweeping. But we like the basic insight very much.

Jankowski: Concerning inward movement of the diaphragm during
inspiration in people with chronic lung disease. First, is there
any mechanical advantage to these people doing this abdominal
paradoxical breathing; and second, should it be corrected in order
to help them to breath or should we just leave them alone?

Goldman: From my perspective in normal subjects, if you squeeze in
the abdomen you create a load underneath the diaphragm but at the
same time you lengthen the diaphragm and give it a greater mechanical advantage. Thus, the diaphragm is uniquely insensitive to abdominal loading. This is why when we breath with our belly muscles
tight most of the time we are not at all compromised, because the
greater the load below, the more effective the diaphragm is as a
pressure generator. I'm not sure just how badly things get in
chronic lung disease. I would suggest that such abdominal paradoxing might give the diaphragm an increased mechanical advantage.
Whether it's good for sick people or not, I don't know. I would
tend to think that it might be, but I don't have the evidence.

Grimby: I think that from what we measure on the outside it is not
easy to interpret what is occurring on the inside. The upwardly
curved diaphragm is favorable for the lung but places the rib cage

muscle in an unfavorable position.

Goldman: I'd like to try to relate all this muscle mechanics to gas exchange. We studied a group of patients who had paralyzed diaphragms from neuro-muscular disease. Ventilation to their lung bases in the upright posture was remarkably less than normal, and I think, therefore, that the distribution of inspired air depends in part not so much on the shape of the thorax and abdomen, but on the local pressures that are developed. Thus, if a patient does breathe with this abdominal paradoxing, and allows his diaphragm thereby to develop a bigger pressure more effectively, it may be that he will increase the regional ventilation to his dependent lung areas and thereby be able to open airways that might have been closed at FRC. So I think there is at least a potential benefit of the paradoxing.

Sutton: Dr. Remmers, you saw different rib cage and abdominal contributions to the tidal volume generated in CO_2 breathing vs. exercise. During exercise there was really very little contribution of the abdominals to ventilation at all. Was this due to the way you perform the exercise, i.e., supine compared with upright, or the rate and intensity of the exercise?

Remmers: When you're not using your respiratory muscles directly in the exercise process, then CO_2 and exercise stimuli are very different and they don't engage the respiratory muscles in the sam way. I don't have an explanation for these differences.

Goldman: I agree. I want to emphasize that John Remmers' exercise in the supine position involved the lower legs and therefore abdominal musculature was not involved. Also the abdominal muscles in the supine position are flatter and shorter at FRC. Therefore, you don't get much out of them in the expiratory direction. So the differences between John's results and ours in the upright posture are dependent in part upon the different mechanical advantage of the respiratory muscles in the supine position.

Goldman: In summary, I would point out that Dr. Remmers' results during supine exercise are certainly quite different from our subjects exercising in the upright posture. However, these results are consistent with the point of view we have developed regarding the actions of different respiratory muscles when one considers the altered mechanical advantage of these muscles in the supine posture. Nevertheless, I think it would be a mistake to imply that all of the speakers agree on everything that was said this morning. We all have our particular points of view and different biases. In part, this stems from the fact that some of us work primarily with conscious cooperative human subjects, while some work mostly with anesthetized or decerebrate animals. So, without trying to rationalize all of these different perspectives, I will summarize the major points made in this session, as I see them.

If all the separate volume displacements of the different parts of the chest wall are lumped into one volume parameter (namely lung volume change), the actions of important respiratory muscle groups may be overlooked. And we have stressed the importance of partitioning volume displacements between the rib cage and abdomen in order to develop insight into the behavior of thoracic and abdominal muscles. Furthermore, when assessing the mechanical work done by the respiratory muscles, if such volume partitioning is neglected and measurements made only from the Campbell Diagram, an important part of the mechanical load "seen" by the respiratory muscles is missed. That is to say, the respiratory muscles do not act solely upon the lung. In addition they act upon other respiratory structures. Thus, the diaphragm sees both the abdomen and rib cage as a load in addition to the lung. And the abdominal muscles act upon the diaphragm and rib cage as well as the lung.

The major difference between the measurement of mechanical work utilizing the separate rib cage and abdominal contributions and that determined from the Campbell Diagram is the elastic distortional work which does not appear on the Campbell Diagram. In normal subjects, chest wall distortion is associated with distortion of both the rib cage and the abdomen, so that both structures may participate in the increased elastic distortional work done. As noted by Dr. Grimby, however, patients with chronic lung disease are forced to increase their FRC as well, in order to increase their expiratory flow rates. Thus, they must do additional elastic work using the inspiratory muscles of the rib cage and the diaphragm.

Dr. Remmers has pointed out the differences between supine and upright exercise. And he has stressed the importance of reflex pathways. In our human experimentation, we have been more impressed by the importance of voluntary muscle acts. Volitional and metabolic "drives" are superimposed in the control of respiratory muscles, and these pathways are separate neuroanatomically. In studying conscious human subjects, the effects of volition may be dramatically visible. Reflex effects are somewhat less easily demonstrable in human subjects, and this in large part accounts for the different perspectives put forth by Dr. Remmers and our own group.

Finally, Dr. Grodins has demonstrated that mathematical modelling of the respiratory system is a very powerful analytical tool. It seems to me that the challenge of such modelling is its demand for the explicit articulation of concepts and assumptions in very precise language. The reward offered by the model--namely, useful insights into how the respiratory system works--is achieved by the very process of meeting this challenge.

Part II
Mechanisms of Exercise Hyperpnea

6

Mechanisms of Exercise Hyperpnea: Introduction

Alfred P. Fishman

Included in Barcroft's monograph "Features in the Architecture of Physiological Function", published almost forty years ago, is a chapter entitled "Every Adaptation is an Integration" (Fig. 6.1). About half way through the chapter he turns to a consideration of exercise based on the approach used by Murray and Morgan (Fig. 6.1) which, in turn, is rooted in the thinking and experimental experience of L.J. Henderson, D.B. Dill and their associates (2, 4, 5, 9).

This approach rests on the ability of the subject to adjust his metabolic rate at will simply by resorting to exercise. Using a quadrangle for graphic representation, Murray and Morgan illustrated the interplay of some physiological changes evoked by the shift from rest to exercise. The physiological factors that they elected to illustrate in this diagram are rate of blood flow, oxygen capacity of the blood and diffusing capacity. Clearly, other quantifiable biological features could be incorporated into this system and carbon dioxide could be substituted for oxygen (6). The apparent simplicity of this type of representation is deceptive since each of these physiological parameters represents, per se, a complex system of integration. Indeed, one way to regard today's session on the regulation of ventilation during exercise is as a detailed examination of one quadrant of a Murray-Morgan representation.

However, for the different physiological factors to be related meaningfully using the Murray-Morgan approach, and for relevant samples of blood and gas to be drawn, a "steady-state" must be achieved, both at rest and during exercise. That this goal of a steady state has been achieved can be shown by proving that oxygen consumption in the tissues, across the alveolar-capillary barrier and measured oxygen uptake at the mouth are identical (3). Only then will the respiratory exchange ratio determined at the mouth and in the arterial blood truly reflect the substrates that are being consumed metabolically. Much of the literature dealing with exercise either presupposes, or purports to have achieved, a steady state and is therefore confined to one particular phase of exercise.

But it is now recognized that an understanding of the control of breathing during exercise must not only account for observations made during the steady state, but also for adaptations that occur at the moment of start of exercise, the end of exercise and during

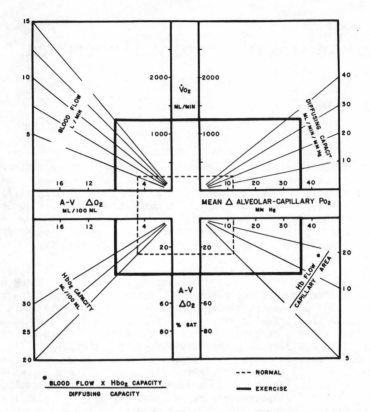

Fig. 6.1. Nomogram illustrating the respiratory and
circulatory interplay involved in delivering an adequate
supply of oxygen to the arterial blood.

the period of recovery. Whether the same physiological mechanisms
are operative during these successive phases, and which mechanism
predominates at each phase, remain to be put into proper perspective.

The earliest workers were careful to distinguish the consecu-
tive phases of exercise. For example, the classical paper by Krogh
and Lindhard in 1913 specified that "we propose to describe the
changes in ventilation, blood flow, pulse rate, respiratory exchange,
and alveolar CO_2 tension taking place in man during the first few
minutes of light or heavy work" (7, 8). Limitations in techniques
then prevented exploration of events at the instant of start or
stop of exercise. But, they did appreciate the need of a steady
state for valid measurements and took this requirement into serious
account in their attempts to unravel the circulatory adjustments
that occurred at the start of work. For their determinations, they
relied on oxygen uptake measured at the mouth as a measure of oxygen
uptake across the alveolar-capillary barrier and as an index of pulmonary blood flow. They concluded that the adaptation of the respiratory and circulatory systems to sudden muscular exertion was
very rapid "though not instantaneous". The "rise in ventilation
like the increase in heart rate" was attributed to irradiation of
impulses from the motor cortex rather than to reflex activity. Finally, with respect to the ventilation, an increase in the excit-
ability of the respiratory center towards hydrogen ions was held
responsible for the barrage of impulses.

Today, more than sixty years later, the propositions of Krogh
and Lindhard are still timely. In particular, serious attention is
being paid, not only to the ventilatory, but also to the circulatory, adaptations that occur with the start of exercise. It has
been shown that the right side of the heart does not have to wait
for an increase in venous return in order to deliver more blood to
the gas exchanging surface of the lungs (10). Instead, increased
myocardial contractility, resulting in improved cardiac emptying,
eliminates the conceptual need to invoke a delay time before ventilation and circulation can be matched. Still uncertain is the
relationship between respiratory rate and tidal volume on the one
hand, and heart rate and stroke volume on the other in making the
necessary adjustments. Also unclear is the extent to which synchronization of the ventilatory and circulatory adjustments involves
overlapping or shared physiological mechanisms.

Almost identical questions have to be raised about the integrative mechanisms that are involved in each phase of exercise.
What is the role of nervous influences? Of chemical stimuli in the
blood? Of humors brought to the lungs from afar? What are the relative roles of these diverse stimuli? And these questions have
proved to be formidable. Indeed, they have often proved too complicated to examine under natural conditions under which adaptive mechanisms operate freely. Therefore, refuge is commonly taken in
"open-loop" preparations where the phenomenon of interest can be

unraveled for detailed scrutiny under controlled conditions. From
these experiments, those attempting to understand the coordinated
regulation of ventilation under natural conditions are inevitably
left with two other problems to solve: 1) what is the physiological
meaning of a response that is elicited under the artificial experimental conditions, and 2) to what extent does the careful experimental control exaggerate, minimize or uncover duplicating mechanisms so that the proportionate contribution of the stimulus under
study is distorted from its role in natural life? In building the
bridge between the experiment and natural life, new complexities
have to be taken into account. How does the experimental situation
involving its own special background of hormones and pharmacologic
agents influence the effectiveness of either neurohumoral or chemical stimuli to ventilation? Does the elimination of one form of
control automatically augment the role of the other? Certainly, as
ventilation is increased during CO_2 breathing, the increase in ventilation must stimulate the flow of nervous information from the
chest bellows to the brain. Also, the state of wakefulness is ex-
ceedingly effective in modifying ventilatory responses to a wide
number of conventional nervous and chemical stimuli. Since it is
rarely possible to weigh all of these variables accurately, "open-
loop" preparations generally do more to disclose potential mechanisms than to provide information about the extent to which these
mechanisms operate spontaneously under natural conditions.

     Barcroft was convinced that exercise is the natural condition
with which physiologists should be concerned. "The condition of
exercise is not a mere variant of the condition of rest, it is the
essence of the machine." He is impressed by the "majesty" of the
locomotive standing "by the platform of a railway station". But,
to understand the concept of a locomotive, he preferred to examine
it with respect to the maximal activity that it was designed to
perform (1). He dismissed the idea of a machine that was designed
to operate at rest. He posed the challenge that the design of the
lungs, the organization of the respiratory system and the coordin-
ating mechanisms that relate respiration and circulation can only
be appreciated when the engine is taxed to the utmost.

     The concept of moving from rest (the stage of the idling en-
gine) to maximal activity redirects the attention of physiologists
to new and fundamental questions. Are the conventional stimuli
that are held to control the resting ventilation the same as those
which control the ventilation during exercise? What is the contribution of chemical stimuli to the control of breathing during exercise? What is the relationship between increased CO_2 delivery to
the lungs by airway, as in the course of determining ventilatory
response curves, and the same quantity of the CO_2 delivered to the
lungs by the blood due to increased metabolic production of CO_2
during exercise?

     These opening remarks are not intended to discourage the pur-
suit of information about the regulation of ventilation during exer-

cise. Instead, they are intended to remind us of the large conceptual framework within which experimental observations have to be
incorporated, particularly if our thinking is to extend beyond the
boundaries of the regulation of ventilation to the coordinated response of the individual as a whole. At this meeting we are engaged in simultaneous attempts at dissection and conceptualization.
From this dissection and conceptualization, new models and hypotheses for testing may emerge. As long as each dissection preserves
sufficient physiological landmarks to allow proper orientation with
respect to natural systems, we will draw closer and closer to a
clear understanding of the control of the ventilation during exercise. It is from this point of view that I look forward to the
papers that follow.

REFERENCES

1. Barcroft, J. Cambridge, University Press, 1934, pp. 1-368.

2. Bock, A.V., D.B. Dill, H.T. Edwards, L.J. Henderson, and J.H.
   Talbott. J. Physiol. 68:277-291, 1929.

3. Fishman, A.P., J.H. McClement, A. Himmelstein, and A. Cournand.
   J. Clin. Invest. 31:770-781, 1952.

4. Fishman, A.P. In: The Handbook of Physiology, Circulation,
   edited by W. F. Hamilton and P. Dow. Washington, D.C., Am.
   Physiol. Soc., 1963, p. 1672, sect. 2.

5. Henderson, L.J. New Haven, Yale University Press, 1928, pp.
   1-397.

6. Jones, N.L., E.J.M. Campbell, R.H.T. Edwards, and D.G.
   Robertson. Philadelphia, W.B. Saunders, 1975, pp. 1-214.

7. Krogh, A., and J. Lindhard. Skand. Arch. Physiol. 27:100-125,
   1912.

8. Krogh, A., and J. Lindhard. J. Physiol. 47:112-136, 1913.

9. Murray, C.E., and J. Morgan. J. Biol. Chem. 65:419-444, 1925.

10. Sarnoff, S.J. Physiol. Rev. 35:107-122, 1955.

7

The Peripheral Neurogenic Drive: An Experimental Study

Frederick F. Kao

Although we began our studies on the mechanisms of exercise hyperpnea with simple assumptions and performed our experiments without new research techniques, they produced some unique experimental results, which with proper interpretation yielded a valid and a definitive conclusion, namely -- There is certainly a peripheral neurogenic drive which must be considered as the, or one of the mechanisms of exercise hyperpnea.

Our experimental study of the mechanisms involved in the regulation of ventilation during muscular exercise followed the publications of Gray in which he exposed his multiple factor theory (14, 15, 16). This theory was refreshingly stimulating to the minds of students who have intrinsically a polytheistic attitude towards science. The monotheistic philosophy of "either-or" changed with Gray's theory to a coexisted, "both or all". Since the chemical regulators for ventilation (namely arterial Po_2, Pco_2, pH) could not account for exercise hyperpnea on the observational level, an additional mechanism was postulated which was named for convenience the exercise stimulus. Grodins published a review article in 1950 (17) in which he exposed convincing argument that an additional factor for exercise hyperpnea must be looked for, and he charted some of the immediate urgent exploratory routes for fruitful experimentation.

The existing hypotheses at the time when we began our experimental studies on the problem of exercise hyperpnea were very conventional, and they include those proposed by Geppert and Zuntz in 1888 (13) which consisted of an exercise impulse from the brain to the respiratory centers to augment ventilation synchronically with exercise (which later supported by Krogh and Lindhard (42, 43) who named it the cortical irradiation), and/or an impulse from the working muscles, which was transmitted to the central respiratory regulatory apparatus in the brain, via the blood stream (the humoral pathway) or reflexly (the neural pathway). Gray, in addition, mentioned the possibility of "chemoreceptors on the venous side of the circulation may respond to changes in Pco_2, pH and Po_2 of the venous blood returning from the exercising region" (16, p 65).

It would not be possible, within the scope of this article,

71

to present the details of a review of all the experimental work
done up to the time when we began our studies. We refer the
interested readers to our earlier publications (25, 28). We
will limit our present communication in some detail to three
major topics: 1. The validity of induced exercise, 2. The
experimental design and results, and 3, the nature of the
peripheral neurogenic exercise stimulus.

I. THE VALIDITY OF INDUCED EXERCISE

Since our experiments were mainly performed with induced
exercise in anesthetized dogs, it is necessary to make some
general statement about the validity of our experimental pro-
cedures. It seems to be self-evident that the exercise stimulus
produced artificially must be similar or nearly so to the one
generated under "normal" conditions, and that no de novo phenomenon
is produced by the experimentally designed procedure for the generation of muscular exercise.

Exercise can be voluntary or involuntary. Under normal
conditions exercise is produced by voluntary impulses originated
in the motor area of the brain. Involuntary exercise can be induced (43). Exercise can also be classified under the headings
of active and passive. Active exercise is defined as that which
produces oxygen consumption, and passive exercise as that which
produces no oxygen consumption. Both active and passive exercise
can be theoretically produced by voluntary and involuntary means.
Passive exercise, such as those produced by means of moving the
limbs passively in man, is actually a mild form of active exercise,
for the oxygen consumption increases during such a maneuver (4, 25).
Even simple intermittent pressure on the calf muscle in man can
increase its oxygen consumption (32).

Induced exercise, such as we employed (40), is a form of
active exercise, for there is an increase in oxygen consumption.
Ventilation, during the steady state of induced exercise, increased
proportionately to the oxygen consumption up to a magnitude when
$\dot{V}O_2$ increased about 5 or 6 times of its resting levels (28, 40).
Furthermore, the slope relating the ventilation and oxygen consumption during induced exercise under the steady state condition
is of the same magnitute as that obtained in data observed in
trained dogs (40). Under transient state, or in the very
beginning of the induced exercise a direct muscle stimulation
caused a slightly greater overshoot of ventilation than when
stimulation was applied of the distal end of one or two severed
spinal motor nerve roots innervating the muscles of the hind
limbs (40). Judging from the oxygen consumption and ventilatory
responses, steady state of induced exercise can be reached within
3 minutes (40).

In all of our experimental studies of the mechanisms of
exercise hyperpnea, we used oxygen consumption of the total

animal or of the exercising hindlimbs as the index of the intensity of the exercise stimulus. This was based on the observation that in mild exercise, whatever the exercise stimulus or stimuli may be they must collectively produce an effect which is proportionate to the oxygen consumption. And during the steady state of moderate exercise ventilation increases in direct proportion to oxygen consumption in man and in dogs (28). In severe exercise, the additional ventilation increase, or the hyperventilation, can be accounted for and explained by the increase in the arterial blood acidemia (17).

The validity of the induced exercise in our experimental studies, was strengthened by the observation that CO_2 interaction with induced exercise in dogs behaved similarly to that as observed in man, namely that there was a parallel shift to the left of the $\dot{V}$-Pco_2 response lines (35). Thus, it can be stated with confidence that the induced exercise such as we produced can be considered as comparable to that of normal voluntary non-induced exercise.

Under anesthesia in dogs, induced exercise produced a $\dot{V}$-$\dot{V}o_2$ relationship similar in slopes as those obtained in trained dogs without anesthesia (40). Therefore, it can be stated that, under steady state at least, induced exercise in anesthetized dogs, when done properly, can be considered as a useful means for studying exercise hyperpnea, for the exercise induced in anesthetized animals in such a controlled fashion is comparable to that of "normal" exercise.

II. EXPERIMENTAL DESIGN AND RESULTS

1. Decerebration Experiments

Induced exercise imposed to the hindlimbs of the decerebrate dogs (39) at the midcollicular level revealed some different responses when compared with that observed in nembutalized dogs during the transient state. In the beginning of exercise, both oxygen consumption and ventilation increased in an hyperbolic fashion to attain a steady state. This is in contrast to the transient or the beginning response of oxygen consumption and ventilation in anesthetized dogs in which there was a sudden overshoot of ventilation. The overshoot of ventilation immediately after the induced exercise again disappeared in decerebrate dogs (39), which resembled the data of Schneider and Clark (51) observed in man. During the steady state, however, the ventilatory response to induced exercise in the decerebrate dogs and anesthetized dogs showed similar slopes of $\dot{V}$-$\dot{V}o_2$ relationship. Arterial Pco_2 and pH remained essentially unchanged during exercise up to an oxygen consumption level of nearly 400 ml/min STPD.

Krogh and Lindhard (42, 43) claimed that a neural component

of the exercise stimulus must be involved, since humoral agents, because of the delay in transport, cannot explain the sudden onset of the increase in ventilation during exercise. They also advanced the idea that the possible neural factor may originate in the muscles as claimed by Geppert and Zuntz (13) or in the cerebral cortex. Our decerebration experiments did not support this cortical irradiation hypothesis, nor did the experiments of Asmussen et al (3), employing induced exercise in man, support the same hypothesis. Evidently there is a pathway from the cortex to the respiratory centers, a mechanism which can affect ventilation, as in the case of voluntary hyperventilation. It would be very convenient if such a pathway existed from the cortex to the respiratory neurons, and especially if it acted in such a fashion to stimulate ventilation proportionally to the oxygen demand during exercise. Obviously, if such a pathway existed, and if it were functional during exercise, it would not be the only mechanism involved, as evidenced by our results obtained in decerebrate dogs.

2. The Relationship of Cerebrospinal Fluid to Exercise
   Hyperpnea

Leusen (44) suggested that during exercise lactic acid may pass into the CSF and act as an additional and hitherto unsuspected stimulus to respiration, since intracranial receptors sensitive to changes in CSF pH can affect ventilation (47). A series of experiments was performed in anesthetized dogs with induced exercise. During severe exercise there was a slight decrease of the arterial Pco_2, pH and HCO_3 indicating that exercise was accompanied by a mild metabolic acidemia. There were, however, no significant changes in the pH, Pco_2 or HCO_3 of the cerebrospinal fluid (41).

In another series of experiments, the ventilation-CO_2 response lines were determined in dogs at rest and during exercise. Instead of using the conventional $\dot{V}$, P_aco_2, variables, ventilation was plotted as a function of CSF H^+. During CO_2 inhalation, ventilation is related to CSF H^+ and, while a similar relationship existed during CO_2 inhalation in exercise, exercise increased ventilation at constant CSF H^+ in an additive fashion. Therefore, it seems justifiable to conclude that, in mild exercise at least, the central H^+ does not play a role in exercise hyperpnea. although it is still possible that a severe metabolic acidemia might stimulate ventilation through central receptors as well as through the arterial chemoreceptors (45) during severe muscular activity.

3. The Perfusion of Arterialized Blood During Exercise to
   the Head of the Recipient Dog

Although during moderate exercise, arterial Pco_2, Po_2, pH do not alter and therefore cannot be considered as "steady

state" exercise stimuli (17), there might be other unknown
arterial agents which could cause exercise hyperpnea (18). In
order to investigate the effect, if any, of the arterialized
blood generated during exercise, on ventilation in an animal
without exercise, experiments were performed in which the
arterialized blood of the exercising dog was perfused into the
head of a second dog via their carotid and/or vertebral arteries
(26). Both dogs were induced to exercise separately but their
ventilation, oxygen consumption and blood pressure were observed
simultaneously.

Since ventilation of the dog receiving arterialized blood
of the exercising dog remained absolutely unchanged, it was
necessary to conclude that there were no humoral factors
produced which would cause hyperpnea. It should be noted, and
can be understood easily, that, if the exercising dog did not
have a normal response, such as under severe anesthesia which made
its blood hypercapnic, during exercise, then the dog receiving
the arterialized blood of the exercising dog may show an increased ventilation. This can explain the work of Heymans et al
(20) in which the twitching on the larynx was used as an index
of ventilation changes. The frequency of the recipient's
twitching increased when the donor dog was induced to exercise,
and the authors concluded that humoral factors must have existed.
It was likely that the exercising dog had a "deep" anesthesia.
Also ventilation was not measured in their experiments, hence any
conclusion drawn in regard to ventilation seems hazardous.

Furthermore, it should be pointed out that our studies limited
to moderate exercise in which some humoral factors such as
catecholamines changed very little. It seems likely that in
severe exercise, some unknown humoral agents related or unrelated
to catecholaimine might appear and affect ventilation during
severe exercise (17).

It should be noted that when the tubes leading the perfusing
blood from the donor dog to the recipient   dog's head was changed
in length (from 3 ft to 9 ft) there was no change in either dog's
ventilation when both were at rest. During exercise of the
donor dog its ventilation responded similarly to that of the single
dog, and ventilation of the recipient dog remained always unchanged.

We also performed experiments in single dogs in which the
exteorized carotid arteries were lengthened using plastic tubings
before they reentered back into the brain. The ventilatory reponse
to induced exercise was the same as in those dogs without exterior-
ized lengthened carotid arteries. The same was true when both
carotid arteries and both vertebral arteries were exteorized and
lengthened (35).

4. The Role of the Carotid Chemoreception in the Regulation of
    Ventilation During Exercise

In a series of experiments, the carotid apparatuses of one
dog (recipient) were perfused exclusively with blood from a second
dog (donor). When the donor was induced to exercise its ventilation
changed which was similar to that of intact anesthetized dogs.
The recipient dog which received exercising blood in its carotid
apparatuses did not show any change in its ventilation. The
"intactness" of the carotid apparatuses of the recipient dog
perfused with the donor dog's blood, was tested by means of
injections of lobeline and/or cyanide to the donor's blood
perfusing these carotids and it was found that the ventilatory
response to such injections was similar as those observed in intact
dogs (33).

Additional experiments with this preparation were performed
in which the recipient dog was exercised but the donor dog was
given hypoxic gas mixture to breathe. It was found that the
hypoxic drive of these perfused carotid apparatuses produced an
additional effect to ventilation during exercise. The carotid
plays an essential role for such an interaction of hypoxia effect
with induced exercise, although the evidence presented here
alone cannot validate whether this hypoxia and exercise interaction
is at the carotid sites, or elsewhere in the brain (33). A
valid conclusion can be drawn, however, with regard to the role
of the carotid apparatus for exercise hyperpnea, namely the
carotids play no primary role in exercise hyperpnea under normal
conditions at sea level.

5. The Separation of the Neurohumoral Pathways from the Limbs
   to the Central Respiratory Regulatory Apparatus

Our experimental study of the exercise hyperpnea with the
separation of the neurohumoral pathways began in 1950 when the
author was working in the laboratory of Drs Gray and Grodins.
Looking back after a quarter of a century, I truly believe that
sometimes experiments happen as accidents. The first pair of
cross-perfusion experiment with dogs was done on a Saturday and
was without witness. But the results were just as exciting, for
when the perfused hindlimbs of the recipient (neural dog) was
exercised, both the humoral (donor) and the neural dogs showed
an increase in ventilation (25, 31, 37).

The experimental design was of a simple nature. In order
to separate the neural and humoral pathways from the exercising
limbs, a simple cross perfusion technique was used. The hindlimbs
of one dog were perfused with blood exclusively from a second dog
via the abdominal aortae to the first dog's hindlimbs and the
venous blood of the perfused hindlimbs coursed back to the second
dog via the inferior venae cavae. The exercising limbs of the
first dog were connected to its respiratory regulatory apparatus
only through the neural pathways, hence it was named the neural
dog. The second dog received the exercising blood of the neural
dog's hindlimbs hence it was named the humoral dog.

If there was a neural pathway operating during exercise, the neural dog's ventilation should respond to exercise and if the humoral pathway was involved, then the humoral dog's ventilation should respond to exercise. The fact that ventilation of both the neural and the humoral dogs responded during exercise pointed to the possibility that there should be both neural and humoral pathways. In other words, both neurogenic and blood borne factors should be responsible for exercise hyperpnea.

An analysis of our data revealed that the neural dog, while its hindlimbs were induced to exercise, showed a hypocapnic body, with respiratory alkalemia. The humoral dog, however, had a hypercapnic (arterial) body with respiratory acidemia. Immediately two questions were raised. First of all, if the perfusion of blood was "poor" in the exercising hindlimbs acidemic condition would be produced while exercising. Then the blood from the exercising hindlimbs perfusing the humoral dog would be acidotic and the respiratory acidemia would be complicated with metabolic acidemia. This is the common "error" in an experimental procedure involving blood perfusion. The pH of the perfusing blood had to be measured if we study the ventilatory response. This we did and in addition we measured the blood flow of exercising hindlimbs (34).

The second question raised in this experiment was the different responses in ventilation when CO_2 was introduced exogenously (e.g. CO_2 inhalation) or endogenously (e.g. perfusing CO_2 rich blood to an animal). The hindlimbs cross-perfusion experiment was actually an ideal method of introducing endogenous CO_2 to the humoral dog.

The advantage of using two dogs, instead of one dog and one machine (perfusing apparatus with excorporal blood) lies in the fact that the body handles many unknown factors which might have been produced during the cross-perfusion procedure, and therefore, no "extra load" of unknown de novo factors could have been produced. While in the case of employing machine for perfusion, the unknown factor generated by the machine could not be "de-toxicated" by the natural animals organs.

6.   Ventilatory Responses in the Neural Dog with an Isocapnic Head

A three-dog cross-perfusion experiment was performed in which the neural dog was made isocapnic by perfusing its head with blood from a third dog (the supporting dog) in similar arrangement as described in I, 3 under the heading of The Perfusion of Arterialized Blood During Exercise to the Head of the Recipient dog (26). In this trial experiment, the neural dog had hypercapnic limbs, hypocapnic trunk, and isocapnic head when its hindlimbs were induced to exercise. The data from a series of such experiments

showed that when the hindlimbs of the neural dog with isocapnic
head was induced to exercise its ventilation behaved similar to
that of the intact single anesthetized dogs. There was no more
respiratory alkalemia in the head of the neural dog, although its
trunk was in a hypocapnic state. Its head and hence the central
regulatory apparatus for ventilation, however, was similar to
that of the intact dogs (28). It seems justifiable to state
that since the neural dog (if its head was isocapnic) behaved in
a similar fashion as the intact dog, the neurogenic exercise
stimulus alone in the working tissues can account for the total
ventilatory response during induced muscular exercise.

7. Perfusing Exercising Blood from the Exercising Hindlimbs
   to the Chest of the Humoral Dog With its Head Remained
   Isocapnic

A three-dog cross-perfusion experiment was performed in
which the humoral dog was supported by blood from a supporting
dog arranged in a similar fashion as for the neural dog. The
blood which became hypercapnic, hypoxic, and hyperacidemic,
during exercise, was perfused to the humoral dog's chest, but
not its head. In 6 pairs of such experiments it was found that
the neural dog had an increase in ventilation during the time
when its legs were induced to exercise, but there was no increase
in its oxygen uptake, hence resulted in an increase in its ventilatory equivalent for oxygen. The humoral dog showed an increase
in oxygen uptake alone, for its blood was supporting the exercising
hindlimbs of the neural dog. The supporting dog, however, showed
no change in ventilation or in oxygen uptake. The humoral dog
with an isocapnic head but with a chest which was receiving
exercising blood, did not show any increase in ventilation when
the neural dog was induced to exercise (28). This series of
experiments was of special interest because it did not support
the existence of the venous receptors which might have been
responsible for exercise hyperpnea.

It is understandable that in perfusion experiments involving
two or three dogs simultaneously, hemorrhage may be produced.
First of all, hemorrhage can be avoided if careful surgery is
done. Secondly, hemorrhage alone does not change the normal
exercise response (27).

8. Transient Studies in Man

A series of experiments was performed in man employing the
breath-by-breath recordings of ventilation during exercise. The
plot of ventilation as a function of alveolar Pco_2 was instant-
aneously displayed by means of an XY plotter (29). The behavior
of such a plot for CO_2 inhalation exhibited a loop which we named
the $\dot{V}$-Pco_2 loops, different in character from the $\dot{V}$-Pco_2 lines.
When such a plot was attempted employing data obtained in
man during exercise, the steady state response of ventilation

as function of the alveolar Pco_2 showed a straight upward move
of the line. This was expected since there is no change in
alveolar Pco_2 during the steady state of exercise, unless the
work intensity becomes severe (17). In the beginning of exercise,
however, there was a transient decrease in Pco_2, hence there was
a small loop travelling from the normal point of the $\dot{V}$-Pco_2 plot
to the left and then coming back to the normal isocapnic line.
At the termination of the exercise, there was an increase in Pco_2, so
the transient response after the termination of exercise looped
to the right and then gradually restored to the normal resting
point, which again fell on to the isocapnic line. This finding
is of special interest, because it is a further validation of the
neurogenic drive, which happened immediately after exercise. This
hyperventilation effect lasted about one minute. After the CO_2
produced in the exercise limbs was transported to the chest,
the refilling just made up what had been lost during hyperventilation; hence the combined effects of neural drive and the CO_2
refilling resulted in an alveolar isocapnia.

9. The Interaction of Exercise Stimulus (Induced) with
   Known Respiratory Stimuli

   A. Exercise and Exogenous CO_2

The study of the interaction of CO_2 with the induced exercise
was to establish whether the exercise such as that we produced
was similar or not to the "normal" exercise stimulus. If the
induced exercise is similar to normal exercise, then the interaction of CO_2 stimulation with exercise must be similar to
that as observed in man which showed that the "rectilinear part
of the stimulus response curves at rest was displaced to the
left with exercise, and the more so the higher the work intensity.
The steepness of the curves was in the majority of cases about the
same" (2).

Experiments with the recipient dog's head perfused by blood
from a donor dog exclusively were performed. $\dot{V}$-Pco_2 lines were
established while the recipient was at rest and during exercise, and
while the donor dog was given different mixtures of CO_2 to breathe.

The results showed that at rest the recipient dog demonstrated a normal $\dot{V}$-Pco_2 response line while the donor dog was given
CO_2 to breathe. When the same procedure was carried out while
the recipient dogs hindlimbs were induced to exercise, a parallel
left shift of the $\dot{V}$-Pco_2 response line was obtained (34, 35).

There are two points of interest. First of all, the exogenous
CO_2 produced a $\dot{V}$-Pco_2 response line with similar slopes as those
obtained with endogenous CO_2, such as those obtained in the
humoral dog's response while the neural dog was induced to

exercise. Secondly, our finding did not support the oscillatory
hypothesis of Yamamoto, which claimed valid experiments can only
be obtained in the presence of an intact arterial pathway. In
our recipient dog, the arterial pathway from the lungs to the
head was interrupted but ventilation responded in a manner similar
as in intact dogs during exercise (55).

10. Further Evidence Supporting the Neural Genesis of the Exercise Stimulus

A. Partial Chordotomy Experiments

Partial chordotomy experiments were performed in order to
identify the neural pathways by means of which the exercise
stimulus travelled for the augmentation of ventilation during
exercise (36). Partial chordotomy was performed in the neural
dog at T-11. It was discovered that cutting the dorsal columns
had little effect on the response to induced exercise, but after
the severance of the lateral columns, the ventilatory response to
exercise was absent. Data were presented in detailed in a later
publication (28). The question arises that since the lateral
columns also convey temperature, these findings were in favor
of temperature as one of the exercise stimuli. But this should in
no way exclude the existence of other unidentified, and perhaps
unidentifiable (at the present time with our limited means of
investigation at least), exercise stimulus which might travel
to the central respiratory regulation apparatus via these spinal
columns. Our finding was not in favor of the proprioceptive
tracts for the mediation of the exercise stimulus and hence,
it might be argued, that propioception, which might be important
in positioning, was not responsible for conveying the exercise
stimulus from the exercising muscles to the central respiratory
apparatuses (9, 53).

B. Afferent Nerve Stimulation Experiments

It follows naturally and it seems to be axiomatic, that
since there is a neural pathway in exercise hyperpnea the
stimulation of the afferent nerve fibers in the muscles must
augment respiration. This is based on the similar maxim that
in identifying the stimulus for any condition, the stimulus
must be presented during the condition studied, and that the
factor or the stimulus alone without the condition studied must
also produce similar response. In other words, if neural
stimulus causes a change in respiration in exercise, the stimulation of such nerves without exercise should also augment
ventilation.

The gastrocnemius, the femoral, or the sural nerve of the hindlimbs of cats, dogs, intact, or in cross-perfused (circulation of
hindlimbs were separated from the body) was cut and the cephalic end
of the nerve was stimulated by means of a stimulator with 60 cycle

AC at a modulation frequency of 120/minute. The results showed
that when stimulating currents of 0.01-3 μA were used, the skin
branch stimulation showed no ventilatory response unless there
was a spread of current to the adjacent muscles. With the stimulation of the muscle nerve, a very small current caused a change
in ventilation. The latent period was short, but not actually
measured (23, 28).

When curare was given to the donor animal (humoral) considerably more current was necessary to stimulate the nerves of
the neural dog for the same ventilation increment. This was
corroborated by the findings of Assmussen et al (1) who used
curare in man.

Recently, Paulev (49) studied the ventilatory changes during
muscle contraction and correlated the time response rate with
the changes in ventilation and EMG. He concluded that the
ventilatory latency, being shorter than the pulmonary effector
period, excluded a peripheral trigger mechanism. It seems difficult
to measure the time of transmission in ventilation not only because
many factors can complicate the situation, but also ventilation
itself is an integrated slow frequency response. More work seems
necessary in this area.

III. THE NATURE OF THE PERIPHERAL NEUROGENIC STIMULUS OF EXERCISE HYPERPNEA

The nature of the exercise stimulus is at present still elusive.
At least two steps must be accomplished in identifying the factor(s).
(1) an identification of the factor(s) during exercise must be
carried out, and (2) the same factor(s) should increase ventilation without exercise. It is very difficult to assess if a factor
(to mimic that as actually occurred in exercise) is exactly identical
to that as generated during exercise. Many of the suggested factors
are difficult to produce without the actual process of muscular
contraction. We have done several types of experiments and the
results are in favor of a multiple of factors produced in the
muscles during exercise which are responsible for the total
response of exercise hyperpnea.

1. Stretch Receptors

Experiments involving the stretch of the freed Achilles
tendon with a displacement of one or two inches at a frequency
of 120, 240, and 360 per minutes by means of a home-made solenoid
operated by a Grass stimulator failed to demonstrate any changes
in ventilation. The same failure was observed in both intact
single cats, dogs, and in the neural dogs (22, 28).

2. Chemoreceptors (pH, Pco_2, and Po_2)

Perfusing blood of one dog during rebreathing to the hind-

limbs of a second dog, did not change the latter dog's ventilation.
We inferred from this observation that in the working tissues,
there were no chemoreceptors which are responsive to CO_2, O_2 and
pH. This experiment, however, did not exclude the possibility
of other chemoreceptors which might be responsible for exercise
hyperpnea. Other chemicals have been used for identifying
peripheral chemoreception but some of the chemicals used were
not known to be produced in exercise (12).

3. Thermoreceptors

During muscular exercise, body temperature rises and a rise
of body temperature without exercise increases ventilation.
Naturally one would assume that body temperature must play a
role in exercise hyperpnea. Some experiments which we did,
support this view. First of all muscle temperature is best
correlated with the changes in ventilation as compared with
rectal temperature, carotid temperature, and cutaneous temperature
which all changed during induced exercise (24, 30, 48). The
difficulty for this type of experiment is the fact that how
can one produce the same temperature changes (both in the temporal
response and in intensity) as it occurs during exercise. Heating
from outside is a very poor method, for exogenous heat affects
the outside skin first, and in exercise heat is generated from
the inside of the body, which affects the muscles first. It
seems that unless new experimental methods were designed, a
quantitative study of the partial effect of temperature on
ventilation would not be possible (10, 28).

4. Mechanoreceptor

In the work which we published in 1971 (32) we demonstrated that a simple pressure on the calf muscles mimicking the
contraction pressure during actual muscular exercise increased
little oxygen uptake, but a great deal of ventilation. The
increase in ventilation was immediate which was accompanied
with alveolar hypocapnia. When CO_2 was added to the inspired
air to maintain an isocapnic state, ventilation increased further
to a considerable magnitude. The ventilation-Pco_2 response line
of the subject during squeezing, shifted to the left, in a
similar fashion as occurred in voluntary muscular exercise, which
was known to have a parallel left shift. It seems inevitable
to conclude that the intra-muscular pressure developed during
muscular contraction may be an important contributor to exercise
hyperpnea (8, 11, 32).

The problem again arises. How can one quantify the pressure
produced in the experimental condition and that during actual
muscular exercise, although we found in our experiments that
there was summation effect of area and tempo of the pressure
on ventilation? Since oxygen consumption is rectilinearly related to muscular exercise in moderate exercise, how can the

amount of pressure be quantitatively related to oxygen consumption? All these problems have to be answered before we can assign a definitive role of pressure as one of the stimuli of exercise hyperpnea.

In 1952 we named the hypothetical receptor in the working tissues the "ergoreceptor", a term   coined with a combination of Latin and Greek, which was violently opposed by the monotheistic schools which believed that there should be no mixing of Latin and Greek in making new words (23, 25).

5. Metaboloreceptor

Gray and Grodins as early as in 1951 named this peripheral muscle receptor for exercise hyperpnea "metaboloreceptor", again a term with a mixing of Latin and Greek. Ramsay in 1953 employing the neuro-humoral dog design and found that 2:4-dinitrophenol could increase ventilation and oxygen consumption and the regression lines related ventilation as a function of oxygen consumption were almost identical when the animal was either anesthetized, decerebrated or decerebrated and anesthetized (50). These regression coefficients were found also to be similar to those found in dogs during exercise (28).

We have also tried to use chemical stimulants for the increase of ventilation including dinitrophenol, but failed to achieve a steady state even the dosages used were small. It was also necessary to monitor temperatures at various sites of the body. But this may be an interesting area to explore.

6. Some Speculations

The design of the human body is evidently equipped with multiple monitoring receptors and loops from the muscle to the central levels of the nervous system. The demand of ventilation to cope with muscular exercise necessitates information pathways from the muscles where the energy is spend during work. It seems logical that such a peripheral neurogenic drive should exist for the gas exchange need of the muscles which is supplied by the ventilatory apparatus.

Many investigators studied the peripheral neurogenic drive, ever since Geppert and Zuntz (13) mentioned its possible role in exercise hyperpnea (5, 6, 19). The interested readers are referred to Matthews' Muscle Receptors 1972, Chapter 7 pp 319-409 for a detailed analysis of the neurological studies of this muscle afferents (46). Others also studied the peripheral neurogenic receptor by means of chemicals (12, 54), or direct nerve stimulation (7, 21, 23, 52, 53).

Although it seems evident that the peripheral neurogenic drive originated from the working muscles must be involved in

exercise hyperpnea, a wide gap still exists between the neurological evidence which is based on nerve stimulation (a useful
but limited means of study, because of the polymodel nature of
nerves) and the actual identification of the nature of the
receptors, and the agent(s) which are responsive to exercise
hyperpnea.

Increase the oxygen consumption in the muscles without
exercise is an attractive means of approach (38), but a quantitative
comparison of the induced hypermetabolism with that of exercise
is not without hazard. Perhaps what we need is a new methodology
to study this elusive mechanism of exercise hyperpnea.

Summary

Employing a series of various cross perfusion techniques,
we have obtained results which definitely pointed to the
necessity of postulating a local reception mechanism in the working
tissues which is mediated to the central ventilation regulatory
apparatus via a neural pathway for exercise hyperpnea. This
peripheral neurogenic drive does not seem to be a single or a simple
factor. Furthermore, from our experimental results it was necessary
to postulate the existence of a polymodel nature of this
peripheral neural drive of exercise hyperpnea.

ACKNOWLEDGMENTS

The author wishes to express his appreciation to all of
his collaborators, visitors, and graduate students who participated
in research in his laboratory in the past years. The names of
these people are listed in the bibliography. We express our
special appreciation to Sarah S. Mei who has been working in our
laboratory since 1961, and to our comparatively new contemporary
collaborators, especially Anthony Babich. This study was supported
in part by a grant (HE-4032) from the National Institute of Health,
U.S. Public Health Service.

REFERENCES

1. Asmussen, E., S.H. Johnansen, M.I. Jørgensen, & M. Nielsen.
   Acta physiol. Scand. 63:343-350, 1965.

2. Asmussen, E and M. Nielsen. Acta physiologica Scand 39:27-35,
   1956.

3. Asmussen, E., M. Nielson, and G. Weith-Pedersen. Acta Physiol.
   Scand. 16:168-175, 1943.

4. Bahnson, E.R., S.M. Horvath, and J.H. Comroe, Jr. J. applied
   physiology 2:169, 1949-1950.

5. Besson, P., P. Dejours, and Y. Laporte. J Physiol (Paris) 51:400-
   401, 1959.

6. Comroe, J.H., and C.F. Schmidt. Am J Physiol 138:536-547, 1943.

7. Coote, J.H., S.M. Hiton, and J.F. Perez-Gonzalez. J Physiol
   (London) 201:34-35p 1969.

8. Coote, J.H., S.M. Hilton, and J.F. Perez-Gonzalez. J Physiol.
   215:789-804, 1971.

9. Dejours, P., Y. Labrousse and A. Teillac. Compt Rend Acad.
   Sci 248:2129- 2131, 1959.

10. Dejours, P., A. Teillac, F. Girard, and A. Lacaisse. Rev. Fr.
    Etud. Clin. Biol 3:755, 1958.

11. Flandrois, R., J.R. Lacour, J. Islas-Maroquin, and J. Charlot.
    Respiration Physiol. 2:335-343, 1967.

12. Gantier, H., A. Lacaisse, P. Pasquis and P. Dejours. J Physiol
    (Paris) 56:560-561, 1964.

13. Geppert, J., and N.Zuntz. Pflieger's Arch. ges. Physiol. 42:
    189-245, 1888.

14. Gray, J.S. AAF School of Aviation medicine, Research Project
    No. 386, 1945.

15. Gray, J.S.Science 103:739, 1946.

16. Gray, J.S. PULMONARY VENTILATION AND ITS PHYSIOLOGICAL REGULATION
    Springfield, Charles C. Thomas 1950.

17. Grodins, F.S. Physiol Rev. 30:220-239, 1950.

18. Haggard, H.W. and Y. Henderson. J. Biol Chem 43:3, 1920.

19. Harrison, W.G., Jr., J.A. Calhoun, and T.R. Harrison. Am J.
    Physiol 100:68-73, 1932.

20. Heymans, C., J. Jacob, and G. Liljestrand. Acta Physiol Scand
    14:86-101, 1947.

21. Hodgson, H.J.F. and P.B.C. Matthews. J Physiol 194:555-563, 1968.

22. Hornbein, T.F., S.C. Sørensen, and C.R. Parks. J Applied
    Physiol 27:476-479, 1969.

23. Iaria, C.T., U.H. Jalar and F.F. Kao. J. Physiol (London)
    148:49-50, 1959.

24. Kao, F.F. Master Thesis, Northwestern University Medical School,
    Chicago, 1950.

25. Kao, Frederick F. Summaries of Doctoral Dissertations, North-
    western University. 20:616-620, 1952.

26. Kao, Frederick F. Am. J. Physiol. 185:145-151, 1956.

27. Kao, Frederick F. Fed. Proc. 15:104, 1956.

28. Kao, Frederick F. In: REGULATION OF HUMAN RESPIRATION. Editors:
    D.J.C. Cunningham and B.B. Lloyd. Blackwell Scientific Publication
    Oxford. pp. 461-502, 1963.

29. Kao, Frederick F., Anthony M. Babich, Sarah S. Mei, and Carol
    Wang. Acta Neurobiologiae Experimentalis 33:163-175, 1973.

30. Kao, Frederick F. and Fred S. Grodins. Fed. Proc. 10:72, 1951.

31. Kao, Fred, and Fred S. Grodins. Fed. Proc. 11:80, 1952.

32. Kao, Fred. F., S. Lahiri, S. Mei, G. Schwartz, and H. Tucker.
    In: RESEARCH IN PHYSIOLOGY, Editors: Frederick F. Kao, Kiyomi
    Koizumi and Mario Vassalle, Aulo Gaggi Publisher, Bologna, pp 729-
    740, 1971.

33. Kao, Frederick F., S. Lahiri, C. Wang, and Sarah S. Mei. In:
    PHYSIOLOGY OF MUSCULAR EXERCISE. Editor: C.B. Chapman. American
    Heart Association Monograph No. 15, Supplement 1 to Circulation
    Research, Vols. XX and XXI, 1-179 - 1-191, 1967.

34. Kao, F.F., C.C. Michel and S.S. Mei. J. Appl. Physiol. 19:1075-
    1080, 1964.

35. Kao, F.F., C.C. Michel, S.S. Mei and W.K. Li. Annals of the New
    York Academy of Sciences. 109:696-710, 1963.

36. Kao, F.F., and Louise H. Ray. XIX International Physiological Congress, Montreal, p. 500, 1953.

37. Kao, Frederick F., and Louise H. Ray. Am. J. PHysiol. 179:249–254, 1954.

38. Kao, Frederick F., and Barbara B. Schlig. Am. J. Physiol. 195:229–232, 1958.

39. Kao, Frederick F., Barbara B. Schlig and Chandler McC. Brooks. J. Appl. Physiol. 7:379–386, 1955.

40. Kao, Frederick F., and Eustace E. Suckling. J. Appl. Physiol. 18:194–196, 1963.

41. Kao, F.F., C.W. Wang, S.S. Mei, and C.C. Michel. IN: CEREBRO-SPINAL FLUID AND THE REGULATION OF VENTILATION. Editors: C.McC Brooks, F.F. Kao and B.B. Lloyd. Blackwell Scientific Publications, Oxford. pp. 269–275, 1965.

42. Krogh, A., J. Lindhard. J. Physiol (London) 47:117–136, 1913.

43. Krogh, A., and J. Lindhard. J. Physiol (London) 51:182–201, 1917.

44. Lensen, I. In: THE REGULATION OF HUMAN RESPIRATION. pp. 207–222 Editors: Cunningham, D.J.C., and B.B. Lloyd, Oxford, Blackwell, 1963.

45. Lensen, I. In: CEREBROSPINAL FLUID AND THE REGULATION OF VENTI-LATION pp. 55–89. Editors: Brooks, C. McC. F.F. Kao, and B.B. Lloyd, Oxford, Blackwell, 1965.

46. Matthews, P.B.C. MAMMALIAN MUSCLE RECEPTORS AND THEIR CENTRAL ACTIONS. The Williams and Wilkins Comp. Baltimore, 1971.

47. Mitchell, R.A., H.H. Loeschcke, W.H. Massion, and J.W. Severing-haus. J. Applied Physiol. 18:523, 1963.

48. Morgan, D.P., F. Kao, T.P.K. Lim, and F.S. Grodins. Am. J. Physiol. 183:454–458, 1955.

49. Paulev Poul-Erik. Journal of Applied Physiology 34:578–583, 1973.

50. Ramsay, A.G. J. Applied Physiology 14:102–104, 1959.

51. Schneider, E.C., and R.W. Clarke. Am. J. Physiology 74: 334, 1925.

52. Senapati, J.M. J. Appl. Physiol. 21:242–246, 1966.

53. Sipple, J.H., and R. Gilbert. J. Appl. Physiol. 21:143–146, 1966.

54. Wildenthal, K., D.S. Mierzwial, N.S. Skinner, and J.H. Mitchell. Am. J. Physiol. 215:542-548, 1968.

55. Yamamoto, W.S. J. Applied Physiology 15:215-219. 1960.

8

Ventilatory Response to Drug-Induced Hypermetabolism: Possible Relevance to Exercise Hyperpnea

Sanford Levine

INTRODUCTION

During moderate muscular exercise in man and animals, the increase in ventilation is proportional to the increment in metabolic rate (i.e., oxygen consumption, carbon dioxide production) (2-4, 6, 14). The mechanism underlying this correlation is not fully understood. However, previous workers have demonstrated that conventional chemical stimuli in arterial blood (i.e., increments in arterial PCO_2, decrements in arterial pH and decrements in arterial PO_2) can not account for this correlation between tissue metabolism and pulmonary ventilation (2-4, 6, 14).

Previous investigators have attempted to elucidate the relationship between tissue metabolic rate and pulmonary ventilation by infusing 2, 4-dinitrophenol (DNP), an uncoupler of oxidative phosphorylation, into animals (1, 9, 10, 12, 15). All workers have reported that increases in ventilation accompany increases in oxygen consumption elicited by DNP; these increases in ventilation occur in the absence of conventional chemical stimuli to ventilation in arterial blood (vide supra).

In experiments designed to uncover the mechanism by which DNP stimulates ventilation, Ramsay (10) administered DNP to the limb of a dog (experimental animal) which was entirely perfused with blood from another dog (donor animal); an increase in ventilation was observed in the experimental animal. Therefore, Ramsay (9) concluded that DNP elicits increases in V̇E by stimulating metabolic receptors in muscles; he hypothesized that these receptors transmit information to the respiratory center via neural pathways.

Subsequent work by Bailen and Horvath (1) challenged Ramsay's conclusions. Their work suggested that the increase in ventilation, which was noted in Ramsay's limb perfusion experiments, was due to leakage of DNP into the central circulation of the experimental animal. However, Bailen and Horvath did not attempt to identify the mechanism by which leakage of DNP into the central circulation elicits an increase in ventilation.

In an attempt to elucidate the mechanism underlying the

89

increase in ventilation elicited by DNP, Williams et al. (15) infused DNP into peripheral chemoreceptor denervated animals (i.e., dogs who had undergone bilateral carotid sinus denervation and bilateral vagotomy); the increases in ventilation, which followed DNP infusion, were similar to those observed in intact animals. Therefore, these authors suggested that stimulation of intracranial sensors by DNP accounts for the major portion of the ventilatory increment which follows DNP infusion. However, the communication by these authors provides no direct evidence in support of this conjecture.

At the present time, considerable controversy exists regarding the receptors which mediate increases in $\dot{V}E$ elicited by DNP (vide supra). The present paper demonstrates that the major portion of the increase in $\dot{V}E$ elicited by DNP is mediated by extracranial receptors other than the carotid and aortic bodies. This paper also demonstrates that a similar extracranial mechanism can account for the increase in $\dot{V}E$ elicited by ethyl methylene blue, another uncoupler of oxidative phosphorylation which differs from DNP in chemical structure (Fig. 8.1).

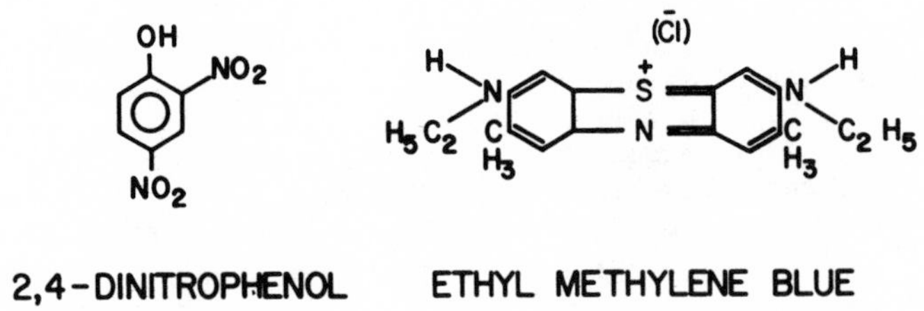

2,4-DINITROPHENOL   ETHYL METHYLENE BLUE

Fig. 8.1.   Structural formulae of uncouplers of oxidative phosphorylation. Ethyl methylene blue (EMB) differs from 2,4-Dinitrophenol (DNP) in chemical structure.

METHODS

General

Two types of experimental preparations were used in this study; intact dogs and head-perfused dogs. Intact dogs were used to establish the effect of uncouplers of oxidative phosphorylation (i.e., DNP or EMB) under the present experimental conditions. Head-perfused dogs were used to demonstrate that these drugs stimulate ventilation via an extracranial mechanism other than the carotid and aortic bodies.   The following measurements were made: oxygen consumption, ventilation, arterial oxygen saturation, arterial PCO_2, arterial [H+] activity, and rectal temperature.

Anesthesia was induced in all animals with methoxyflurane and anesthesia was maintained with chloralose (60 mg/kg). In each animal, a tracheal cannula was placed and a catheter was positioned in the right femoral artery; this catheter was used for sampling arterial blood and for administration of drugs (i.e., DNP or EMB).

Intact Animals

Drug-infusion experiments. Two types of drug-infusion experiments were carried out in intact animals: DNP-infusion experiments EMB-infusion experiments.

DNP-infusion experiments. Six DNP-infusion experiments were carried out in six intact animals. The dose of DNP was 2.5 mg/kg; this dose was infused into the right femoral artery. These experiments indicated that DNP infusion elicited sustained increments in ventilation and oxygen consumption. A steady state with respect to ventilation, oxygen consumption, arterial PCO_2, arterial pH and arterial oxygen saturation was achieved eight minutes after the completion of DNP infusion; these steady state relationships generally remained unchanged for the subsequent fifteen to twenty minutes. Data in the results section refer to determinations carried out in the time interval extending from ten to twenty minutes after the termination of DNP infusion.

EMB-infusion experiments. Six EMB-infusion experiments were carried out in six intact animals. The dose of EMB was 8-15 mg/kg. The experimental protocol was identical to the DNP-infusion experiments.

Head-Perfused Animals

Experimental Preparation. In these experiments, the head of the experimental animal was perfused with arterial blood from a support dog via both carotid and both vertebral arteries (Fig. 8.2). Blood was drained from the head via the external jugular veins to a reservoir; a pump was used to return this venous blood to the support dog. To ensure vascular separation between the perfused head and the remainder of the experimental animal, nerves, muscles, and blood vessels in the neck were cut and tied and an occlusive collar was placed around the bony spine. The spinal cord remained intact. Completeness of vascular separation between head and body was tested by injection of Evans blue dye into the body; after such injections, no dye was demonstrable in external jugular venous blood draining from the head. In these head-perfused animals, the carotid bodies lay within the region of the perfused head. The aortic bodies, which lay outside the perfused head, were denervated via cervical vagotomy. We (7) have previously demonstrated that head-perfused animals prepared in

this manner demonstrate virtually no increase in $\dot{V}E$ coincident
with arterial hypoxemia or arterial hypercapnia of the body.

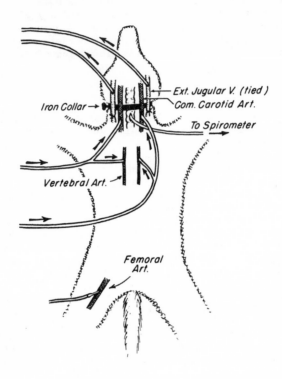

Fig. 8.2. Diagram of a head-perfused animal. The head of
the experimental animal was completely perfused with blood from
a support dog via both carotid and both vertebral arteries.

Arterial blood perfusing the head of a head-perfused animal
(i.e., support-dog arterial blood) generally had a PCO_2 of 35
mmHg, a [H+] of 40 nmol/liter and a PO_2 of 80 mmHg. These parameters remained constant during the transition from control to
test periods. (Control measurements were made subsequent to
initiation of the head perfusion.)

Initial head-perfused animal experiments demonstrated that
increases in ventilation and increases in oxygen consumption
followed the infusion of DNP or EMB into the body (See Drug administration to body). To assess the head-perfused animal's ventilatory response to increases in oxygen consumption (of the body)
elicited by non-pharmacologic techniques, we studied the head-
perfused animal's ventilatory response to muscular exercise of

the hind-limbs (see Muscular Exercise). To evaluate the possibility that DNP or EMB can elicit increases in ventilation via stimulation of receptors within the region of the perfused head, these drugs were selectively administered to the head (see Drug administration to head).

Drug administration to body. DNP (2.5 mg/kg) was infused into the body of four head-perfused animals. EMB (8-15 mg/kg) was infused into the body of four head-perfused animals. The experimental protocol was identical to the intact animal drug-infusion experiments.

Muscular Exercise. Six muscular exercise experiments were carried out in six head-perfused animals. Exercise was induced by direct stimulation of hind-limb muscles with electric pulses of 3/s frequency, 5 ms duration, and 60 V intensity. These pulses were delivered by a Grass SD5 stimulator (Grass Instrument Co., Quincy, Mass.) for a period which varied from 6 to 10 minutes. A steady state with respect to oxygen consumption and minute ventilation was achieved after four minutes of exercise. Experimental observations were made during the final two minutes of muscular exercise.

Drug administration to head. DNP or EMB was selectively administered to the head of four head-perfused animals. Since the support-dog would be exposed to these drugs, the dose of DNP or EMB was computed per kilogram of support-dog body weight (i.e., 2.5 mg/kg DNP or 8-15 mg/kg EMB). The weight of the support dog always exceeded the weight of the experimental animal.

In these experiments, the dose of DNP or EMB was infused into a jugular vein of the support dog or into the common catheter which carried blood to the vertebral and carotid arteries. In all experiments, ventilation in the experimental animal reached a steady state seven minutes after the termination of drug infusion: this steady state persisted for 10-20 minutes. Experimental observations were made in the time interval extending from 8 to 25 minutes after the completion of drug infusion.

Analytical Techniques

In all experiments, animals breathed 100% oxygen from a spirometer which was fitted with a CO_2 scrubber; oxygen consumption and ventilation were measured during the course of rebreathing. In most experiments, pH, PO_2, and PCO_2 were directly measured with a Radiometer PHM 71 acid-base analyzer and appropriate electrodes--E 5021, E 5032, E 5046 (The London Co., Cleveland, Ohio). These electrodes were maintained at 37°C. Arterial oxygen saturation was computed by standard nomograms (11). In some experiments, PCO_2 was computed from blood carbon dioxide content, hemoglobin and pH. We (7) have previously described the methodology utilized in these analyses.

Data Analysis

Data are described in this manuscript by the mean and standard error of the mean (SE). In each type of experiment, the significance of differences between control and experimental values was determined by using paired t-tests (13). A measured difference was considered a chance occurrence unless its significance would be demonstrated at the 0.05 level.

RESULTS[1]

Intact Animals

Control measurements in arterial blood. Arterial PCO_2 was 41 + 2 mmHg and arterial [H+] was 47 + 1 nmol/liter; arterial oxygen saturation was 100% in all animals.

DNP-infusion experiments. DNP infusion elicited hypermetabolism in the absence of motion; oxygen consumption increased 100 + 2% and ventilation increased 122 + 22%. Figure 8.3 shows the individual data points. Arterial PCO_2, arterial pH and arterial oxygen saturation remained constant.

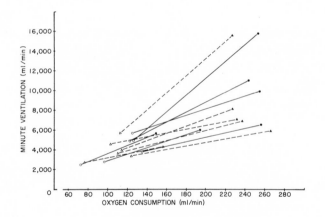

Fig. 8.3. Intact animal drug-infusion experiments. Open circles = prior to DNP; solid circles = after DNP. Open triangles = prior to EMB; closed triangles = after EMB.

EMB-infusion experiments. EMB infusion also elicited hypermetabolism in the absence of motion; oxygen consumption increased 110 + 5% and ventilation increased 93 + 17%; figure 8.3 shows the

[1]Table I of our previous publication contains a statistical summary of all data contained in the present paper.

individual data points. Arterial PCO_2, arterial pH and arterial
oxygen saturation remained constant.

Head-Perfused Animals

Control measurements in arterial blood (of body). Arterial
PCO_2 was 26 ± 2 mmHg and arterial [H+] was 44 ± 1 nmol/liter.
Arterial oxygen saturation was 100% in all animals.

DNP administration to body. DNP infusion into the body
induced hypermetabolism in the absence of motion; oxygen consumption increased 97 ± 15% and ventilation increased 129 ± 41%.
Figure 8.4 shows the individual data points. Arterial PCO_2,
arterial pH and arterial oxygen saturation (of the body) remained
constant.

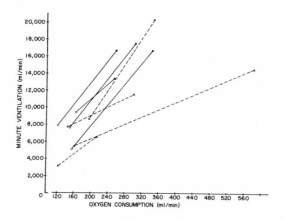

Fig. 8.4. Head-perfused animal drug administration to body experiments. Open circles = prior to DNP; solid circles = after DNP.
Open triangles = prior to EMB; closed triangles = after EMB.

EMB administration to body. EMB infusion into the body likewise induced hypermetabolism in the absence of motion; oxygen
consumption increased 130 ± 45% and ventilation increased 116 ±
25%. Figure 8.4 shows the individual data points. Arterial PCO_2,
arterial pH and arterial oxygen saturation (of the body) remained
constant.

Muscular Exercise. Electrical stimulation of the hind-limbs
induced muscular contraction and hypermetabolism; oxygen consumption increased 120 ± 18% and ventilation increased 126 ± 3%.
Figure 8.5 shows the individual data points. Arterial PCO_2,

arterial [H+] and arterial oxygen saturation remained constant.

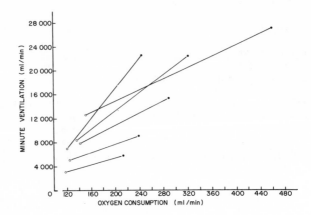

Fig. 8.5. Head-perfused animal muscular exercise experiments.
Open circles = control observations; solid circles = experimental
observations during muscular exercise of the hind limbs.

DNP administration to head. DNP administration to the head
failed to elicit significant increases in ventilation. Figure 8.6
compares the ventilatory changes which were observed upon administration of DNP to the head and to the body of a head-perfused
animal.

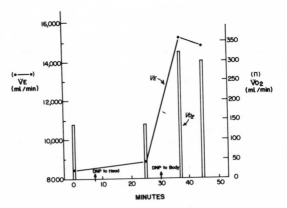

Fig. 8.6. A comparison of the ventilatory and metabolic
changes which were observed upon administration of DNP to the
head and to the body of a head-perfused animal. DNP to the

head produced no change in oxygen consumption of the body; a 500 ml/min increase in ventilation was observed. When the same dose of DNP was given to the body, a twofold increase in oxygen consumption and a 6,600 ml/min increase in ventilation occurred.

EMB administration to head. EMB administration to the head elicited modest increases in ventilation [30 ± 7%]; these increases in ventilation are significant at the 0.05 level.

Analysis of Relationship between Oxygen Consumption and Ventilation

Table 8.1   presents control and experimental ventilatory equivalents for oxygen (i.e., $VEO_2 = VE/VO_2$) for all experiments. In each type of experiment, paired analysis of differences in VEO_2 failed to reveal a significant difference.

Type of Expt	Control	Experimental	P
Intact animals			
DNP infusion	36 ± 3	40 ± 5	>0.1
EMB infusion	38 ± 3	36 ± 7	>0.1
Combined DNP & EMB	37 ± 2	38 ± 4	>0.1
Head-Perfused animals			
Drug administration to body			
DNP infusion	51 ± 7	56 ± 3	>0.1
EMB infusion	39 ± 6	38 ± 7	>0.1
Combined DNP & EMB	45 ± 5	47 ± 5	>0.1
Muscular exercise of the body	55 ± 8	56 ± 9	>0.1

Table 8.1. Values are means ± SEM. P values represent the probability of the difference between control and experimental observations occurring by chance; a paired t-test was used to compute these P values.

DISCUSSION

The DNP and EMB intact animal experiments confirm previous work (1, 5, 8, 15) that these drugs stimulate ventilation by a mechanism other than conventional chemical stimuli in arterial blood (i.e., arterial PCO_2, arterial pH and arterial oxygen saturation.) The head-perfused animal drug administration to body experiments demonstrate that these drugs stimulate ventilation via extracranial receptors other than the carotid and aortic bodies.

Comparative role of intracranial and of extracranial receptors in mediating increases in ventilation elicited by uncouplers of oxidative phosphorylation. The drug administration to head experiments demonstrate that selective administration of the full

dose of these drugs to the head elicited only modest increases in
ventilation. Since these increases in $\dot{V}E$ were appreciably smaller
than those elicited by infusion of these drugs into the body, this
comparison suggests that extracranial receptors mediate the major
portion of the intact animal's ventilatory response to uncouplers
(i.e., DNP or EMB). The results of those experiments in which
DNP or EMB were selectively administered to both head and body of
the same animal (e.g., figure 8.6) support this conclusion.

Nature of the extracranial receptors. We (7) have previously demonstrated that the head-perfused animal exhibits a markedly
attenuated ventilatory response to increments in arterial PCO_2
and to increments in arterial [H+] of the body. We have also
shown that the head-perfused animal displays no increase in $\dot{V}E$
coincident with arterial hypoxemia of the body (i.e., an arterial
PO_2 of 32 mmHg). Therefore, the head-perfused animal drug administration to body experiments suggest that the extracranial
receptors, which mediate increases in $\dot{V}E$ elicited by uncouplers
of oxidative phosphorylation, are poorly responsive to increments
in arterial PCO_2, increments in arterial [H+], and to decrements
in arterial PO_2.

Location of the extracranial receptors. The present study
did not localize the extracranial receptors which mediate the
increases in ventilation elicited by infusion of uncouplers of
oxidative phosphorylation. The data are compatible with Ramsay's
concept (10) of multiple scattered tissue receptors, (i.e.,
metaboreceptors). Our data are also compatible with the hypothesis
that a sensor in the central circulation mediates the ventilatory
response to uncouplers of oxidative phosphorylation; this receptor
may respond to some aspect of uncoupler-induced tissue hypermetabolism or to direct stimulation by these drugs.

Communication between extracranial receptors and respiratory
center. It is reasonable to assume that the extracranial receptors
which mediate the ventilatory response to uncouplers of oxidative
phosphorylation, transmit information to the respiratory center.
Since the spinal column constitutes the sole communication between
head and body in the head-perfused animal, the drug administration
to body experiments suggest that the uncoupler-induced stimulus to
$\dot{V}E$ is transmitted to the respiratory center via afferent pathways
of the cervical spinal cord.

Relevance of drug-induced hypermetabolism to exercise hyperpnea. The present work demonstrates that head-perfused animals
exhibit similar ventilatory responses (i.e., unchanged $\dot{V}EO_2$ and
unchanged arterial PCO_2) to drug-induced hypermetabolism and to
exercise-induced hypermetabolism. These comparisons suggest that
a similar mechanism may be operative in both conditions. Therefore, the extracranial receptors which mediate the ventilatory
response to drug-induced hypermetabolism may play a role in eliciting the hyperpnea of muscular exercise.

Summary

1. Two chemically different uncouplers of oxidative phosphoryla-
tion--i.e., 2,4-dinitrophenol (DNP) and ethyl methylene blue
(EMB)--elicited both increases in ventilation [107 $\pm$ 14%] and
increases in oxygen consumption [105 $\pm$ 3%] in anesthetized dogs.

2. At the drug doses employed in the present study, the increments
in ventilation elicited by these drugs were accompanied by an
unchanged arterial PCO_2 and by an unchanged arterial pH.

3. In order to explore the possibility that DNP and EMB stimulate
$\dot{V}E$ via an extracranial mechanism, heads of dogs were completely
perfused with blood of unvarying gas composition from a support
dog via both carotid and both vertebral arteries. The carotid
bodies lay within the region of the perfused head; the aortic
bodies, which lay outside, were denervated.

Infusion of DNP or EMB into the body of these head-perfused
animals elicited both increases in ventilation [123 $\pm$ 22%] and
increases in oxygen consumption [113 $\pm$ 23%].

4. When similar doses of DNP or EMB were selectively administered
to the head region of head-perfused animals, increases in $\dot{V}E$ were
limited to 21 $\pm$ 6%.

5. It is concluded that extracranial receptors other than the
carotid and aortic bodies mediate the increase in $\dot{V}E$ elicited by
representative uncouplers of oxidative phosphorylation.

These receptors may play a role in mediating the hyperpnea of
muscular exercise.

ACKNOWLEDGMENTS

The experiments described in this publication were carried out
in collaboration with Dr. William Huckabee. Ms. Geraldine Hill
provided invaluable assistance in assembling the manuscript.

REFERENCES

1. Bailen, H.N. and S.M. Horvath. Am. J. Physiol., 196:467-469,
   1959.
2. Comroe, J.H. Physiology of Respiration, Chicago: Year Book
   1965, p. 192.
3. Dejours, P. In: Handbook of Physiology, Respiration.
   Am. Physiol. Soc., 1964, Sect. III, Vol. II, Chapt. 25,
   p. 631-648.
4. Grodins, F.S. Physiol. Rev., 30:220-239, 1950.
5. Huch, A., D. Kotter, R. Loerbroks, and J. Piiper. Respr.
   Physiol., 6:187-201, 1969.

6. Kao, F.F. In: Regulation of Human Respiration, edited by
    D.J.C. Cunningham and B.B. Lloyd. Oxford: Blackwell, 1963,
    p. 461-502.
7. Levine, S. and W.E. Huckabee. J. Appl. Physiol., 38:827-833,
    1975.
8. Liang, C.S. and W.B. Hood. J. Clin. Invest., 52:2283-2292,
    1973.
9. Ramsay, A.G. J. Appl. Physiol., 14:102-104, 1959.
10. Ramsay, A.G. (Abstract) J. Physiol., London 127:30p, 1955.
11. Severinghaus, J.W. In: Handbook of Physiology, Respiration,
    Washington, D.C.: Am. Physiol. Soc., 1964, Sect. III. Vol.
    II, Chapt 61, p. 1478.
12. Shen, T.C.R. and W.H. Hauss. Arch. Intern. Pharmacodyn.
    63:251-258, 1939.
13. Snedecor, G.W. and W.G. Cochran. Statistical Methods,
    Ames, Iowa: Iowa State Univ. Press, 1967, p. 91.
14. Wasserman, K. and B.J. Whipp. Am. Rev. Resp. Dis., 112:219-
    249, 1975.
15. Williams, T.F., R.W. Winters, J.R. Clapp, W. Hollander, and
    L.G. Welt. Am. J. Physiol., 193:181-188, 1958.

DISCUSSION

Sampson: What was the time course of the increase in ventilation after 2,4-DNP injection? Where do you think these metabo-receptors are located?

Levine: In response to your first question, we infused 2,4-DNP intra-arterially for two minutes; $\dot{V}E$ and $\dot{V}O_2$ increased over the initial 7-10 minutes after infusion. A steady state with respect to both $\dot{V}E$ and $\dot{V}O_2$ was achieved between 10 and 20 minutes after infusion. In response to your second question, the data that I have presented do not localize the extracranial receptors which mediate increases in ventilation elicited by DNP. However, some recent work by Liang and Hood (Circ. Res., 38:209, 1976) indicates that receptors innervated by lower lumbar and sacral spinal afferents mediate some portion of the increase in $\dot{V}E$ elicited by DNP. In order to quantitate the contribution of these receptors to the intact animal's ventilatory response to DNP, I have recently infused DNP into L-1 spinal transected animals; following DNP infusion, these L-1 spinal transected animals exhibited increases in $\dot{V}E$ similar to intact animals. This comparison suggests that the receptors of Liang and Hood do not play a quantitatively important obligatory role in mediating the ventilatory response elicited by DNP.

Eldridge: Won't some of the drug you are injecting reach the medulla? Even if not, there may be an alternative explanation to your findings. Your drug is going to the whole body including the spinal cord and spinal cord metabolic rate will increase and therefore the firing of spinal cord neurons will probably increase. Do we have to, then, postulate any sort of special metabolic receptor?

Levine: I have demonstrated that administration of the full drug dose to the head region elicits only modest increases in ventilation (see Fig. 8.6). This piece of evidence makes it unlikely that leakage of small amounts of drug from body to head accounts for the head-perfused animal's ventilatory response to drug-induced hypermetabolism. In response to your second point, the data that I have presented do not exclude the possibility that uncouplers are eliciting increases in ventilation by direct stimulation of the spinal cord. However, some recent work from my laboratory (Levine, S., Rev. Resp. Dis., 113:218, 1976) indicates that the body of the head-perfused animal contains receptors which respond to humoral agents released by muscular exercise. The possibility exists that these receptors may also respond to humoral agents released by drug-induced hypermetabolism.

Filley: You said that neither cardiac output nor lactic acid concentration in blood increased with the drug injections. However, mixed venous PCO_2 must have increased and PO_2 decreased; did they not in these drug induced studies?

Levine: Yes, mixed venous PCO_2 increased and PO_2 decreased.

9

CO_2 Flow to the Lungs & Ventilatory Control[1]

Karlman Wasserman, Brian J. Whipp,[2] Richard Casaburi,
William L. Beaver,[3] & Harvey V. Brown

In spite of the long interest by physiologists in the mechanism of the control of breathing during exercise, and its obvious biological importance, the mechanism of the hyperpnea of exercise remains obscure. The neurohumoral hypothesis (5), which is most often invoked to explain the hyperpnea of exercise, does not adequately account for the experimental observations of gas exchange during exercise.

The neurohumoral hypothesis stipulates that the abrupt increase in ventilation which occurs at the start of exercise in many (but not all) subjects must have its origin in a neurogenic stimulus. Gas exchange measurements, however, suggest that humoral mechanisms can account for the initial exercise hyperpnea. Breath-by-breath measurements of end-tidal CO_2 ($P_{ET}CO_2$), minute ventilation ($\dot{V}_E$), CO_2 output ($\dot{V}_{CO2}$), O_2 uptake ($\dot{V}_{O2}$) and the respiratory gas exchange ratio (R), during the transition from rest to exercise are shown in Figure 9.1 for a typical normal subject who demonstrated an abrupt increase in V_E. These measurements show that, despite the hyperpnea, there is neither a decrease in $P_{ET}CO_2$ nor an increase in R, in contrast to what would be expected if ventilation increased out of proportion to the increase in pulmonary blood flow.[4]

---

1. Supported by PHS Grants HL-11907, HL-05916, HL-14967 and HL-17107.
2. Established Investigator of the American Heart Association.
3. Department of Electrical Engineering, Stanford University, Stanford, California.
4. In fact, $P_{ET}CO_2$ increases and R decreases following a short delay. After the early seconds of exercise, the alveolar phase of the CO_2 concentration is no longer a plateau as it is at rest, but is sloped upward with time. This increase in slope reflects the appearance at the lung capillaries of CO_2 produced during exercise. Thus, the end-tidal P_{CO2} increases relative to the mean alveolar tension.

The decrease in R at this time must reflect the difference between the rate of change in tissue CO_2 and O_2 stores as the tissue P_{CO2} and P_{O2} change after exercise begins.

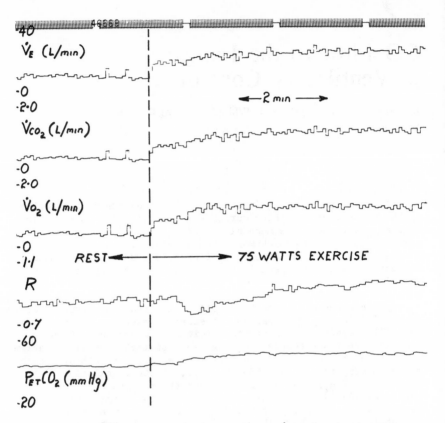

Fig. 9.1   Change in minute ventilation, ($\dot{V}_E$), CO_2 production ($\dot{V}_{CO_2}$), O_2 consumption ($\dot{V}_{O_2}$), gas exchange ratio (R) and end-tidal CO_2 ($P_{ET}CO_2$) breath-by-breath at the onset of exercise.

In interpreting these results, it is apparent that a significant amount of CO_2 manufactured in the muscle at the start of exercise could not have had time to reach the lungs within the first 10-15 seconds. However, a rapid increase in venous return and cardiac output at the onset of exercise, charged with resting values of CO_2 and O_2, could result in an increase in CO_2 flow to the lungs sufficient to account for the increase in $\dot{V}_{CO_2}$ noted at the onset of exercise (Fig. 9.1). If $\dot{V}_E$ did not increase appropriately for the increased CO_2 flow, there would be an imbalance of alveolar ventilation ($\dot{V}_A$) relative to perfusion. This would result in an altered P_{CO_2} on the arterial side of the circulation. A sensitive CO_2 control mechanism could keep arterial P_{CO_2} relatively constant following an abrupt increase in delivery of venous blood at the start of exercise by effecting a matching increase in $\dot{V}_A$. In fact, the only way that both P_{CO_2} and R would not change when $\dot{V}_E$ increased at the start of exercise would be if venous blood, charged with resting values of CO_2 and O_2, perfused the lungs at an increased rate, and $\dot{V}_E$ increased appropriately to maintain the overall alveolar ventilation-perfusion ratio the same as that at rest.

The observations in gas exchange noted above and previously reported (1), suggest that sensitive chemoreceptors on the arterial (high P_{O_2}) side of the pulmonary circulation function to change $\dot{V}_E$ pari passu to any change in CO_2 flow to the lungs. To examine this hypothesis, we changed CO_2 flow to the lungs by a variety of methods to determine its effect on breathing. In this presentation, we shall report on the ventilatory response to changes in CO_2 flow induced by: a) increasing (14), and b) decreasing cardiac output (2), c) venous loading of CO_2 (13), d) progressively incremented work rate exercise (15), e) sinusoidally varying work rate exercise (3,18) and f) dietary manipulation (17). We shall conclude by describing our current understanding of the chemoreception responsible for the ventilatory response to CO_2 flow.

Effect of Increase in CO_2 Flow to the Lungs by Increasing Cardiac Output

To study the effect of abruptly increasing cardiac output on $\dot{V}_E$, we stimulated cardiac output with a bolus injection of isoproterenol in doses of 2 to 10 µgm into the superior vena cava in awake and lightly anesthetized dogs (pentobarbitol-25mgm/KBW). We continuously measured expiratory flow, $P_{ET}CO_2$, breathing rate, heart rate and cardiac output. We integrated the expiratory flow signal to obtain $\dot{V}_T$ and $\dot{V}_E$ breath-by-breath.

When boluses of isoproterenol were injected into the superior vena cava to increase cardiac output, $\dot{V}_E$ abruptly increased with no change or only a slight increase in $P_{ET}CO_2$ (Fig. 9.2). The increase in $\dot{V}_E$ did not occur unless cardiac output increased; we term this ventilatory increase a "cardiodynamic hyperpnea". Excess anesthesia or beta-adrenergic blockade with propranolol resulted in proportional reductions in cardiac output and $\dot{V}_E$ (Fig. 9.3). In doses of propranolol which partially block the cardiac output increase induced by the isoproterenol injection (Fig. 9.3) the increase in $\dot{V}_E$ was also partially blocked. Complete blockade of the heart rate increase by propranolol completely eliminated the isoproterenol induced hyperpnea.

Injection of isoproterenol into both common carotid or left subclavian (vertebral) arteries, resulted in a relatively attenuated and delayed ventilatory response (Fig. 9.4) compared with an identical injection into the superior vena cava. This is most likely due to loss of the drug in the tissues of the head and the circulatory delay before the drug can reach the heart and effect an increase in cardiac output.

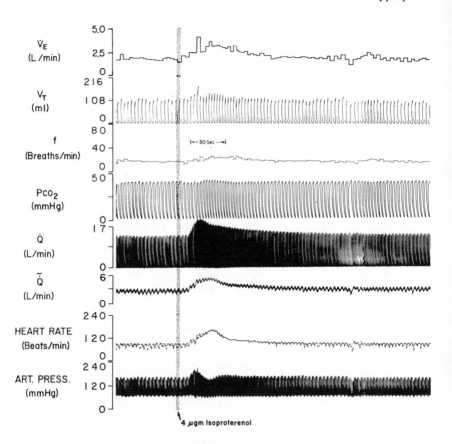

Fig. 9.2   Effect of 4µg of isoproterenol (stippled bar) injected into the superior vena cava on minute ventilation ($\dot{V}_E$), tidal
volume (V_T), respiratory rate (f), end-tidal CO_2 (P_{CO_2}), aortic flow
(Q), mean aortic flow (Q), heart rate and arterial pressure during
air breathing in an awake dog.

    The persistence of the response with 100% O_2 breathing and
the lack of enhancement of the response during 11% O_2 breathing
(Fig. 9.5) suggests that the carotid bodies are not required for
this "cardio-dynamic hyperpnea". Furthermore, removal of the
carotid bodies does not eliminate the isocapnic cardiodynamic
hyperpnea (14). The aortic bodies and vagal afferents from the
lungs also do not appear to be involved, since the hyperpnea
following isoproterenol bolus injections is also present following
bilateral cervical vagotomy and following simultaneous sectioning
of the vagi and resection of the carotid bodies (14).

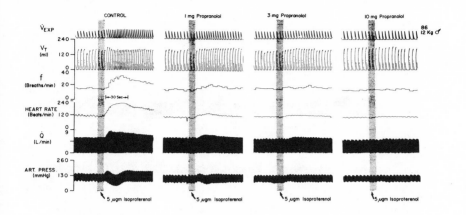

Fig. 9.3 Effect of 5μg of isoproterenol (stippled bars) injected into the superior vena cava on expiratory flow ($\dot{V}_{exp}$), tidal volume ($\dot{V}_T$) respiratory rate (f), heart rate, aortic flow (Q) and arterial pressure during a control period and following the cumulative intravenous dose of 1, 3, and 10mg of propranolol in an anesthetized dog.

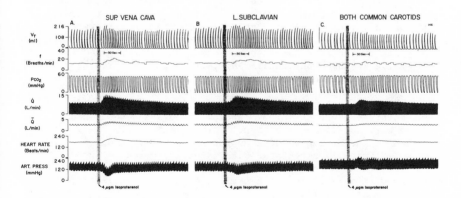

Fig. 9.4 Effect of 4μg of isoproterenol injected into the superior vena cava (A), 4μg into the left subclavian artery, from which the left vertebral artery originates (B), 2μg simultaneously injected into each common carotid artery (C). Stippled bars are the injection period. Symbols are same as those for Figure 9.3.

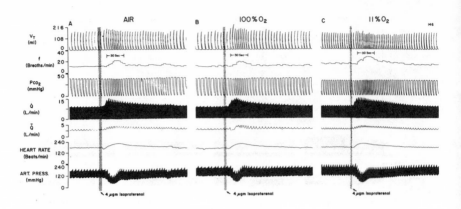

Fig. 9.5 Effect of 4μg of isoproterenol (stippled bars) injected
into the superior vena cava on tidal volume (V_T), respiratory
rate (f), end-tidal CO_2 (P_{CO_2}), aortic flow (Q), mean aortic
flow (Q̄), heart rate and blood pressure during air, 100% O_2 and
11% O_2 breathing in an anesthetized dog.

     To determine whether an abrupt increase in cardiac output
can induce an hyperpnea in the presence of hypocapnia, we injected
a bolus of isoproterenol into the superior vena cava following
mechanical hyperventilation and compared the ventilatory
response with that observed after hyperventilation alone (Fig. 9.6).
In spite of the increase in cardiac output following isoproterenol
injection in the hyperventilated state, the dog's breathing
pattern remained unaltered.
     To determine if the cardiodynamic hyperpnea could be induced
by other than pharmacological means, stimulating electrodes were
put into the right atrial myocardium of dogs and their heart
rates were increased by pacing. Unfortunately, this is a poor
method of increasing cardiac output since the increase in heart
rate is typically associated with a reduced stroke volume.
However, in dogs whose heart rates happened to be relatively
low we were able to induce a small increase in ventilation
during cardiac pacing (14).
     In summary, the hyperpnea resulting from a bolus injection
of isoproterenol is isocapnic or slightly hypercapnic. It is
very reproducible in a given animal and can be repeated, without
evidence of tachyphylaxis as soon as the effects of the previous
dose have worn off (approximately 5 minutes). This phenomenon
has been demonstrated in dogs, cats and rabbits. Experimental
animals which are too deeply anesthetized or traumatized and
unable to maintain respiratory homeostasis, may not demonstrate

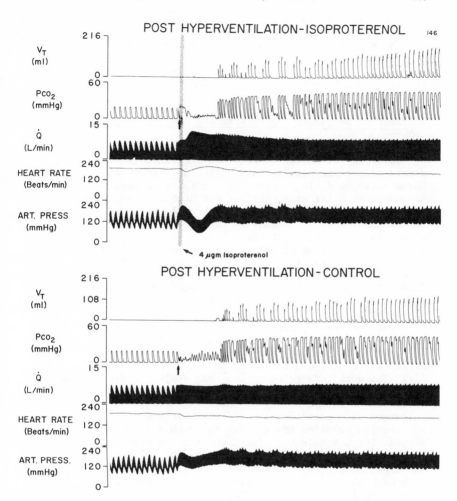

Fig. 9.6 Effect of prior hyperventilation, with a mechanical
respirator, on the isoproterenol-induced hyperpnea. The stippled
bar indicates time of injection of 4μg of isoproterenol into the
superior vena cava. Lower panel is a control study in which isoproterenol was not injected. Arrow indicates time of discontinuing
the hyperventilation. CO$_2$ tension to the left of the arrow is a
measure of the CO$_2$ tension in the expired air during the
mechanical respiration.

the response. If the experimental animal cannot maintain a
physiological pH, it appears that all of the responses to normal
humoral stimuli for ventilation become depressed. Therefore,
we feel that is is important to report measurements of arterial
pH and blood gases, as well as the ventilatory response to bolus
isoproterenol injection, in any animal preparations used to
investigate ventilatory control.

Effect of Decreased CO_2 Flow to the Lungs by Decreasing Cardiac Output

Epstein, et al (6) showed that propranolol hydrochloride,
a beta-adrenergic blocker, administered intravenously to normal
human subjects during sub-maximal exercise, caused sustained
decreases in heart rate, cardiac output and pulmonary arterial
oxygen saturation, while $\dot{V}_{O_2}$ and arterial oxygen saturation
remained unchanged. Because of the relatively high solubility
of CO_2 in the tissues, it would be expected that the acute
reduction in cardiac output induced by beta-adrenergic blockade
should cause a transient reduction in CO_2 flow to the lungs.
When the tissue CO_2 tension is sufficiently increased to raise the
venous CO_2 content to a level which would bring the rate of CO_2
flow to the lungs back to the pre-propranolol level, CO_2 homeostasis would be re-established.

To test the CO_2 flow hypothesis, we studied the effect
of the acute lowering of cardiac output during exercise on $\dot{V}_E$
in normal subjects, by injecting propranolol (0.2mg/KBW) over a
period of about 1 minute during moderate, steady-state exercise
(2). The work rate selected for each subject's exercise test
was at a level which was approximately 80% of his anaerobic
threshold as determined by an incremental exercise test
performed on a previous day. After a minimum of six minutes
of exercise to allow the subject to reach a steady-state,
propranolol was injected intravenously. There was no evidence
that the subject was aware of the time that he was receiving
the drug. $\dot{V}_E$, f, $\dot{V}_T$, $P_{ET}CO_2$, $\dot{V}_{O2}$ and $\dot{V}_{CO2}$ were measured breath-
by-breath as previously described (1). The exercise was con-
tinued for 10 minutes after the injection of the drug.

For purposes of analysis, the study was divided into three
experimental periods with respect to the drug infusion: the
pre-infusion phase, the response phase and the post-infusion
phase (Fig. 9.7). The pre-infusion phase comprised the 2 minutes
immediately prior to propranolol injection. In order to select
a time when cardiac output was decreasing, the response phase
was defined from the time at which heart rate started to decrease
to the time at which the heart rate had undergone 80% of its
total change to the new reduced "steady-state" value following
the propranolol injection. This period was about 3 minutes in
duration. The post-infusion phase comprised the 6th and 7th
minutes following injection of propranolol, by which time the
heart rate had stablized to its new value. Mean values for
each variable during each phase were determined by averaging

individual breath-by-breath measurements. Since the difference between the pre- and post-infusion phases were not appreciable, their averaged values were used as a control for comparison with the response phase (period of decreasing heart rate).

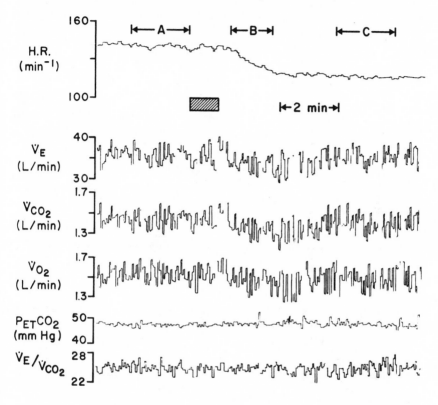

Fig. 9.7 Breath-by-breath measurement of heart rate (HR), minute ventilation ($\dot{V}_E$), CO₂ output ($\dot{V}_{CO_2}$), oxygen uptake ($\dot{V}_{O_2}$), end-tidal CO₂ tension ($P_{ET}CO_2$) and ventilatory equivalent for CO₂ ($\dot{V}_E/\dot{V}_{CO_2}$) in subject H.M. during steady-state exercise. The bar indicates the time during which propranolol was injected intravenously. The exercise period shown is divided into: 1) pre-infusion phase (A), 2) response phase (B) and, 3) post-infusion phase (C).

All subjects had a reduction in heart rate following the propranolol similar to that shown in Figure 9.7. Coincident in time with the fall in heart rate was a decrease in $\dot{V}_{CO_2}$ and $\dot{V}_E$ (Fig. 9.7). The start of these decreases as   coincident with the start of the heart rate decrease and reached a nadir when the rate of heart rate decrease was most marked. Both

$\dot{V}_{CO2}$ and $\dot{V}_E$ increased back to the pre-propranolol levels after approximately 3 minutes of the onset of heart rate decrease. A smaller transient change occurred in $\dot{V}_{O2}$. The parallel change in $\dot{V}_E$ and $\dot{V}_{CO2}$ is reflected by the failure of the ventilatory equivalent for CO_2 to change during the response period. $P_{ET}CO2$ increased less than 0.5mmHg during the response period, suggesting close coupling of $\dot{V}_E$ and $\dot{V}_{CO2}$.

All subjects showed a significant decrease in $\dot{V}_E$ during the response phase, averaging 9.6% of their exercise control values (Fig. 9.8). In all instances, the fall in $\dot{V}_E$ was coincident with the subject's decrease in heart rate and $\dot{V}_{CO2}$. After the nadir was reached both $\dot{V}_E$ and $\dot{V}_{CO2}$ returned to pre-infusion levels despite the persistent reduction in heart rate. $P_{ET}CO2$ was unchanged during the response phase in three subjects (Fig. 9.9). In the remaining five, end-tidal CO_2 tension increased. However, the magnitude of the increase for the group was small and averaged .71mmHg. $\dot{V}_{CO2}$ demonstrated consistent decreases in each subject during the response phase (Fig. 9.10) which correlated well (r=0.85; p<.005) with a corresponding decrease in $\dot{V}_E$ (Fig. 9.11). In contrast, $\dot{V}_{O2}$ showed no significant change in five subjects and diminished slightly in the remaining three (Fig. 9.10). There was a poorer correlation (r=0.67; .05>P>.01) between the decrease in $\dot{V}_E$ AND $\dot{V}_{O2}$ (Fig. 9.11). The magnitude of the transient decrease in $\dot{V}_{CO2}$ was consistently greater than the decrease in $\dot{V}_{O2}$.

The hypopnea, after an exercise steady-state was established, is consistent with our hypothesis that a change in CO_2 flow to the lungs will be associated with ventilatory adjustments necessary for the maintenance of arterial isocapnia. A sudden decrease in cardiac output during steady-state exercise would have the immediate effect of creating a transient discrepancy between the amount of CO_2 produced metabolically and the CO_2 flow to the lungs. If alveolar ventilation were kept constant by artificial means during the period of decreasing cardiac output, there would be a decrease in arterial (and alveolar) P_{CO2} as described by Farhi and Rahn (7). The present studies indicate that, unlike the controlled ventilation situation, $P_{ET}CO2$ does not decrease under conditions of acutely decreasing cardiac output. Thus respiratory control mechanisms in man appear to sense the reduced CO_2 flow to the lungs and cause a reduction in ventilatory drive, despite a continued constant rate of exercise.

This study also addresses itself to the role of postulated muscle metaboloreceptors (8) which might affect $\dot{V}_E$ in man. When cardiac output decreases during constant work rate exercise, tissue PO_2 decreases and P_{CO2} and hydrogen ion concentration increase, while CO_2 flow to the lungs decreases. Thus, the reduction in cardiac output transiently uncouples tissue metabolism from CO_2 flow to the lungs. The observation that $\dot{V}_E$ changes in a direction opposite to that which would be expected if tissue metabolite concentrations were important stimuli for the exercise hyperpnea, argues against the importance of these postulated metabolorecetors in the normal respiratory control of man.

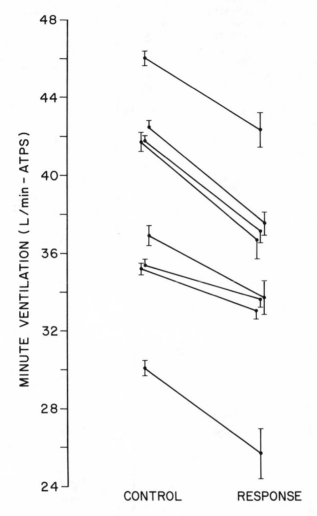

Fig. 9.8 Change in ventilation during the period of decreasing heart rate (response phase) compared with the exercise control. The points shown are the mean values of the total number of breaths averaged during each period. The vertical bars are ± one S.E.M. All of the decreases during the response phase are significant ($P > .05$).

Fig. 9.9 Change in end-
tidal CO_2 tension during
the period of decreasing
heart rate (response
phase) compared with the
exercise controls. The
points have the same
significance as de-
fined in the legend for
Figure 9.8. Non-
significant changes
(P ⊁.05) are
asterisked.

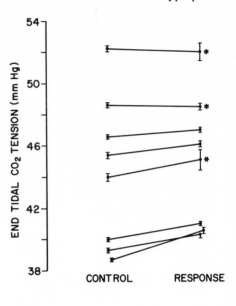

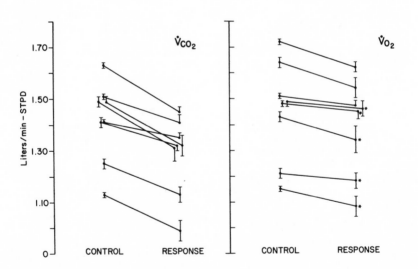

Fig. 9.10 Change in CO_2 output ($\dot{V}_{CO_2}$) and O_2 uptake ($\dot{V}_{O_2}$) during
the period of decreasing heart rate (response phase) compared
with the exercise control. Points and vertical bars have the
same significance as defined in the legend of Figure 9.8. Non-
significant changes are asterisked.

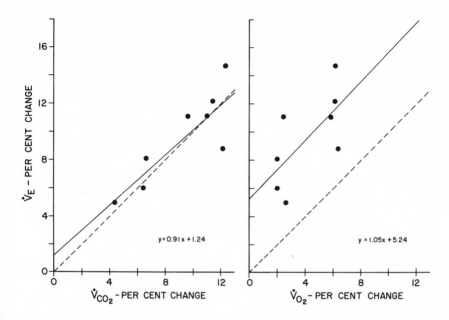

Fig. 9.11 Correlation of percent decreases in $\dot{V}_E$ and $\dot{V}_{CO_2}$ (left panel) and $\dot{V}_E$ and $\dot{V}_{O_2}$ (right panel) in each subject during the response phase. The correlation coefficient for the $\dot{V}_{CO_2}$-$\dot{V}_E$ plot is 0.85 (P < 0.005) and for the $\dot{V}_{O_2}$-$\dot{V}_E$ plot is 0.67 (P < .05). The solid line is the least squares regression line for the data. The dashed line is the line of identity. The standard error of the estimate for the $\dot{V}_{CO_2}$-$\dot{V}_E$ plot is 1.85 and for the $\dot{V}_{O_2}$-$\dot{V}_E$ plot is 2.63.

The proprotional change of $\dot{V}_E$ with $\dot{V}_{CO_2}$ with an approximate isocapnia reinforces the concept that receptors for respiratory control functionally sense CO_2 flow to the lungs. The <u>transient</u> nature of the ventilatory response is predictable from the CO_2 flow hypothesis since the acute reduction in cardiac output causes only a transient reduction in CO_2 flow.

<u>Effect of Increasing CO₂ Flow to Lungs on Ventilation by Venous CO₂ Loading</u>

To determine the effect of increasing mixed venous CO_2 on ventilation, we returned to the dog as an experimental model (13). Dogs were anesthetized with chloralose-urethane anesthesia

(75mg alpha-chloralose and 40mg urethane/KBW) after pre-
anesthesia with ketamine (10mgm/KBW). The femoral artery was
cannulated and attached to a membrane gas exchanger through which
femoral artery blood flow was diverted. The blood from the gas
exchanger was returned to the femoral vein on the ipsilateral slide.
To minimize cardiovascular effects, the blood flow to the gas
exchanger was limited to 250ml/min. The gas ventilating the blood
in the gas exchanger was equilibrated with CO_2 and N_2 in various
proportions to obtain 2 or 3 different levels of venous CO_2 loading above that of the control, during which the blood was
equilibrated with 5% CO_2 in air. Each level of venous loading
was maintained for 10 minutes in order to allow for complete
wash-out of the reservoir system with the newly equilibrated
blood and to obtain steady-state conditions. Changes in $\dot{V}_E$ and
$PaCO_2$ from the control level were measured during the 9th and
10th minutes as previously described (13).

The responses of one dog to venous loading are shown in
Figure 9.12. The femoral and pulmonary artery CO_2 tensions and
$P_{ET}CO_2$ are plotted on the same scale. Both the $P_{ET}CO_2$ and $PaCO_2$
indicate that the ventilatory response is such that arterial
isocapnia is maintained.

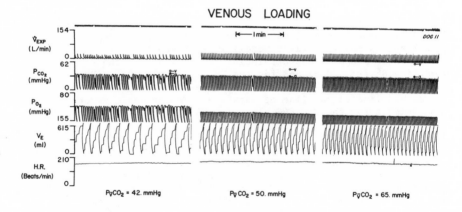

Fig. 9.12 Last two minutes of the recordings of the control
period and of the response to ten minute exposures to two levels
of venous CO_2 loading. The channels, from the top down, are
expired air-flow, airway, arterial (-a) and venous (-v) P_{CO2},
airway P_{O2}, expired volume and heart rate.

The slopes of the venous CO_2 loading studies are compared
with those for inhaled CO_2 loading determined from steady-state
(10 minute) ventilatory responses to 3, 5 and 7% CO_2 in the
inhaled gas, in the same dogs (Fig. 9.13). The venous CO_2

loading slopes are not significantly different from infinity, whereas the inhaled CO2 loading slopes are clearly finite.

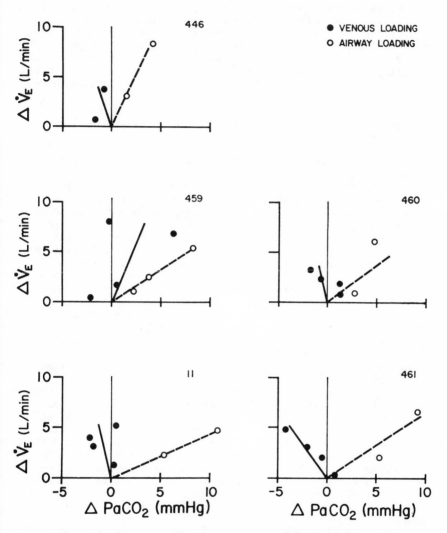

Fig. 9.13 Comparison of ventilatory response to airway (○) and venous (●) CO2 loading in five dogs as related to changes in PaCO2. Lines of best fit to airway (---) and venous (——) loading are shown.

Dr. Stremel has now repeated these studies in unanesthetized dogs in our laboratory using a directly recording indwelling

arterial PCO_2 electrode with essentially the same results
(manuscript in preparation). During these studies, he
discovered that high blood flow rates through the gas exchanger
(those in excess of 400ml/min for 20kg dogs) results in a small
but significant $PaCO_2$ elevation which was not evident at lower
flow rates. We suspect that altered hemodynamics played a
role in the ventilatory response at these higher exchanger
blood flows. On the other hand, we cannot rule out the possibility that the dogs become aware of their hyperpnea with the
increased CO_2 load of high flow, and consciously restrain their
breathing effort.

Effect of Progressive Increase in CO_2 Flow (Incremental Exercise) on $\dot{V}_E$

We previously reported that a closer relationship existed
between $\dot{V}_E$ and $\dot{V}_{CO_2}$ than between $\dot{V}_E$ and $\dot{V}_{O_2}$ during incremental
exercise tests (12). The results for ten normal male subjects
are shown in Figure 9.14. Each work increment lasted for four
minutes and the measurements of $\dot{V}_E$, $\dot{V}_{CO_2}$ and $\dot{V}_{O_2}$ were made during
the 4th minute of each work rate. The smaller inter-subject
variation in the relationship between $\dot{V}_E$ and $\dot{V}_{CO_2}$ than between
$\dot{V}_E$ and $\dot{V}_{O_2}$ is apparent. In addition, we noted that the regression
line of the $\dot{V}_E$ and $\dot{V}_{CO_2}$ relationship extrapolated through the
origin. This observation was difficult to reconcile with the
hypothesis that a portion of the ventilatory response to muscular
exercise is due to neurogenic mechanisms. We expected to observe
a positive intercept on the $\dot{V}_E$ axis to account for the neural,
non-humoral portion of the ventilatory stimulus. A third
interesting observation was a more linear relationship between
$\dot{V}_E$ and $\dot{V}_{CO_2}$ than between $\dot{V}_E$ and $\dot{V}_{O_2}$, i.e., $\dot{V}_E$ remained
linearly correlated with $\dot{V}_{CO_2}$ through a higher work level than
with $\dot{V}_{O_2}$.

We demonstrated that $\dot{V}_{O_2}$ increases linearly with progressively
increasing work rate while $\dot{V}_{CO_2}$ increases curvilinearly (15).
The curvilinearity of $\dot{V}_{CO_2}$ is due to the significant amount of
CO_2 output being derived from bicarbonate buffering of lactic
acid (10) above a certain work rate (the anaerobic threshold (15)).
We took advantage of this decoupling and created a continually
increasing rate of CO_2 flow and O_2 demand by progressively increasing the work rate on a cycle ergometer at a rate of 15 watts
per minute (Fig. 9.15). This procedure permitted measurement of
the ventilatory response when CO_2 production and O_2 demand became
disparate.

Figure 9.15 demonstrates that $\dot{V}_{O_2}$ retains the expected
linear relationship to work rate up to the maximal $\dot{V}_{O_2}$ at which
time it levels off. $\dot{V}_E$ and $\dot{V}_{CO_2}$ start to increase above the anaerobic threshold in a curvilinear manner with the two precisely
matched so that $P_{ET}CO_2$ does not change. Because $\dot{V}_E$ increases
out of proportion to $\dot{V}_{O_2}$, the difference between inspired and end-
tidal oxygen narrows, i.e., the subject hyperventilates with
respect to O_2. Thus, the $P_{ET}O_2$ increases without a simultaneous

decrease in $P_{ET}CO_2$. This period of isocapnic buffering is again
consistent with the concept of $\dot{V}_E$ being primarily responsive to
CO_2 flow and that $\dot{V}_E$ is responding non-linearly because of the
excess CO_2 produced from the reaction of lactic acid with $NaHCO_3$.
At still higher work rates, $\dot{V}_E$ increases even more rapidly than
$\dot{V}_{CO_2}$. As the metabolic acidosis becomes longer lasting and more
severe, the increased H^+ becomes sensed. At this point, the
ventilatory drive increases out of proportion to CO_2 flow,
facilitating partial respiratory compensation for the acidosis.
The sensor which transmits the increased H^+ signal has been shown
to be the carotid bodies in man (16).

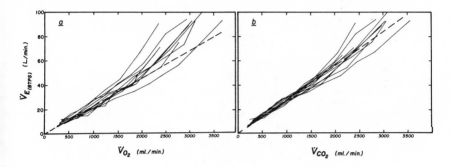

Fig. 9.14 Minute ventilation ($\dot{V}_E$) as related to O_2 consumption
($\dot{V}_{O_2}$) (left panel) and CO_2 production ($\dot{V}_{CO_2}$) (right panel) for 10
normal male subjects. Each curve is made up of five or more work
rates with the measurements being made during the fourth minute of
each work rate (12).

Effect of Continually Varying CO₂ Flow (Sinusoidal) Exercise on $\dot{V}_E$

We studied the dynamic relationships between ventilation and
gas exchange variables breath-by-breath using sinusoidal perturbation   of work rate of 0.7, 1, 2, 4, 6 and 10 minute periods
on a cycle ergometer at a constant pedal rate of 60 rpm (3). Each
sine wave frequency was studied for 30 minutes and no more than
one period was studied on a given day. Steady-state measurements
were also made at the peak (80% of the subject's anaerobic threshold) and the trough (25 watts) of the sinusoidal perturbation.
Figure 9.16 illustrates the protocol used and the type of results
obtained from the continuous breath-by-breath measurements for
three (10, 4 and 2 minutes) of the sine wave periods studied.

To establish the amplitude and phase angle relationships between a given response variable and the input work sinusoid, the responses to each stimulus period were superimposed. The averaged responses of one subject to the 2, 4 and 10 minute periods are shown in Figure 9.17. It should be noted that, for all but the irregular responses in end-tidal gas tensions, a progressive increase in stimulus frequency engenders progressively smaller amplitudes and larger phase lags. When plotted on a Nyquist diagram (Fig. 9.18) it can be seen that, for $\dot{V}_E$, $\dot{V}_{CO_2}$, $\dot{V}_{O_2}$ and HR that the locus of points describes a semicircle with the high frequency assymptote approaching zero amplitude and a 90° phase lag. Such responses are characteristic of a first order, linear relationship between these variables and the perturbing work rate. It is thus possible to describe these response dynamics by a time constant.

The time constant for the ventilatory response to the sine wave work perturbation is compared to the time constants for the $\dot{V}_{O_2}$ and $\dot{V}_{CO_2}$ responses for each of 5 subjects (Fig. 9.19). This plot shows that the time constant for the $\dot{V}_{O_2}$ response is considerably shorter than that for $\dot{V}_E$ and $\dot{V}_{CO_2}$. The correlation between the time constants for $\dot{V}_E$ and $\dot{V}_{O_2}$ is not significant. More interesting, however, is the highly significant correlation between the time constants for $\dot{V}_{CO_2}$ and $\dot{V}_E$. Of major significance is the observation that the time constant for $\dot{V}_{CO_2}$ is uniformly slightly shorter than the time constant for $\dot{V}_E$, suggesting that the increase in $\dot{V}_E$ is not the cause of the increase in $\dot{V}_{CO_2}$, but rather $\dot{V}_{CO_2}$ is leading $\dot{V}_E$. This is also consistent with the observation that when $\dot{V}_E$ increased to its peak response, $P_{ET}CO_2$ was at its highest level, and not its lowest, although the slope of the alveolar phase may play some part in end-tidal P_{CO_2} fluctuations. These studies provide further support for a primary role of CO_2 flow to the lung in the exercise hyperpnea.

Because we are interested in the precise humoral stimulus for the change in $\dot{V}_E$ during the sinusoidal work rate studies, we measured the arterial P_{CO_2} in two of the subjects over the course of the six minute period sinusoidal studies (18). For each subject, arterial blood samples were drawn every 30 seconds over a 15 second period for the four six-minute sine wave studies (48 arterial blood measurements). The four PaCO2 values for each of the 12 points on the six minute sine wave periods were averaged (Fig. 9.20). While the measurements in $\dot{V}_E$ and gas exchange described a sine wave pattern for the six minute sine wave work perturbation, the PaCO2 values did not demonstrate systematic fluctuation for either of these two subjects. Thus, despite constantly changing work rate, ventilatory response seems to be rather precisely coupled to $\dot{V}_{CO_2}$ so that a relatively constant PaCO2 is assured.

Effect of Varying CO_2 Production by Diet on Exercise $\dot{V}_E$

By dietary manipulation, it is possible to alter the rela-

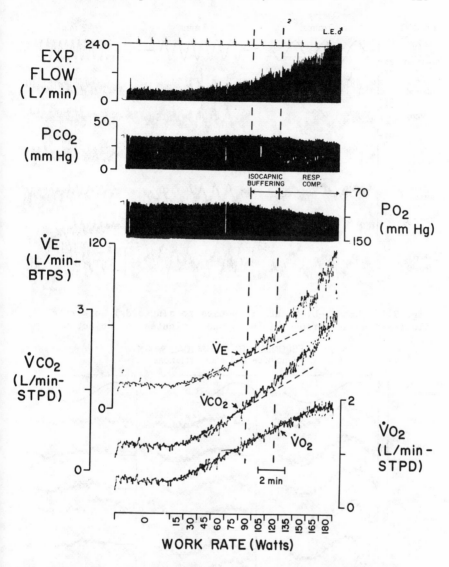

Fig. 9.15 Effect of one minute incremental work rate test on expired flow, P_{CO_2} and P_{O_2} in the respired gas, $\dot{V}_E$, $\dot{V}_{CO_2}$ and $\dot{V}_{O_2}$ in a 43 year old male subject. "Isocapnic buffering" refers to the period when $\dot{V}_E$ and $\dot{V}_{CO_2}$ increase curvilinearly relative to $\dot{V}_{O_2}$, while retaining a constant $P_{ET}CO2$ (period between vertical dashed lines). The vertical dashed line on the left denotes the anaerobic threshold. Following the period of isocapnic buffering $P_{ET}CO2$ decreases reflecting respiratory compensation for the metabolic acidosis of exercise.

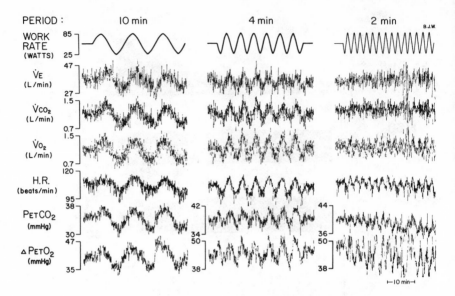

Fig. 9.16 Breath-by-breath responses to sinusoidal work rate
fluctuations at periods of 10, 4 and 2 minutes in subject BW.

RESPONSES TO SINUSOIDAL WORK
Amplitude and phase relations

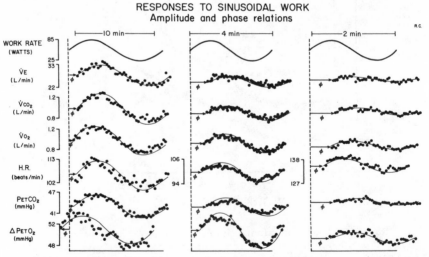

Fig. 9.17 Amplitude and phase relations with respect to the sinusoidally varying work rate at periods of 10, 4 and 2 minutes for
subject RC. Points are the average responses for 2, 6 and 10 work
rate periods, respectively. The curves are sine waves of best fit
to the response data.

FREQUENCY RESPONSE TO SINUSOIDAL WORK
Nyquist Plots

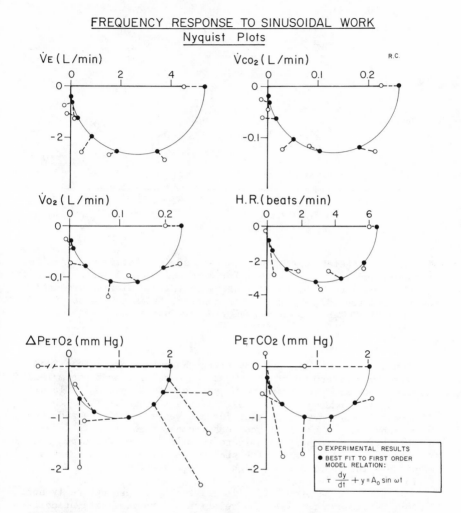

Fig. 9.18 Nyquist plots of the ventilation, carbon dioxide production, oxygen consumption, heart rate and end-tidal gas tension
responses for subject RC. Open circles are experimentally observed
responses; closed circles represent, for each work rate fluctuation
period, the best fit to a first order model relation.

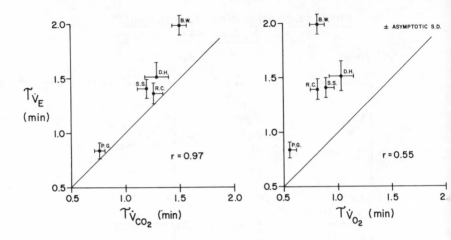

Fig. 9.19 Relation of time constant of $\dot{V}_E$ relative to $\dot{V}_{CO2}$ (left panel) and $\dot{V}_{O2}$ (right panel) for each subject. Illustrated is the close coupling between ventilatory and carbon dioxide production dynamics (r=0.97, P $\leq$ .002). In contrast, time constants of ventilation and oxygen consumption are poorly correlated (r=0.55, N.S.).

tionship between $\dot{V}_{CO2}$ and $\dot{V}_{O2}$ (17). When fats are metabolized, only seven molecules of the CO_2 are evolved for each ten molecules of O_2 consumed. But, for carbohydrate metabolism, one molecule of CO_2 is produced for each O_2 molecule consumed. Thus, the CO_2 output is considerably higher for a given metabolic demand when carbohydrate is the fuel source as compared to fat. To determine the degree of coupling of minute ventilation to CO_2 output and O_2 uptake, normal subjects were studied during periods of controlled dietary intake of normal, high carbohydrate-low fat and high fat-low carbohydrate foods.

When minute ventilation is related to oxygen uptake (ventilatory equivalent for O_2), the relationship varies systematically. A greater ventilation is required for each liter of O_2 consumption when the R.Q. is increased (Fig. 9.21). On the other hand, $\dot{V}_E$ retains a constant relationship to $\dot{V}_{CO2}$ regardless of the R.Q. (Fig. 9.21).

These studies provide further evidence that $\dot{V}_E$ during exercise can vary with respect to $\dot{V}_{O2}$, but the relation to $\dot{V}_{CO2}$ is relatively fixed. The primary manipulation of CO_2 flow by diet effects predictable changes in $\dot{V}_E$ with respect to the work rate being performed.

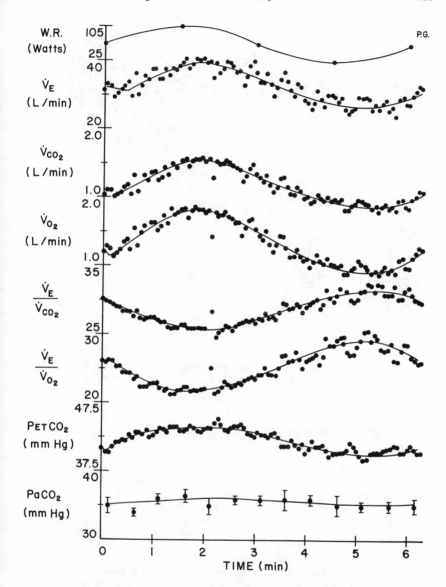

Fig. 9.20 Ventilation and gas exchange during sinusoidal exercise. The response represents the mean of four sine wave work oscillations.

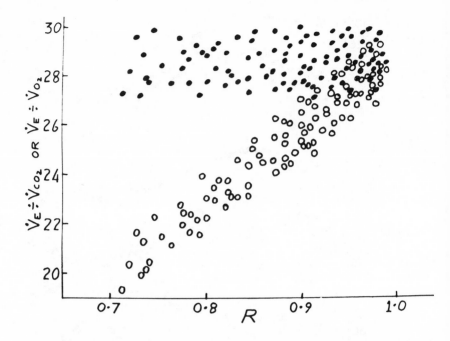

Fig. 9.21 The steady-state gas exchange ratio during exercise
(R=R.Q.) and the ventilatory equivalent for CO_2 (•) and O_2 (○)
(17).

The Carotid Bodies and the Ventilatory Response to Changes in CO_2 Flow

The carotid bodies, located in the main arterial stream, might
be expected to have some role in the ventilatory response to
humoral stimuli which are produced during exercise. Thus, we
studied the breath-by-breath ventilatory response to two levels of
constant work rate cycle ergometer exercise, of five subjects with
history of bronchial asthma, whose carotid bodies had previously
been removed (CBR) and five age and sex matched normal subjects
(16). At the time of this study, the CBR subjects were asymptom-
atic and had normal or near normal respiratory function studies.
The two levels of work studied were 70% and 150% of the
subject's anaerobic threshold. The duration of the exercise was
30 minutes or to tolerance, whichever came first. All subjects
were able to complete 30 minutes of the below anaerobic threshold

work. None of the subjects were able to complete 30 minutes of
exercise for the above anaerobic threshold work.

The results for each individual subject for the work rate
studies below the anaerobic threshold are shown in Figure 9.22,
and the responses above the anaerobic threshold are shown in
Figure 9.23. The average time to reach 25, 50, 75 and 90% of the
asymptotic $\dot{V}_E$ value are shown on the bottom of each figure. The
immediate increase in ventilation is not different for the two
groups at either work intensity. Some subjects in each group have
a significant abrupt increase in $\dot{V}_E$ at the start of exercise, while
others do not. On the other hand, the subjects without carotid
bodies had a significantly slower increase in $\dot{V}_E$ to steady-state
after the exercise was underway for both above and below anaerobic
threshold work intensities. Thus, the carotid bodies seem to
influence the ventilatory drive during the period of increasing
CO_2 flow to the lungs.

The apparent sluggishness of the ventilatory response of the
CBR subjects during the transition from the start to the steady-
state of exercise is reflected by a concomitant overshoot in end-
tidal and arterial CO_2 tension during these early minutes of
exercise (Fig. 9.24). As the CBR subjects continue to perform
exercise to steady state, $P_{ET}CO_2$ and $PaCO_2$ decrease. For below
anaerobic threshold work, the CBR subjects have a steady-state
$P_{ET}CO_2$ and $PaCO_2$ which is not significantly different from that
of the control group. Above the anaerobic threshold the $PaCO_2$
and $P_{ET}CO_2$ of the CBR subjects are significantly higher than
those for the control population. This persistent elevation in
P_{CO_2} is caused by the failure of the CBR subjects to develop a
ventilatory response to metabolic acidosis.

From these studies, it appears that the carotid bodies are
important for the transient increase in $\dot{V}_E$ from the resting to
steady state level. While other mechanisms are available to effect
the necessary increase in ventilation during exercise, the carotid
bodies appear to be needed for the tight coupling of $\dot{V}_E$ with CO_2
flow in man.

In conclusion, we now feel that sufficient data are available
to indicate that the neurohumoral hypothesis is not an adequate
explanation of the ventilatory control mechanism during exercise
in man. In its place, we would propose an hypothesis which links
ventilatory drive to CO_2 flow to the central circulation (Fig.
9.25). This hypothesis would state that a sensitive chemoreceptive
mechanism is active at a site beyond the pulmonary capillary which
causes ventilation to increase in proportion to CO_2 flow thus maintaining an approximate arterial isocapnia. This concept is not
particularly new for it was one of several possible mechanisms
suggested by Comroe (4).

The carotid bodies appear to have a role in stimulating
breathing to maintain CO_2 homeostasis during periods of transient
changes in CO_2 flow. However, we are not yet aware of the CO_2-stat
receptor site and precise manner of transduction of the CO_2 flow
signal during steady-state exercise.

Figure 9.25 illustrates, schematically, factors which are

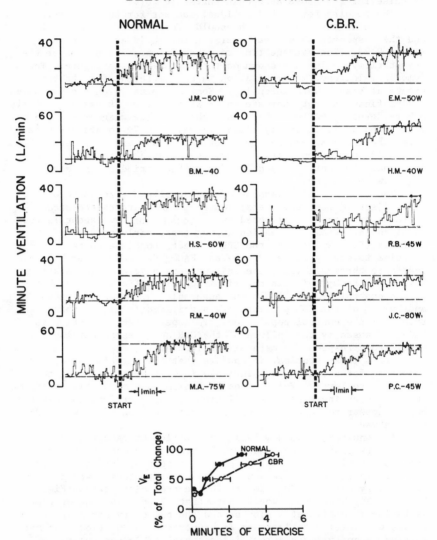

Fig. 9.22. Minute ventilation for normal and CBR subjects for 30 minutes of constant load exercise <u>below</u> the anaerobic threshold. Work rate for each subject is shown in watts. Dashed line at bottom of each panel indicates average resting $\dot{V}_E$ while dashed line at top of each panel indicates exercise $\dot{V}_E$. Bottommost plot is the average time ($\pm$ 1 SEM) required to reach 25, 50, 75 and 90% of the steady-state $\overline{\dot{V}}_E$.

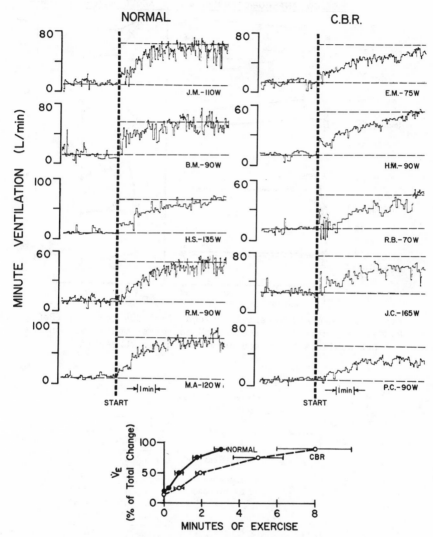

Fig. 9.23. Minute ventilation for normal and CBR subjects for 30 minutes or less of constant load exercise <u>above</u> anaerobic threshold. Work rate for each subject is noted in watts. Dashed lines have the same significance as in Figure 9.22. Bottommost plot is the average time ($\pm$ 1 SEM) required to reach 25, 50, 75 and 90% of steady-state $\dot{V}_E$. CBR patients require significantly more time to reach 50, 75 and 90% of steady-state value.

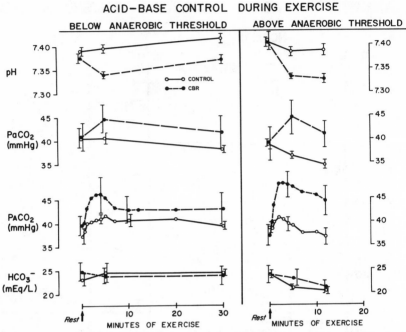

ACID–BASE CONTROL DURING EXERCISE

Fig. 9.24 Average arterial and end-tidal CO_2 tensions ($PaCO_2$ and P_ACO_2, respectively), arterial pH and bicarbonate for control and CBR subjects below and above anaerobic threshold.

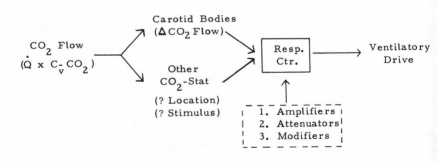

Fig. 9.25 Diagram of determinants of ventilatory drive during exercise.

known to amplify or attenuate ventilatory drive. During exercise, we are mainly concerned with the superposition of the amplifying effects of increasing arterial H$^+$ concentration and decreasing O$_2$ tension. Our studies on subjects without carotid bodies indicate that these receptors are necessary to obtain the ventilatory adjustments in response to hypoxemia or to the acute metabolic acidosis of exercise (9,16).

As suggested by the studies of Phillipson et al (11), pulmonary mechanoreceptors function primarily as modifiers of breathing pattern but have little effect on ventilatory drive during exercise. However, the mechanism by which altered respiratory mechanics might affect ventilatory drive, independent of humoral effects, needs further clarification.

The normal ventilatory control system operates with sageness and versatility to provide diversified, but yet appropriate responses. Thus, special ventilatory responses which result from acute changes in acid-base balance and from hypoxemia are accomplished. However, independently or in concert with these special ventilatory demands, the respiratory control mechanism attempts to achieve its primary function as a precise homeostatic regulator of arterial CO$_2$ tension.

SUMMARY

Ventilation and gas exchange measurements during exercise are presented which indicate that the neurohumoral hypothesis is an unlikely explanation for the hyperpnea of exercise. Breath-by-breath measurements of gas exchange reveal that the ventilatory response is closely linked to the rate at which carbon dioxide is delivered to the lungs. This response is so precise that arterial isocapnia is maintained, except when metabolic acidosis stimulates the carotid bodies to cause a reduction in PaCO2. To evaluate the hypothesis that ventilatory drive is linked to the rate of CO2 flow to the central circulation, the ventilatory responses to changes in CO$_2$ flow induced by a) increasing and b) decreasing cardiac output, c) venous loading of CO2, d) progressively incremented work rate exercise, e) sinusoidally varying work rate exercise, and f) dietary manipulation were studied. The results of all of these studies strongly point to the existence of a sensitive chemoreceptive mechanism which causes ventilation to increase in proportion to CO2 flow, thus maintaining PaCO2 essentially constant. The carotid bodies appear to play some role in the ventilatory response to changing CO2 flow, but the precise control mechanism to account for the total response remains unclear.

REFERENCES

1. Beaver, W.L., K. Wasserman and B.J. Whipp: J. Appl. Physiol. 34:128-132, 1973.
2. Brown, H.V., K. Wasserman and B.J. Whipp: J. Appl. Physiol. In Press.
3. Casaburi, R., B.J. Whipp, S.N. Koyal and K. Wasserman: Fed. Proc. 34:431, 1975.
4. Comroe, J.H.: Physiology of Respiration. Chicago, Year Book Medical Publishers, Inc. 1965. p 194.
5. Dejours, P.: The Regulation of Breathing During Muscular Exercise in Man. A Neurohumoral Theory. In: The Regulation of Human Respiration. Ed. D.J.C. Cunningham and B.B. Lloyd, Oxford, Blackwell, 1963. pp. 535-547.
6. Epstein, S.E., B.F. Robinson, R.L. Kahler and E. Braunwald: J. Clin. Invest. 44:1745-1753, 1965.
7. Farhi, L.E. and H. Rahn: J. Appl. Physiol. 7:472-484, 1955.
8. Levine, S. and W.E. Huckabee: J. Appl. Physiol. 38:827-833, 1975.
9. Lugliani, R., B.J. Whipp, C. Seard and K. Wasserman: N. Eng. J. Med. 285:1105-1111, 1971.
10. Naimark, A., K. Wasserman and M.B. McLlroy: J. Appl. Physiol. 19:644-652, 1964.
11. Phillipson, E.A., R.F. Hickey, C.R. Bointon and J.A. Nadel: J. Appl. Physiol. 29:475-479, 1970.
12. Wasserman, K., A.L. Van Kessel and G.G. Burton: J. Appl. Physiol. 22:71-85, 1967.
13. Wasserman K., B.J. Whipp, R. Casaburi, D.J. Huntsman, J. Castagna and R. Lugliani: J. Appl. Physiol. 38:651-656, 1975.
14. Wasserman, K., B.J. Whipp and J. Castagna: J. Appl. Physiol. 36:457-464, 1974.
15. Wasserman, K., B.J. Whipp, S.N. Koyal and W.L. Beaver: J. Appl. Physiol. 35:236-243, 1973.
16. Wasserman, K., B.J. Whipp, S.N. Koyal and M.G. Cleary: J. Appl. Physiol. 39:354-358, 1975.
17. Whipp, B.J., G.A. Bray, S.N. Koyal and K. Wasserman: Exercise Energetics and Respiratory Control in Man Following Acute and Chronic Elevation of Caloric Intake, in Obesity in Perspective, G.A. Bray, Ed. Washingron, D.C., U.S. Government Printing Office, 1975, pp. 157-163.
18. Whipp, B.J., R. Casaburi, S.N. Koyal and K. Wasserman: Fed. Proc. 34:431, 1975.

DISCUSSION

Fishman: At the start of exercise and then in the steady state of exercise, which receptor do you think is the most important to the ventilatory response? Is the receptor site you are proposing in the lungs or is the carotid body an important site of reception?

Wasserman: Our studies indicate that the carotid bodies are important for the respiratory compensation of the metabolic acidosis of heavy exercise and probably as a fine controller for the normal tight coupling of $\dot{V}E$ with CO_2 flow.

Filley: Dr. Wasserman, your intriguing hypothesis is that $\dot{V}E$ is stimulated by CO_2 flow from blood to alveolar gas. Now, the opposite should occur, it seems to me, if a man breathes CO_2 for one breath (especially in N_2O), i.e. that breath should be depressed. In Figures A and B, we see the records of subjects on a treadmill, each breathing one breath of 5-6% CO_2 in N_2 or N_2O. As seen, the inspiratory flow rate is invariably slowed. So CO_2 by the airway depresses ventilation just as would be required by your CO_2 flow hypothesis.

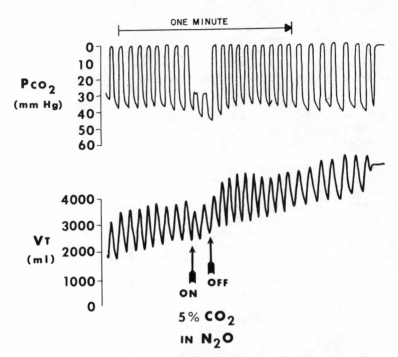

Fig. A. Subject 1, after reaching a reasonably constant respiratory
rate and tidal volume (V_T) during exercise was switched to 5% CO_2
in N_2O at the end of an expiration (first arrow). The two breaths
while breathing this mixture were clearly reduced in volume compared
to previous breaths. Four seconds after the CO_2 was removed, beginning with the second breath, ventilatory stimulation, presumably via
the carotid body, occurred for 25 seconds (9 breaths).

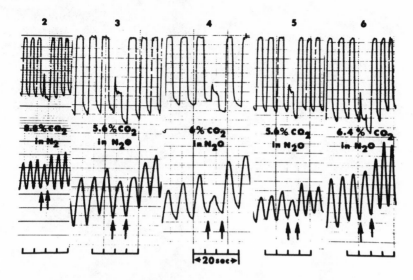

Fig. B. Single breath exposures in the other 5 subjects. Subject 4 had a very marked _slowing_ of inspiration even showing a discontinuity but the slowing toward the end of inspiration is clearly visible in Subjects 3 and 5 as well. The test breath in Subject 6 was actually greater than previously (2.6 vs. 2.21 liters) but he showed the usual reduction in the rate of inspiration (V'_I = 0.94 vs. $\bar{V}'_I$ = 1.11 liters/sec). The tracing on Subject 2 illustrates the fact that higher CO$_2$ concentrations were needed to depress V_I and V'_I when administered in N$_2$ rather than in N$_2$0 (Filley, G., Trans. Amer. Clinical & Climatalogical Assoc., Vol. 87, 1976).

10

Looking at the Regulation of Ventilation as a Signalling Process

William S. Yamamoto

The premises, on which the class of studies I shall review are based, are few. First, that pulmonary ventilation in the intact animal is regulated on the basis of _informative signals_ delivered to (received at) an appropriate sensory mechanism inside the body which in turn manages the machinery of the pulmonary gas exchange. Second, all known signals which transmit information are _time series_ of symbols. If to these we add the notion that ventilation is not inconsequentially related to the signal such that message and action are finely coordinated to accomplish a goal, we form the basis for study.

One should recognize that the problem in abstract is a generic problem of physiology and is a problem of aggregates. It requires a more or less arbitrary choice in each specific instance of a sufficient organ system with sensors, pathways, motormechanisms, and an attributable purpose. We choose chemoreceptors, both neural and humoral connections of brain to lung, the mechanism of the chest, and homeostasis of CO_2 respectively.

Thus, we may state our premises as follows: A goal of the organism is to adjust pulmonary ventilation to a magnitude such that based upon a performance signal delivered from the lung to the brain, the influx and outflux of CO_2 from the body are, on the average, equal. Note that we use the indefinite article to begin the statement, and that the dimension, time, is buried in the words "flux" and "average". To get to the experimental level we need to make further sometimes justifiable but nevertheless arbitrary identification. We choose as a symbol string the CO_2 tension in the body at various sites: alveolus, artery, extracellular space, neuronal space. We accept implicitly the general idea of encoding; thus hydrogen ion, chloride ion, membrane potentials, neural impulses are all potential if not actual forms of the same message. Ultimately we seek to identify the message independently from the medium.

Now, I can justify for you the relationship between the individual experimental studies that make up the quest for a signal in the humoral pathway. With immodesty appropriate to a dispassionate scientist, much of what I will here report is our own work.

137

It is probably incontestable that the hyperpnea of exercise and the similar "isocapnic" hyperpneas due to various natural and induced processes are brought about by multiple mechanisms. However, in the implicit philosophy of parsimony, many physiologists have sought for single mechanisms, which seem sometimes to be sufficient while at other times demonstrably unnecessary. The issue of course is simply resolved by invoking a multiple factor concept. Multiple factor analysis unhappily has its root notions in the additivity of variance. The equations of Gray (10) best portray this hidden root, even when non linear expressions are introduced as by Lloyd, the situation does not improve completely. It seems to me that the difficulty is not with the multiple mechanism view but by an inadequate ability to formalize rigorously Sherrington's concept of occlusion. That is, the appearance of any surface activity like the adjustment of pulmonary ventilation may in any given instant depend upon the merging of alternative, equivalently powerful mechanisms by a "policy" maker mechanism that adapts the output ventilation by adding, compromising, or ignoring signals pertinent to several conflicting goals of the organism.

We are in this session concerned with exercise hyperpnea, which is at once the most dramatic and puzzling of the isocapnic hyperpneas. Many characteristics of such hyperpnea are familiar to all in this audience, one need not recount the many facets of evidence which have contributed to the puzzle. Suffice it to say that ventilation is linearly related to exercise to the metabolism, however measured (12). If we select CO_2 flux as the measure of metabolism we find that a similar relation holds for the other isocapnic hyperpneas. This must follow whenever the inspired air has zero carbon dioxide tension and there is material balance in the organism. This of course is tautological.

The limited time available to develop this discussion will not allow me to pay adequate recognition to two very important classes of effort which deal with the issue of the nature of the message. Not all of this effort is recent but in this audience most of it is familiar.

There has been and will continue to be a need for recording the humoral CO_2 signal in transit. For it may be the spot sampling of Pa_{CO_2} that leads to the whole enigma. We do not have today a fast dissolved CO_2 sensor. Most significant continuous methods use hydrogen ion as the surrogate for CO_2 tension. The best example to my mind is still the data of Band, Cameron and Semple (1, 2), who measured pH oscillations in the blood stream. Their data showed the computable prediction that the peak to peak amplitude is depressed during inhalation of CO_2 mixtures. The end tidal CO_2 is elevated, as is the mean. I was and am a little surprised that this recording could be produced. The left ventricle is a digital filter operating theoretically at a sampling rate that is, at rest, the minimum necessary to pass the respiratory frequency. Most biological mechanisms function within more comfortable margins of safety.

After failing ourselves to produce a nice small intravascular pH electrode, but also because we were not convinced that the prin-

cipal signal frequency was that of the chest we attempted some indirect attacks. We decided to take advantage of reported slow
potentials by C. Von Euler (9) and at the blood brain barrier by
R. Tschirgi (18). Tschirgi and Taylor (18) showed that cortical-
jugular bulb potential differences on inhalation of CO_2 followed a
time course not unlike the respiratory response to CO_2 (Fig. 10.1).
Dr. William Raub (14) and I decided to record at expanded bandwidth,
ventilatory movement along with the potential between the blood in
the jugular bulb and a micro electrode in the caudal brain stem.
There are, as you know, many movement artifacts to overcome so we
used a narrow hypothesis. The power spectra of these signals are
shown in Figure 10.1. The airflow is recorded by pneumotach which
is unfortunately a high pass device. Most of the spectral power is
at respiratory frequency. The auto correlogram always shows long
range coherence.

The correlogram and power spectra of the blood brain barrier
potential difference also show long range correlation, but negligible power at respiratory frequency. Because of technical limitation
and choice we sampled 20 times a second for 1440 sec, remembering
these experiments were performed on the rat with a resting rate of
90 per minute or 1.5 hertz. Our bandwidth of effective estimation
was only from 0.1 hertz to perhaps 10. Both the correlograms and
the power spectra during IV CO_2 infusion or CO_2 inhalation were to
the eye similar and dissimilar and even for the narrow hypothesis
of amplitude modulation did not fall clearly out of the experiment.
In fact, it looked as though the most interesting power components
lay in the vicinity of 0.1 hertz or less--that is below the range
of our analysis. 0.1 hertz, let me hasten to remark, is for breath
groupings of 10-15 breaths in this test animal.

There obviously was not going to be a simple feedback loop formulation. At any rate unlike the direct recordings reported from
the blood we could find no brain stem biopotential at respiratory
frequency but signal power well below the respiratory frequency.
We were then delighted when Lenfant (13) published a paper showing
a much wider spectrum of respiratory gas exchange (Fig. 10.2).
Three spectral regions were notable: (1) fast, 2-6 breath grouping,
(2) medium, 25-50 breaths most conspicuous in hyperventilation, and
(3) slow, 150-200 breaths. The oscillations produced a continual
change in ventilation/perfusion ratio ranging from .8 to 1.20.
Similar results were recorded by Goodman (8, 9) and others. The
paper apparently triggered no interest among others, and our group
didn't know where to go from the findings. It became obvious to
me about a decade ago that the "transmitted" signal was not going
to yield to any simplistic adaptation of continuous wave communication theory to the humoral CO_2 signal (is such it was).

Along with others, who still continue in the effort we tried
to simulate various "stylized" signals mostly through inhalation
maneuvers to produce some signal and by recording the response from
it, to deduce the stimulus for exercise hyperpnea. We were not
alone, There were signle breaths, sinusoidal breaths, end tidal
clamps,gas injection into the air way, cyclical-exercise and numerous others that fill the literature today and puzzle the mind with

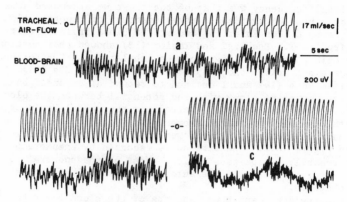

Fig. 10.1.   Tracheal air flow and blood brain P.D.   Rat #30.
(a) inhalation of 100% O_2 (b) intravascular CO_2
loading   (c) inhalation of 5% CO_2 in O_2 (14).

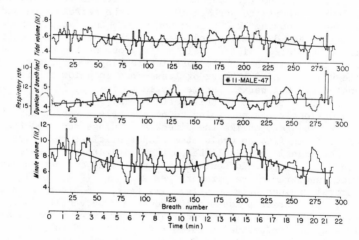

Fig. 10.2.   Time dependent variation of pulmonary gas exchange
in normal man at rest (13).

the realization that any ultimate and correct analysis of respiratory control by CO_2 must account for all of them. I am reminded of a story my mother told me of her first days in America. Using the medium vocal sound, she tried to buy bread, but knew not the word. Knowing Japanese would be of no avail she tried one of the few French words she knew "pain" and with a look of relief the grocer produced a skillet. And so it might be with CO_2 and the central controller--we have the medium but not the message--and we just might be ending up with skillets. Among the odd things we tried was, that of reversing the process of electrical recording by electrical forcing--that was in the fad period when Terzuolo and Bullock (17) showed impulse modulation by slow potentials, and Bishop (3) wrote an enchanting review about the natural history of the nerve impulse. Dr. Richard O. Davies (5, 6) and I tried almost as a lark to drive various sites in the caudal brain stem with biased sinusoidal electric current (Fig. 10.3). To our happy dismay ventilatory movement synchronized immediately to the electrical signal over a wide range of frequency. In the rat which normally breathes about 90 per minute, synchronization followed up to 8 hertz and down to 0.1 hertz. In addition the tidal volume was observed to increase at lower frequency, the maximum observed was from a V_T of 1.4 to 8 ml in an animal synchronized at 1 hertz. The pleasure because at current densities employed, low frequency signals of an electrochemical nature applied extracellularly can produce dramatic respiratory change...Dismay because we found synchronization rather than modulation, but didn't make a simple next logical step...Today I may have some ideas to try, but my obligations and commitments--lie elsewhere.

One experiment that Arthur Guyton (11) did long ago intrigued me then, and still does. He interposed a long tube in the arterial circuit between lung and brain of the dog, 140 to 650 ml, such that all the cerebral flow was delayed. Under these conditions 10 of 30 dogs developed, without initiation, significant 2 to 10 minute oscillations in ventilation. Simplistically these might be called "phase shift" oscillation in a feedback loop, and was proposed as evidence on the mechanism of Cheyne Stokes respiration. To me it raised another issue--and, pursuing the idea that a humoral pathway is a communication channel, we decided to look at the physical channel again. We had considered it only mathematically before. We said to ourselves--if the message is a time sequence in a flowing fluid stream and lengthening it makes communication go badly out of step what happens if we don't lengthen greatly but deliberately try to erase any messages by putting a chamber between lung and brain and mixing it up. On the one hand we might end up with a permutation message. For example, a man lives up stream from another and sends messages to his down stream neighbor by throwing alphabet soup letters into the stream, the neighbor then reads the letters and reassembles the message. If the first man sends BREATHE and the second man should respond, but if while the message is in transit a large paddle boat travels up stream, the second man might read THE BEAR and his response would bear no relationship to the original message.

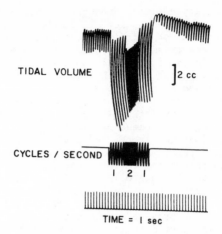

Fig. 10.3. A synchronized hyperpnea, elicited by a stimulus of
            -30 μa dc plus a sinusoid with an amplitude of +75
            μa and a frequency of 1 and 2 cycles/sec (6).

    Dr. Maurice DuBois (7) and I tried the erasure experiment.
We decided not to try for permutation but for erasure. Using rats
we cross connected the abdominal aortas and recorded the central
arterial pressure at the cross connection. Both brains thus see a
common blood. The ventilation was recorded from both animals.
To open the loop, in the recipient, a balloon catheter was inserted
into the right ventricle, and a pump assisted venous drainage was
set up using a multiperforate catheter in the inferior vena cava.
This assured us there was no pulmonary blood flow in the recipient.
Its ventilation was presumably nearly all dead space. The devices
that were placed in the circuit included a direct connector which
was essentially a short piece of polyethylene and a small stirring
chamber with a volume of 1.5 ml. Mathematically, I am sure you
recognize, these are both low pass filters, which we checked physically by colorimetric methods. Unfortunately the short connection
still gives 25% attenuation at respiratory frequency--and the
chamber attenuates nearly 100% at less than 5 per minute.

    What happens is shown in Figure 10.4. Typically, each animal
is metabolizing and excreting CO_2. When the connection is made the
donor excretes CO_2 equivalent to both animals and has a minute volume
equal to both. The recipient rat continues to breathe (regardless
of connection) but exchanges no CO_2. If the recipient inhales CO_2
there is no response. If the donor does both respond, but the recipient's response is significantly smaller than expected. We now
exercise the donor electrically and do the obvious permutation.
This figure shows the response. Finally the experiment demonstrated

that the recipient's ventilatory response to exercise in the donor
is significant when the connection is direct and not significant
when the connection is a stirred one. We conclude a message got
through. At rest it appears to be quantitative, at exercise we can
erase a good piece of it but not resoundingly--only statistically
significant.

Our joy, however, is severely tempered by the magnitude of the
change. Even though the change is statistically significant, it was
not a resounding demonstration. Something got erased--i.e., there
is a time series involved but it is not again apparently a simple
continuous wave kind of message.

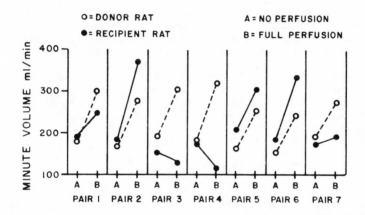

Fig. 10.4 Ventilation of the donor and recipient rats during
          (A) the unperfused state and (B) the perfused state.

By now it had become plain to me that my research had wandered
pretty far from the orthodoxy of respiratory control physiology. I
could not conveniently ratiocinate about respiratory control without
extensive mathematical modelling. It was plain that bandwidth however used was much narrower than the low pass pattern with a cut-
off at the respiratory frequency. We knew the system had transport
lags and perhaps essential non linearities. The oscillation of the
chest and perhaps of the blood associated with the specific cyclical
process of breathing may be the relatively unimportant part of a
message. The next obvious step away from a simple signal response
relationship is a carrier communication system, AM or FM, or PCM.
The logical thing should be to strip out what confusion the carrier
produces. I had for long been impressed by the old claim that CO_2
inhalation increased the depth more than the rate of breathing and
I began to seek in this claim a method to conceptualize the separation of signal from carrier. This led me to the last things I want

to discuss with you; the problem of looking at the humoral signal
and its response (breathing) as a modulation process which is intrinsically non linear. The trick then would be to demodulate the
response (and perhaps the signal) into whatever number of signal
envelopes that are appropriate. In our case we chose what physiolo
gists have been doing traditionally, amplitude envelope and frequency envelope functions: translated "depth" and "rate".
     Dr. Urs Ruttimann (15, 16) and I pursued the following theory.
The problem is the adjustment not just of alveolar but of total ven·
tilation since the brain stem does not "know" the extensions of the
airway or its peculiarities--as in tube breathing. One can approacl
the problem by a brute force numerical method treating the air flow
(pneumotachograph) as an hybrid (AM-FM) modulated wave V(t)=A(t)
Cos 0_t and a frequency envelope. A more elegant derivation was
derived by Ruttimann by constructing an analytic function of the
complex variable such that the physically recorded pneumotachograph
was the real part of its Hilbert Transform. The imaginary part can
be deduced and demonstrated to be simply a convolution of the real
signal with all frequency shift of $-\pi2$, a quadrature filter. This
is physically realizable through computation. Demodulation into
components can then be accomplished by composing the Hilbert pairs
as (recalling that in FM, the argument is the integral of the modulation signal).

$$A(t) = \sqrt{V^2(t) + V_H^2(t)}$$

$$F(t) = \frac{\dot{V}_H(t)V(t) - \dot{V}(t)\dot{V}_H(t)}{2\pi A(t)}$$

Where V is airflow and the subscript H is the imaginary part of the
Hilbert transform.
     We can back track from these continuous functions and show that
the envelopes in fact are reducible to the traditional concepts for
tidal volume, and respiratory rate. Having now a continuous function we could try to relate it to the "sampled" continuous function
represented by end tidal P_{CO_2}'s.
     There are three questions that must be borne in mind that have
haunted all our studies at the most deep conceptual level. The relation between signal and response may not be simple because:
     1. There is extraneous noise present both instrumental and
         biological
     2. The relationship between signal and response is non linear
     3. The response is due not only to the signal in question but
         to other signals which may be conflicting, reinforcing, or
         showing occlusion.
     We therefore sought the tool that abstractly at least will ex-
tract a well defined examinable part of the relationship. We viewed
both signal and ventilation as member function of stochastic processes.

The critical function we used was the ordinary coherency function
(where Sjj is a power spectrum on jj)

$$0 < K_{xy}^2 (f) = \frac{\left| S_{xy} (f) \right|^2}{S_{xx} (f) \, S_{yy} (f)} \leq 1$$

From this and the related spectra we extracted the linearly predictable portion of the relationship between end tidal CO_2 envelope and ventilation envelopes. Adequate statistical methods exist for estimating the coherencies.

After a good bit more complicated analyses, which I am not capable of reviewing here, we came to experiment. Human subjects were allowed breathe through mask and pneumotachogragh. An intranasal catheter collected CO_2 continuously through an infra red analyser. 2, 4, 6% CO_2 mixtures were delivered as seven minute step transients. 10%, 2 breath impulse transients were also used.

Figure 10.5 shows typical results (concentrating only on the upper half of the figure). The step is smeared out by the airway, residual volume and other known phenomena. There is a distinct amplitude envelope response and a less distinct but provable frequency response delayed by 21.6 seconds. Impulse test produces this figure where the observed delays are 6.0 seconds. These differences are explicitly measurable and statistically significant.

To define a sufficient (incomplete) structure relating A(f) and F(t) to C(t) requires three partial coherency functions. Let me illustrate with a sample of a subject responding to a 6% CO_2 step (Fig. 10.5). There appears to be under this model coherency between CO_2 and amplitude but not between CO_2 and frequency. All the rate change can be attributed to the coherency between amplitude and frequency.

These coherencies can be used to construct a linear model which best fits the data taking into account the noise (Fig. 10.6). The codes used are K_a, K_{af}, leading to the two boxes in the figure. K_{cf} does not appear because the coherency is not statistically significant. The figure shows how one input signal, the end-expiratory CO_2 (C(t)), may produce the two outputs A(t) and F(t). As we proceed with this analysis we find that for each of the test conditions (but for all subjects) a different, sufficient linear description of the respiratory control system arises. In all cases our data can be fit to a linear representation shown in Figure 10.7 but for the experiment conditions the Bode plots are different. This circumstance implies intrinsic non linearity or non stationarity. The respiratory system acts like a croquet ball in Alice's Wonderland.

In complexity the analysis necessary has come a long way from the simple concept of stimulus and response. The principle of superposition obviously does not hold and the object studied appears to have sufficient versatility to give a unique answer to unique challenges. It is as though the signal selects the recipient and the response is still always appropriate. If to the appropriate men I send the message "Fire"--one may shoot his gun, another may run in terror from the theater, and the third may discharge his secretary, and the fourth may put on his boots and slide down a brass pole.

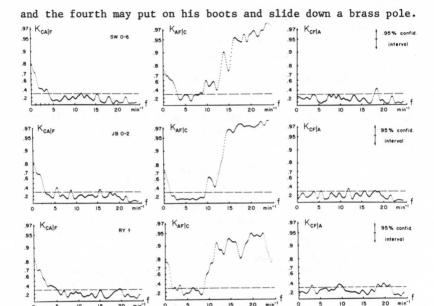

Fig. 10.5 Partial coherency functions for 3 subjects based upon
step transient CO_2 inhalation. Broken horizontal line shows the
level at which the coherency function is statistically significant.
Large values of coherency, above 5 cycles/min. in the middle column
of charts are not significant because of increasing error or estimation in this technique. Observe that while amplitude and CO_2 ($K_{CA/F}$)
and amplitude and frequency ($K_{AF/C}$) are significant. The partial
coherency of CO_2 and frequency ($K_{CF/A}$) is not significant.

There are less colorful but more technical terms to describe
these and even more challenging problems. Suppose for example we
look not just at bandwidth and continuous amplitude, frequency, or
even phase encoded signals but pulse code modulation and its vari-
ants. Suppose the humoral message is a highly compressed code such
as delta modulation, or a Huffman encoding and sending to the sensor
which may be a fixed (or variable) statistical predictive sensor
which needs as messages only the corrections. A similar communication structure is implicit in the model suggested by Cunningham (4).
We may have a mixed message with two sensors which confer. Then the
low bandwidth may still provide enough channel capacity and erasure
may for the most part not be easily accomplished.

Summary

In 1976, I am not sure where we are but I still am convinced
of the correctness of the premises. The problem is not impossible,
just a little more difficult.

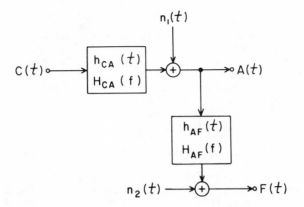

Fig. 10.6. First order approximation of the ventilatory controller.
The fluctuations of the alveolar PCO_2 are considered as forcing
function C(t). The amplitude A(t) and frequency F(t) of the airflow rate are the output functions, n_1(t) and n_2(t) represent
uncorrelated noise.

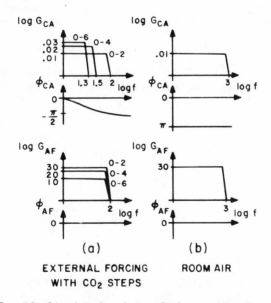

Fig. 10.7. Idealized Bode plots of the estimated transfer functions
H_{CA}(f) and H_{AF}(f) under conditions of (a) applied CO_2 steps, and
(b) room air. The critical observation is that the mechanism of the
response depends on the nature of the stimulus. This observation
implies non linearity certainly, since super position fails; but
may also include an adaptive or predictive controller.

REFERENCES

1. Band, D.M., Cameron, I.R., Semple, S.J. J. Appl. Physiol.,
    26:268-273-1969.
2. Band, D.M., Cameron, I.R., Semple, S.J. J. Appl. Physiol.,
    26:261-267, 1969.
3. Bishop, G.H. Physiol. Rev., 36:376-399, 1956.
4. Cunningham, D.J.C. Nature, 253:440-442, 1975.
5. Davies, R.O. and Yamamoto, W.S. Resp. Physiol., 1:41-57, 1966.
6. Davies, R.O. Doctoral Dissertation, University of Pennsylvania,
    1964.
7. DuBois, R.M. Doctoral Dissertation, University of Pennsylvania,
    1969.
8. Goodman, N. Dissertation, Case Institute of Technology, 1962.
9. Goodman, N. IEEE Trans. Bio. Med. Eng., 11:82-93, 1964.
10. Gray, J.S. Pulmonary Ventilation and Its Physiological Regu-
    lations, C.C. Thomas, Springfield, Illinois, 1950.
11. Guyton, A.C., Crowell, J.W., Moore, J. Am. J. Physiol., 187:
    395-399, 1956.
12. Kao, F.F. The Regulation of Human Respiration, eds. D.J.C.
    Cunningham and B.B. Lloyd, p. 460-502, 1963.
13. Lenfant, C. J. Appl. Physiol., 22:675-684, 1967.
14. Raub, W.F. Doctoral Thesis, University of Pennsylvania, 1965.
15. Ruttimann, U.E. Dissertation, University of Pennsylvania, 1972.
16. Ruttimann, U.E. and Yamamoto, W.S. Ann. Bio. Med. Eng.,
    2:239-251, 1974.
17. Terzuolo, C.A. and Bullock, T.H. Proc. Natl. Acad. Sci.,
    U.S., 12:689-694, 1956.
18. Tschirgi, R.D. and Taylor, J.L. Am. J. Physiol., 195:7, 1958.
19. Von Euler, C. and Soderberg, U. J. Physiol., 118:555, 1952.
20. Yamamoto, W.S. J. Appl. Physiol., 25:439-445, 1968.

11

Neural Drive Mechanisms of Central Origin

Frederic L. Eldridge

Despite over a century of studies, chemical stimuli have not provided a full understanding of the control of breathing, especially in exercise. Neural signals have always been an attractive alternate source of stimulation which might provide the necessary answers, but most investigators have not found them to be of sufficient magnitude. However, it has been assumed that changing neural input, whether from neural receptors per se or from chemoreceptors, would be expressed fully and rapidly as a change in respiratory output; the further assumption followed that, because of their very slowness, slow responses could not be neural in origin. The studies that I shall present here show that the assumption of an immediate and full response to the onset and offset of neural stimuli is incorrect, and that it is necessary to add this new element to our considerations of the control of respiration.

Over a century ago, it was noted that animals became apneic when passively hyperventilated. This was consistent with a chemical theory of the control of respiration. It clearly applies as well to passive hyperventilation (HV) in man, provided hypocapnia occurs. In 1905, Haldane and Priestly (9) reported that awake human beings also have post-HV apnea, thereby seeming to confirm the overriding importance of CO_2 as the stimulus to respiration. However, Boothby (2) as early as 1912 showed that post-HV apnea did not always occur after active HV; a number of subsequent investigators (1,8,10,11) have also demonstrated that apnea is not common after active (voluntary) HV in normal subjects, despite the hypocapnia. The absence of apnea has usually been attributed to the effect of wakefulness, thought to provide a neural stimulus sufficient to prevent apnea.

The present studies were based on the hypothesis that the lack of post-HV apnea is not due to wakefulness; rather that there is an intrinsic central neural mechanism which is activated during increased active breathing, which is responsible for maintaining respiration after the cessation of a perturbing stimulus and which may be responsible for an important part of the respiratory response to any kind of respiratory stimulus.

149

FINDINGS

The first study (4) which I wish to report was carried out in spontaneously breathing cats anesthetized with chloralose and urethane. Ventilation, $P_{ET}CO_2$ and arterial pressure were recorded. Hyperventilation was induced for 2 minutes in two different ways: 1) passive (mechanically generated) HV was produced by a volume respirator; and 2) active (neurally generated) HV was induced by carotid sinus nerve (CSN) stimulation or by calf muscle squeezing. Each active HV run was matched by a passive HV run in which an equal duration and degree of hypocapnia was achieved.

In all experiments there was a striking difference between the post-HV breathing patterns of active and passive hyperventilation. Passive HV always led to post-HV apnea (Fig 11.1A): the greater the degree of hypocapnia, the longer was the period of apnea (Fig 11.2). On the other hand, active HV was never followed by apnea in the early recovery period (Fig 11.1B). In only 2 of 28 such

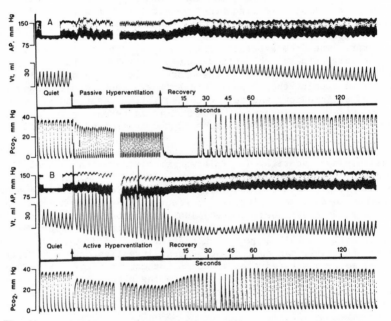

Fig 11.1 Arterial pressure (AP), tidal volume (V_t), and airway P_{CO_2} during quiet breathing, hyperventilation, and recovery from hyperventilation in one cat. A: passive hyperventilation of 2 min duration. Tidal volume not recorded during hyperventilation. There is apnea during the initial 20 sec of posthyperventilation period. B: active hyperventilation (carotid sinus nerve stimulation) of 2 min duration. Hyperpnea is present during initial 15 sec of recovery and apnea does not occur.

Type	No. of Runs	Decrease in P_{CO_2} during HV, mm Hg		Duration of Apnea, sec
		Group	Mean	
Active	17	<8.5	5.7 ± 0.4	None
	28	>8.5	11.9 ± 1	None*
Passive	13	<8.5	6.3 ± 0.4	19.2 ± 3.3
	19	>8.5	12.2 ± 0.7	29.7 ± 3.4

Values are means ± SE.   *Two of these with the greatest
P_{CO_2} decrease (16.6 and 18.4 mm Hg) did develop apnea later in
the first minute of recovery.

Fig 11.2 Duration of apnea after active or passive hyperventilation.

active HV experiments did apnea occur at all; both were in runs
where P_{CO_2} had been markedly decreased (-16.6 and -18.4 mm Hg)
from quiet breathing levels and the apnea occurred between 15-45
seconds of recovery. The immediate post-HV period not only showed
no apnea but rather an hyperpnea which declined on a smooth curve
similar to that of Fig 11.1B.

The presence of intact carotid bodies was not necessary for the
phenomenon to occur, nor were the vagal nerves necessary. Carotid
sinus nerve stimulation was not uniquely responsible, for the same
process appeared after the more physiological calf squeezing stimulus. Circulatory changes were likewise ruled out as causal.

In order to eliminate effects of anesthesia and of higher brain
structures, a second study (7) was carried out in spontaneously
breathing unanesthetized decerebrate cats. Midcollicular decerebration was performed under ether anesthesia. After recovery from
the anesthesia, CSN stimulation was used to produce active hyperventilation in a manner similar to the previous study. A typical
experiment is shown in Fig 11.3. Stimulation of the CSN led to
an increase in ventilation and concomitant decrease in end-tidal
P_{CO_2} (Panel A). At the end of stimulation, ventilation fell with
first recovery breath but never to control level; it then decreased
slowly over the next 15-20 s to or below control. Apnea never occurred after active HV. On the other hand, passive HV which was
associated with a similar degree of hypocapnia always led to a
period of post-HV apnea (Panel B). After active HV, the post-
HV hyperpnea was consistently present whether the vagus nerves
were intact or cut and had no relationship to any changes in arterial pressure.

The studies are interpreted as follows: The apnea of passive
HV is due to a simple decrease in CO_2-H^+ ion stimulus in the classical sense. Since, however, active HV had the same decrement in
chemical stimulus, some other mechanism sustains respiration in
the post-HV period. Thus, the presence or absence of post-HV apnea
is not related to wakefulness but to whether HV is passively or

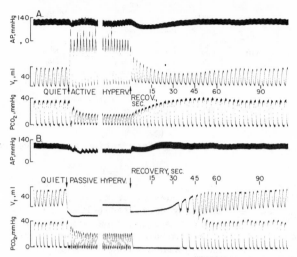

Fig 11.3 Arterial pressure (AP), tidal volume (V_t) and airway P_{CO_2} during quiet breathing, hyperventilation (HV), and recovery in an unanesthetized decerebrate cat. A: active HV due to carotid sinus nerve stimulation of 40 sec. Despite marked hypocapnia apnea does not occur and hyperpnea is present during first 15 sec of recovery. B: passive HV of 62 sec duration is followed by 30 sec of apnea.

actively generated. Active HV must therefore activate a neural mechanism which sustains respiration and decays slowly, thereby overriding the effect of low CO_2. The results in decerebrate cats indicates that it resides in the medulla and pons.

A third study was carried out in awake human beings (13). They were persuaded to hyperventilate voluntarily for a period of 10-15 s, thereby causing a significant degree of hypocapnia. During the recovery their breathing pattern was determined. Two examples in one subject are shown in Plate 11.1. Following the brief voluntary hyperventilation, there is no apnea. Both rate and tidal volume are increased in the post-HV period and gradually decline to control or below only over a period of 40 s. The averaged findings for 16 "naive" subjects are shown in Fig 11.4. Again there is no apnea, the first post-HV breaths are clearly increased over control in spite of the hypocapnia, and there is a gradual return of ventilation to control over the first 10-20 s of recovery. The findings of awake human beings are thus similar to some previous reports (2, 10) and to those of the anesthetized cats. A recent report (12) confirms that posthyperventilatory hyperpnea occurs in most human subjects and lasts even longer when isocapnic conditions are maintained.

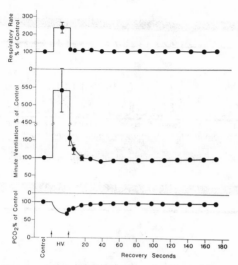

Fig 11.4 Courses of respiratory rate, ventilation, and end-tidal P_{CO_2} in 16 "naive" subjects before, during, and after a brief period of hyperventilation. Vertical bars are $\pm$ SE of the mean. Where they do not appear SE is smaller than size of point. Note brief post-HV hyperpnea and absence of apnea.

A problem with the studies so far reported is that the chemical stimulus (CO_2-H^+) decreased with HV, so there was a mixed effect of that decrease and the neural mechanism in question. For that reason, it was impossible to quantitate the true magnitude or duration of the process. Additional studies were therefore performed in cats that were paralyzed and maintained on a respirator, thereby assuring constancy of arterial P_{CO_2}. The peak level of phrenic activity integrated in 0.1 s episodes was used to quantitate the neural output for each breath (6). "Respiration" was again stimulated by the CSN or by calf-squeezing and the findings on cessation of stimulation were examined breath-by-breath for up to 5 minutes. In some cases, rapid cessation of stimulus input to the brain was accomplished by withdrawal of the physiological output of the carotid bodies by means of cold-blocking (4°C) both carotid sinus nerves.

In the stimulation experiments, both types of stimulation led to an increase in respiratory neural output. At the end of either type of stimulation, output always fell with the first offset breath. However, this accounted for only 30-50% of the previous increase due to stimulation. The remainder of the fall was a slow component which took 3-4 minutes before reaching control output (Fig 11.5). Ninety-seven runs carried out in 28 cats showed that the findings were reproducible under a wide variety of conditions. Carotid body and vagal influences had no effect. Barbituate anesthesia gave the

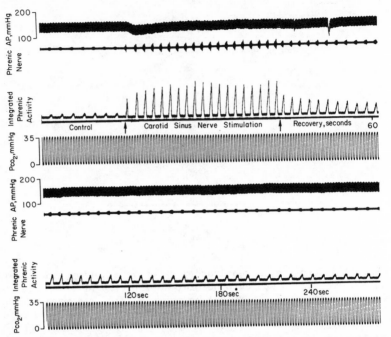

Fig 11.5 Example of respiratory effect of carotid sinus nerve stimulation and of recovery at end of stimulation in cat with sectioned vagi and carotid sinus nerves. Note relative hyperpnea, shown by increased height of phrenic activity, during recovery, and slow decline in respiratory output to control. Top and bottom tracings are continuous.

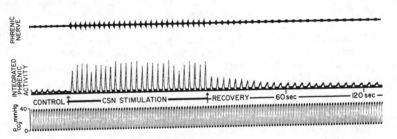

Fig 11.6 Experiment performed in cat with vagi and carotid sinus nerves cut and spinal cord sectioned at C_7-T_1. Poststimulus hyperpnea and slow recovery process not abolished by cord section.

same results as chloralose-urethane. Cutting the spinal cord at C_7-T_1 did not abolish the process (Fig 11.6).

When plotted semilogarithmically, the slow offset process was essentially a straight line, showing that it had an exponential decay with a time constant of approximately 48 s. This function appeared to be independent of the CO_2 level at which the experiment was run.

The same type of studies were again repeated in decerebrate unanesthetized cats. The findings were similar to those just shown.

The effect of stimulus withdrawal following cooling of the CSN was similar to that of cessation of electrical stimulation of the CSN; an immediate small decrease in respiratory output was followed by a prolonged slow decrease over a period of 4-5 minutes. There was also a relatively slow development of the maximal respiratory response when the stimulus was started with CSN warming. It is suggested that this represents the slow build-up of the central process responsible for the findings. In Fig 11.7 the effect of periods of unblocking CSN activity can be seen. When the stimulation is short (7 s, Panel A) so is the magnitude and duration of the slow recovery process; when the stimulation is longer (27 s, Panel C), the slow recovery process is much larger and longer.

DISCUSSION

These studies demonstrate the existence of a central neural process which, once fully activated, sustains respiration for a long period of time after cessation of the primary stimulus. Peripheral input has been ruled out as causal. The process is not related to circulatory changes. It is independent of the CO_2-H^+ stimulus. Since the process occurs in decerebrate animals, its locus must therefore be in the medulla and pons.

The most likely mechanism is that of maintenance of activity in neural circuits in the brain stem due to facilitatory feedback of neurons within the circuits. Once activated, the feedback process ("reverberation", afterdischarge, "fly-wheel effect") itself maintains the activity of respiratory neurons, and the slowly declining respiratory output during recovery reflects gradual decay of activity within the reverberatory circuits. This feedback activity could be in the respiratory neuronal circuits themselves. However, two findings suggest that it lies outside them: 1) the slow activation of the process during stimulation (Fig 11.7) and 2) the finding that large inspirations (sighs) occurring during the slow recovery process have little effect on the overall pattern of the process (Fig 11.8). It is suggested that the most likely locus of the maintained neural activity is the reticular activating system (RAS).

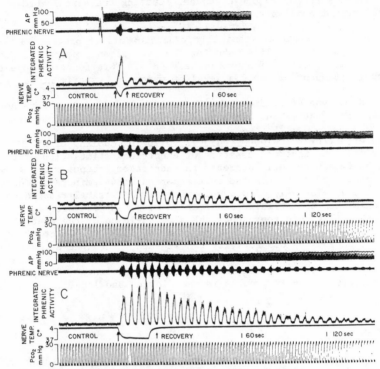

Fig 11.7 Effect on respiratory output of short periods of respiratory stimulation from the carotid body produced by unblocking
carotid sinus nerve (CSN) conduction. In all three panels, control
values were obtained with the CSNs at 4°C and show that cat was
apneic. At first arrow CSN warmed to 37°C and at second arrow
recooled to less than 8°C. Stimulus durations were A: 7 sec.;
B: 13 sec.; C: 27 sec. Slow recovery process shows progressive
augmentation with longer periods of stimulation.

Because the process is activated by a variety of stimuli, including those which are so-called primary ones for respiration and
operates in animals and man, awake or anesthetized, it must be considered an integral part of the respiratory control mechanism. The
process appears to account for approximately 50% of any increase
in respiration secondary to a primary stimulus. The studies are
consistent with the concept that respiration is partially self-
stimulating, or self-amplifying. A significant part of the ventilatory response to any stimulus may therefore be a function of this
central neural effect, and not just a function of the stimulus and
its receptors. The likelihood that the characteristics of the process vary from subject to subject may explain the observed variability of respiratory responses to a variety of stimuli.

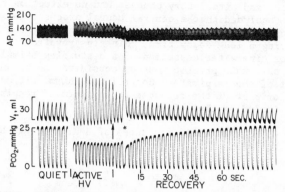

Fig 11.8 Control, active hyperventilation, and recovery after
carotid sinus nerve stimulation in unanesthetized decerebrate cat
with intact vagi. This cat had regularly occurring deep sighing
inspirations, one of which occurred at the third breath (*) of recovery. Note that the smoothly declining inspiratory pattern is not
significantly affected by the sigh.

Finally, I believe that the interpretation of the findings after
any kind of primary respiratory stimulation, whether neural or
chemical, must take this central neural process into account. It
must be considered a potentially important mechanism for part of
the increase in ventilation in exercise, regardless of the primary
stimulus or stimuli. It has been postulated in the past that ventilatory changes at the beginning and end of exercise consist of
an immediate neural component and a slower, humoral component (3).
Since the slow neural component of the present studies mimics that
of exercise, it seems probable that the slow component of exercise
recovery is also neural in origin. Thus, there is no need to invoke humoral mechanisms to explain the findings.

SUMMARY

The breathing patterns during recovery from active (neurally generated) hyperventilation (HV) were compared to those of passive
(mechanically generated) HV in anesthetized cats and in unanesthetized decerebrate cats. After passive HV, apnea always occurred
whereas after active HV there was hyperpnea and a slow return to
control ventilation. Similar results were found in awake human
beings after active (voluntary) HV. In paralyzed cats, anesthetized or unanesthetized and decerebrate, where chemical stimuli
remained constant, the post-stimulation respiratory output was initially substantially higher than control and declined exponentially
to control only over a period of minutes. Vagal and carotid sinus
nerve section, transsection of the spinal cord at C_7-T_1, bilateral

pneumothoraces, and circulatory changes had no effect on the findings. It is concluded that a central neural process, located in
pons and medulla, activated in association with increased respiration and having a long decay time, maintains respiration for a
long period of time after cessation of a disturbing stimulus. It
is suggested that this process must be considered to be an intrinsic component of the respiratory control mechanism. It may be
responsible for part of the response to any form of respiratory
stimulation, including that of exercise.

Supported by USPHS, National Institutes of Health Grants NS09390,
NS11458, and HL17689.

REFERENCES

1. Ashbridge, K. M., S. Jennett, and J. B. North. J. Physiol.,
    London 230:52P, 1973.
2. Boothby, W. M. J. Physiol., London 45:328-333, 1912.
3. Dejours, P. In Handbook of Physiology, Respiration. Washing-
    ton, D.C. Am. Physiol. Soc., 1964. sect. 3, vol. I, 25,
    p. 631-648.
4. Eldridge, F. L. J. Appl Physiol. 34:422-430, 1973.
5. Eldridge, F. L. J. Appl. Physiol. 37:723-735, 1974.
6. Eldridge, F. L. J. Appl. Physiol. 39:567-574, 1975.
7. Eldridge, F. L. J. Appl. Physiol. 40:23-28, 1976
8. Fink, B. R. J. Appl. Physiol. 16:15-20, 1961.
9. Haldane, J. S., and J. G. Priestly. J. Physiol., London
    32:225-266, 1905.
10. Mills, J. N. J. Physiol., London 105:95-116, 1946.
11. Plum, F., H. W. Brown, and E. Snoep. J. Am. Med. Assoc.
    181:1050-1055, 1962.
12. Swanson, G. D., K. A. Aqleh, D. S. Ward, and J. W. Bellville.
    Federation Proc. 35:633, 1976.
13. Tawadrous, F. D., and F. L. Eldridge. J. Appl. Physiol.
    37:353-356, 1974.

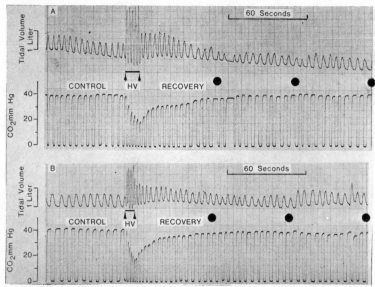

Plate 11.1   Control, voluntary hyperventilation, and recovery in two separate experiments (A and B) in one human subject. Despite decreases of end-tidal P_{CO_2} to below 20 mmHg, hyperpnea and tachypnea persists in the posthyperventilation period for at least 40 sec.

Discussion

Goldman: Dr. Yamamoto, I thought I heard you say that the heart acts as a digital filter and cuts off signals related to respiratory rate. Is this correct?

Yamamoto: Yes, that is approximately correct. The Sampling (Nyquist) Theorem states that if you want to represent (reconstruct or pass) in digitized form a signal with band width w hertz you must sample at a rate of $(2W+1)/\text{sec}$. Now in the physiological context this means that to pass the basic respiratory wave form the heart rate must be at least 3 times as fast as the respiratory rate. In engineering practice a higher sampling rate is always required for noise protection. If you look at people or animals in all kinds of states, a heart rate to respiratory rate ratio of three is the bottom level but not unusual. In exercise the ratio goes up to 16. So at the low ratio we are just at the theoretical limit of transmitting the continuous respiratory CO_2 signal in terms of samples values (Biophysical J., 2:143-159, 1962).

Goldman: Does that presuppose that heart rate and breathing rate are independent? We've observed at rest and during either CO_2 breathing or exercise, that the cardiac artifact comes at a fairly consistent point in the breath. I'm wondering whether this may bear a relationship to phasic CO_2 fluxes within the breath by the cardiac pump action.

Yamamoto: That particular issue is not very critical, because generally when you breath faster your heart beats faster and the ratio tends to stay constant, and its that ratio that determines whether you're passing respiratory frequency or not. Whether its synchronized in one part of the cycle or another is not important.

Eldridge: In a good carotid sinus nerve preparation with normal blood flow to the carotid body (for example, in a cat) you will find that there are small oscillations of carotid body output when the respiratory rate is on the order of 30.

Swanson: I would like the panel to consider an observation concerning CO_2 regulation with exercise when an inspired CO_2 background is present. By regulation, I mean that arterial CO_2 tension does not change (increase) when progressing from rest to moderate exercise. That is the case when breathing room air, as shown in Figure A. Note ventilation increases without an increase in arterial CO_2, yielding perfect regulation. If at rest, an inspired CO_2 of, say 2% is added, the ventilation and arterial CO_2 increase as given by the traditional CO_2 response curve in the steady state. Now if exercise is added to the inspired CO_2 background, the exercise induced hyperpnea is accompanied by an increase in arterial PCO_2 (from the resting value), yielding the loss of perfect regulation as shown. If the inspired CO_2 background is higher, say 4%, then the exercise induced hyperpnea is accompanied by an even larger

increase in arterial CO_2, yielding a still greater loss of regulation. This plot has been abstracted from my own work (Swanson and
Bellville, The Physiologist, 18:413, 1975), that of Menn et al.
(J. Appl. Physiol., 28:663-671, 1970) and that of Lugliani et al.
(New Eng. J. Med., 285:1105-1111, 1971). Furthermore this loss of
regulation can be predicted from theoretical considerations of gas
exchange (Swanson, J. Appl. Physiol., 40:651-657, 1976). I find
it interesting that adding dead space via tube breathing yields a
CO_2 response curve similar in slope to the inspired CO_2 case.
However, when exercise is added to the tube breathing, regulation
of CO_2 at the resting value appears to be maintained, in contrast
to the inspired CO_2 case. Again this result is predictable from
theoretical considerations of gas exchange and is supported by the
study of Jones et al. (Respiration, 28:389-398, 1971). It seems
to me that these observations provide clues as to the structure
of the respiratory controller and I would hope that the panel might
comment.

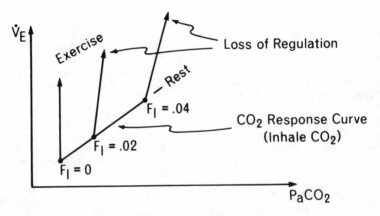

Fig. A. Effect of inspired CO_2 on CO_2 regulation.

Wasserman: This question is pertinent to Dr. Eldridge's experiments
where he raised the volume of the balloon in the right atrium. He
showed ventilation to go up or not change at all. But he didn't
show us what happened to arterial PCO_2.

Eldridge: The blood flow to the lung was close to zero.

Wasserman: Ventilation was the same but alveolar ventilation may
have gone down in response to that reduced blood flow, i.e. physiological dead space increases. When you raised the right atrial
balloon volume, did you increase your arterial to end-tidal PCO_2
difference and did your arterial PCO_2 actually go down?

Fishman: I really want to clarify this one point. If I understand

what Eldridge did, he cut off CO_2 delivery to the lung and found
that ventilation was unaffected. The conclusion has to be either
that the CO_2 delivery to the lung has nothing to do with ventilatory
control or that there is some other mechanism that takes over as
soon as you cut it out. Those are the only two alternatives I can
see.

Eldridge: Or there is discontinuity in the mechanism.

Fishman: That's the one that I am holding in reserve. Is it all
boiling down to either discontinuity in the mechanism, or that some
other mechanism becomes operative when CO_2 delivery is cut off, or
that CO_2 delivery has nothing to do with the control mechanism?

Wasserman: What I'm saying is that the experimental analysis is
incomplete. We have to know whether or not the arterial PCO_2
changed in response to the situation.

Eldridge: I didn't try to answer the issue, all I was trying to do
with that experiment was to show that making such a profound change
as reducing Qc to zero did not produce the kinds of things that I
was showing in the post-hyperventilation period. This was not done
in a rigorous way. I did not measure arterial PCO_2 and I don't
intend to say that it answers all the questions. I do think though
that it does show pretty clearly that what I'm claiming to be a
central neural reverberation or feedback, cannot be explained by
changes in circulation.

Wasserman: With 10 seconds of hyperventilation you're decreasing
$PaCO_2$, but your mixed venous PCO_2 is not changing. But you have
increased cardiac output. Have you ruled out the possibility that
the post-hyperventilation hyperpnea is due to an increased CO_2 flow
to the lung. I know with 2 minutes of hyperventilation, you don't
get the same results.

Eldridge: I don't think that the human experiments are in any way
critical. I merely throw those in to demonstrate that you can
accomplish exactly the same thing in awake humans as you can get in
anesthetized cats where it's done in a fairly rigorous way. As a
matter of fact, the period of hyperpnea in the post-hyperventilation
period in humans, when $PaCO_2$ is allowed to fall, is very much shorter.
The CO_2 dropping is affecting all kinds of things, and furthermore
I suspect that in the 10 second period that it probably had plenty
of time to effect venous circulation.

Fishman: Dr. Swanson, have they succeeded in answering your question?

Swanson: I think it is important to recognize that arterial PCO_2
is well regulated under normal conditions in the sense that it stays
constant with increase in ventilation and that when you add inspired
CO_2 you lose regulation. I think we must explain that.

Eldridge: I can attempt to give you an explanation. That is, the answer may be related to the timing of the oscillating signal that's coming out of the lung and acting at the level of the carotid body. It has been clearly shown now by several investigators that the effect of a signal from the carotid body is primarily important when it occurs during the last 50% of inspiration. And if it occurs at any other time during the respiratory cycle it has little effect on inspiration. If the peak of the carotid body signal occurs during this vulnerable period you're going to have a big effect. If the nadir of that oscillating carotid body signal arrives during this critical period you're not going to have much effect. I have been able to demonstrate this in cats with intact vagi.

Filley: Dr. Eldridge, you're talking about tube breathing, and that's not the issue. As Swanson said, if you breathe CO_2 you lose control; if you have tube breathing you don't lose control.

Eldridge: The CO_2 breathing decreases the oscillation in a very striking way. Tube breathing not only makes it bigger but it changes the time relationship, because you've delayed the pulse of new non-CO_2 containing air to come in until later in the breath.

Filley: We must try to tie together what Swanson has said which is really very important, namely, that CO_2 breathing interferes with the control mechanism. First when you put CO_2 in the airway you clog this mechanism. Secondly, if the $CO2$ not only clogs the mechanism but actually acts as a depressant with every breath you can tip that response slope just the way Swanson has presented. Now we will tie this together with what you have spoken of regarding two types of hyperventilation. Passive hyperventilation leads to apnea, I believe, because the cardiac output and CO_2 flux across the lung are not increased and may even be decreased. But when you actively hyperventilate, the diaphragm--just as at the onset of exercise--squirts blood from your guts into your lung, and hence the $CO2$ flux across the lung is suddenly increased. Hence you get this tremendous drive. It takes about 15 seconds for that drive to dissipate (via recirculation of blood) and appears to have nothing to do with the resonating circuit in your head, which you claim obeys the law of angular momentum but which I've never heard of in the medulla.

Eldridge: Well, now you've heard of it. Sherrington reported the spinal cord after discharge many years ago (Sherrington, Sir C. The Integrative Action of the Nervous System (2nd Ed.), New Haven: Yale University Press, 1947, pg 26-35). The extension of this mechanism to the medulla doesn't seem to be a very large step.

Filley: Anyway, it seems to me that Wasserman's mechanism does very well.

Eldridge: Giles, you haven't gotten around the whole question of why this keeps on going when the spinal cord is cut at C7.

Milhorn: We've also been interested in the transients you see
after hyperventilation; and we've just finished a series of experiments on human subjects. We felt that the reason you didn't see
the apnea in awake subjects was because they didn't breath hard
enough or long enough to get down below the CO_2 threshold centrally.
We decided that we would really stress them and we picked 40 liters
per minute for 4 minutes as the hyperventilation. That gets the
end-tidal PCO_2 down to about 15 mmHg. So if you're going to see
post-hyperventilation apnea you certainly ought to see it under these
conditions. There was certainly no apnea occurring in these actively
ventilated awake human subjects. We also passively hyperventilated
the people at the same tidal volume and frequency and they did the
same thing.

Eldridge: Fink did that too in 1961 (J. Appl. Physiol., 16:15,
1961).

Milhorn: But that wasn't for 4 minutes.

Eldridge: That really doesn't make any difference.

Milhorn: Yes it does!

Eldridge: The problem is that it is virtually impossible for people
stuck on a respirator, unless they are highly trained, to relax and
be passively hyperventilated. The only way you could prove to me
that you were passively hyperventilating your subjects would be by
having electrodes in their diaphragm and intercostal muscles to
prove that they weren't going along with the machine. Fink showed
that active and so-called passively hyperventilated people behaved
the same during recovery. Bainton and Mitchell (J. Appl. Physiol.,
21:411, 1966) also did this and found that subjects had hyperpnea
after the first time they were apparently passively hyperventilated.
But if they came back a number of times, they finally did learn to
relax and become passively hyperventilated. Then they had apnea
after the passive hyperventilation.

Milhorn: Well, that may be, I don't know. I've tried the passive
hyperventilation myself and it's very easy to relax, no problem at
all.

Kao: First, I would like to make a comment on Dr. Swanson's remarks
that when a response to a stimulus is not associated with an increase
in CO_2 there is perfect regulation, as in the case of muscular exercise, and that when a response to a stimulus is associated with an
increase in CO_2, as in the case of CO_2 inhalation, there is a loss
of regulation. This seems to be muddled thinking, but he raised a
fundamental question. If we need "an error", whether steady or un-
steady state, as depicted in the concept of engineer regulators, in
CO_2 inhalation the stimulus is PCO_2 and in exercise the stimulus
must be something else and not CO_2. This is also the basis of Dr.
Yamamoto's oscillation theory. In both CO_2 inhalation and in mus-

cular exercise there is regulation, but for different aims and with different mechanisms. In exercise it is to meet the metabolic demand, to supply oxygen and to remove CO_2; in CO_2 inhalation the purpose is for CO_2 elimination. In relation to the experiments with added dead space via tube breathing, I would like to ask if ventilation rose to the same magnitude with various sizes of added dead space. In your slide, only directional arrows of ventilation were given. The vertical rise of ventilation indicated that there was no change in CO_2 and hence by your definition, and here I quote: "By regulation, I mean that arterial PCO_2 does not change", there was perfect regulation of PCO_2. This can possibly be explained by our experiments which involved an artificially increased resistance in the breathing passageways. With added increased resistance ventilation changed, judging from the ventilation-PCO_2 response lines, but there was absolutely no change in PCO_2, so PCO_2 was regulated at the expense of ventilation, a situation similar to that with added dead space in your experiment, Dr. Swanson. The question to raise perhaps is what is being regulated? PCO_2 or ventilation? It is customary for respiratory physiologists to speak of regulation of ventilation. By Dr. Swanson's definition we should then not speak of regulation of ventilation of muscular exercise, because ventilation is not regulated! Perhaps it is time now we should be more precise in our language and denote exactly what is being regulated. In some situations such as imposed increased resistance and added dead space, we should speak in terms of regulation of PCO_2. I also would like to make a comment on hyperventilation. As we all know well, the work of Nielsen and Smith (Acta. Physiol. Scand., 24:293-305, 1951) has shown that there is a dog-leg phenomenon at low PCO_2, in contrast to our "old" thinking that at low CO_2 (for example, conditions produced by means of hyperventilation) there is "always" apnea. Presumably when anesthesia is used in animal experimentation, the slope of the ventilation-PCO_2 response line is so low that the dog-leg may become imaginary (Michel and Kao, J. Appl. Physiol., 19:1070-1074, 1964). The state of mind or the amount of real and unreal anesthesia is a very important factor for the investigation of apnea, especially that after hyperventilation.

Goldman: I wonder if the following experiments, at least in humans, might shed some light on the question of the effect of CO_2 flow. If you have active hyperventilation or even if you are on a ventilator and presumably not relaxing totally, hyperventilation may increase cardiac output and thereby contribute to an increase in CO_2 flow. Consequently, you see the increased ventilation in the post-hyperventilation period. If one wants to look at the effect of cardiac output, you could take naive subjects and make them breathe against a substantial positive pressure and then let them actively hyperventilate. I would suggest that it's not unlikely that their cardiac output would decrease. If, with positive pressure in the airway, we did not see post-active hyperventilation hyperpnea, then one might believe that this was related to a decrease in CO_2 flux to the lung.

Wasserman: Mike, I haven't tried that experiment, but if I understand it correctly, you would have a reduction in cardiac output
which is essentially a Valsalva type of effect. You also have a
problem of whether or not you're going to increase physiological
dead space. It's clear to us at this particular time, that if we
do certain things to affect physiological dead space, the minute
ventilation won't follow the CO_2 flow, yet $PaCO_2$ stays constant.
We have seen this in sinusoidably varying work rate studies. In
the experiment you describe, I can predict a great increase in
physiological dead space.

Goldman: You could make them ventilate at target volumes. In other
words, they'd have to do a Valsalva against this positive pressure
to keep their FRC and expiratory level constant.

Sampson: Dr. Eldridge, I thought you made a very elegant defense
of your initial thesis and I think it's been well recognized for
many years that there is something to the central excitatory state;
input to the central nervous system can prime a system and render
it more or less excitable. It is a well known physiological phenomenon. I've looked for many years for oscillations in chemoreceptor
discharges and I don't really see them. I've only seen them at very
slow rates of artificial ventilation; never at anything that would
be anywhere near physiological. Perhaps we ought to introduce one
of Comroe's laws and that is when two people differ about an observation they ought to get in the lab at the same time and see if they
can see it together. When you cool the sinus nerve, do you have any
evidence that conduction in the nerve is actually blocked? Have you
stimulated and not evoked any changes in blood pressure or ventilation?

Eldridge: Yes, I have a direct recording of the carotid sinus nerve
showing that all impulses cease within a few seconds of its cooling
to 4°C and return within a few seconds of warming back to normal
temperature.

Sampson: Are these evoked impulses or spontaneous discharges?

Eldridge: In a previous paper I have showed (J. Appl. Physiol.,
37:723, 1974) that carotid sinus nerve cooling completely abolished
carotid sinus nerve conduction; when it's warmed conduction of spontaneous discharge comes right back.

Sampson: Have you ever used more selective stimulation for chemoreceptors by infusing cyanide or hypoxic blood from somewhere else
rather than using electrical stimulation of the nerve, which as you
know stimulates both chemoreceptor and baroreceptor fibres. Not
that that is necessarily central to your argument.

Eldridge: Not for this purpose, because I found that when I was
doing the previous timing studies that if you pull venous blood
directly out of the vena cava and inject it into the ascending

aorta the carotid body functions for about 3 shots and then it quits.
In fact, Band and Semple in one of their studies on timing found
that if they injected high CO_2 materials in saline, the carotid body
seemed to quit. I found the same thing. And the cyanide is another
very funny one. If you give a single shot of cyanide to a carotid
body, it puts out a nice burst of impulses which looks pretty normal,
but by the time you've given about 3 small shots of cyanide it just
starts firing continuously for long periods of time. Therefore, I
think one has to be very careful about the use of cyanide in a carotid body because you've got a very unphysiological and artificial
kind of output from it that has no relationship to what happens
normally.

Edelman: It seems to me that the dog leg phenomenon during hypoxia
makes a very strong argument for the reverberation hypothesis. In
awake, and presumably naive, goats, we regularly got apnea with
mechanical hyperventilation even in combination with hypoxia.
(Edelman, N. et al., Fed. Proc., 28:1223-1227, 1969). The study
was done to look at the difference between reaching a level of
hypoxia and hypocapnia with mechanical hyperventilation as compared
to actively ventilating by being given a hypoxic gas to breathe.
The difference is enormous, although the identifiable stimuli are
the same. It seems to me that the only reasonable way to explain
that discrepancy is a phenomenon similar to the one described by
Dr. Eldridge.

Eldridge: Let me point out one problem for those of you who might
want to study apneic animals. If you place the animal on a respirator and lower the CO_2 to about the level at which the animal ought to
become apneic, it's going to take a few minutes for apnea to appear.
This is because of two factors: one is the slow lowering of arterial
CO_2; the second is that the process of reverberation appears to apply
to onset and offset of the CO_2 stimulus.

Edelman: Yes, that's precisely the protocol we used--hyperventila-
tion to a fixed level for 5 minutes and introduce hypoxia and then
stop the machine. They all get apneic at a point where they wouldn't
be apneic if they were breathing the hypoxic gas mixture.

Dempsey: I think there is only one person on the panel who has a
mechanism which appears to be substantial enough to account for much
of exercise hyperpnea. The studies Dr. Kao has done over the years
have been very convincing to me and Dr. Levine mentioned that he has
confirmed some of them. Dr. Levine, why are you injecting substances
to artificially produce an increase in metabolic rate if the neural
drive is explaining most of what you're looking for? Karl, the CO_2
flow to the lung and especially cardiogenic hyperpnea looks to me to
be a relatively small contribution to the total hyperpnea. Dr.
Eldridge, your central reverberating circuit requires substantial
input from somewhere else; and Dr. Yamamoto you've been looking for
the oscillation signal and its receptor for a long time but is it
any more than a "fine" controller if a strong neural drive exists?

What's wrong with the neural drive hypothesis as explaining most of
the hyperpnea? Is the main objection only that such a stimulus
doesn't appear to have a role in a feedback system with circulating pH or PCO_2?

Yamamoto: If you believe that everybody's experiments are correct
you have a very interesting dilemna. In my opinion, the only analytical way in which you can handle that thesis is through an extensive mathematical model. For example, in regard to Dr. Eldridge's
oscillating mechanism, in 1971 I reviewed the physiological literature on central neural mechanisms of respiration and there were about
1400 papers. We decided that we would select 300 and make a model
on the basis of 17 neural centers and indeed you can produce what
looks like post-hyperventilation hyperpnea for quite a long time.
It really stems from the work; for example, by Ngai and Wang, Cohen
and Huicuhara in Japan and Salmorraghi and Burns who showed that
when you isolate a small slab of brain stem and stimulate it, you
get repetitive breath cycles. So there is a long tradition of
literature that leads up to the possibility. On the other hand,
this is not at all incompatible with the CO_2 flux if you build that
into a breathing model. At the present time we have 3 separate mathematical models; all of them rather gigantic, and each with many
identifiable physiological variables in them. One can perform a
large number of experiments which parallel experiments in the
literature. I don't believe that you can argue or discuss the
compatibility or non-compatability of some of the things that have
been discussed, unless you do it in a context of an idealized system which is at least that complex. In my case, I propose a
mechanism, I'm looking for the signal to which it must respond.
The whole effort is only a very small part of trying to do what I
call synthetic physiology, that is, trying to put together the
findings of many people.

Fishman: Dr. Yamamoto, I can't let you off that easily. You have
a model in your mind and you must put what we have just heard into
some kind of perspective. How can we reconcile Eldridge's neural
drive, Kao's neural mechanism and Levine's humoral mechanism?

Yamamoto: Now remember that I mentioned that we have ignored the
concept of occlusion. That is, you may have many sufficient
mechanisms, each of which in a given, isolated circumstance ex-
plains the whole phenomenon. When they act simultaneously, they
mask each other. Unfortunately, at the present time, and I've
tried for a long time to write a mathematics of systems showing
occlusion and I cannot do so.

Wasserman: I'm looking for the chemoreceptor; I think I have a
mechanism in mind. I'm very impressed with the idea of the occlusion phenomenon in experimental work and I think that this is why
so many of us get different ideas and different experimental results. It's very easy to anesthetize an animal and start doing
experiments and soon have him unresponsive to various chemoreceptor

drives. The animal may allow pH to decrease; that is, initially
he may have a pH of 7.40 and a few hours later he may have a pH
of 7.30. An animal that has normal chemoreceptor drive should
have a pH of 7.40. If it's ignoring that drop in pH, then he
doesn't have responsive chemoreceptors. He's just responding to
the central oscillator (respiration center rhythm) and mechanico-
receptors. The latter may respond even after the animal is dead.
I think that before we start experiments on control of breathing,
we should test whether or not the animals have adequate chemoreceptor drive. We propose that the following tests be done to
evaluate chemoreceptor function: 1) the arterial blood gases be
measured to make sure that they are in the physiological range
and 2) the slope of a CO_2 response be determined; the latter
should be approximately 1 liter/minute per mmHg $PaCO_2$ increase
for a 20 Kg dog. We should also be able to demonstrate an appropriate response to hypoxia and a cardiodynamic hyperpnea. We
find all of these tests to be important.

Eldridge: Karl, I hate to do this, but what I think you're saying
is that when you give too much anesthesia you get depression of
central neurons. You're not really talking about chemoreceptor
drive. You're talking about the way some central structure is
handling impulses that come from chemoreceptors. You're not implying, surely, that the chemoreceptors are damaged somehow by
too much anesthesia.

Wasserman: I don't know if the chemoreceptors are unresponsive or
that the brain's interpretation of the chemoreceptor signal is
depressed.

Eldridge: Alright, but that's neuronal and that's not chemoreceptor
drive. Chemoreceptor drive is what comes out of the chemoreceptors
and you're saying that something is wrong with the brain, it can't
process these signals properly.

Wasserman: What I'm saying is that you have to make sure that
you're dealing with an animal preparation that is capable of responding to chemical stimuli.

Eldridge: I would expand this to say that you've got to be sure
that the animal can respond to any kind of stimulus. Why single
out chemoreceptors!

Fishman: So much depends on the question that is being asked and
the experimental preparation to which the question is being addressed. Isn't much of the apparent discrepancy attributable to the
fact that in reality, the different investigators are asking different questions?

Wasserman: Different laboratories do the same experiments but come
out with different results and that's what bothers me. I would
like to see each laboratory come out with the same results and if

not, explain it or repeat the experiments together.

Fishman: Well, that is certainly a wonderful ambition and I am confident that this goal will be considered later when the topic of standardization of testing is discussed. But, before we close this session, I would like to put one question to Dr. Yamamoto: how does the concept of occlusion phenomena relate to your approach to modelling the control of breathing?

Yamamoto: The concept of modelling is really the attempt to literally translate assertions made from various laboratories in a mutually compatible and executable fashion in terms of the computer language. You, therefore, can aggregate these assertions and at some point you have enough assertions that you can extract consequences through computer execution. You may put in assertions that appear to be mutually antagonistic, then you exercise the model and even if both are simultaneously present you get one result. This is occlusion. For example, I could put in a neural reverberatory circuit and control based purely on CO_2 flow through the lung in the same model and still get what appears to be hyperpnea of exercise in the model, and I would call that occlusion again. That particular thing I have not yet done.

Levine: I believe Dr. Dempsey's question is still on the floor. In response to your blunt question, I'd like to make three points. Firstly, I certainly share your respect for Dr. Kao's work. Secondly, the work of Dr. Kao suggests that extracranial mechanoreceptors elicit the hyperpnea of muscular exercise. My work on the ventilatory response to drug-induced hypermetabolism suggests that these extracranial receptors are responding to some chemical change or conceivably to some physical change such as muscle temperature. Thirdly, I do not believe that Dr. Kao's work eliminates the possibility that humoral agents released by the peripheral tissues play an important role in eliciting the hyperpnea of muscular exercise.

Kao: The fact that the ventilation of both the neural and the humoral dogs increased while the perfused neural dog's hindlimbs were induced to exercise does not necessarily support the humoral theory, because the response in the humoral dog existed only after the neural signals were removed.

Levine: Can I just follow up on Dr. Kao's point. Dr. Kao, I agree that your cross-circulation experiments would argue against the existence of exercise-released humoral factors which stimulate ventilation. However, various workers have transected the spinal cords of animals and have demonstrated that exercise of these denervated extremities still elicits increments in ventilation. During steady state exercise of denervated extremities, the work of Lamb (Resp. Physiol., 6:88-104, 1968-9) would indicate that the increment in ventilation is accompanied by no changes in arterial PCO_2, pH or SO_2. I have recently carried out some experiments which are consistent with these earlier observations of Lamb. Therefore, I would think that failure to show a humoral mechanism in your cross-perfusion experiments, which admittedly are very difficult, really does not eliminate a humoral mechanism.

Kao: Grodins and Morgan (Am. J. Physiol., 162:64-73, 1950) performed experiments with induced exercise in dogs following transection of the spinal cord. If no de novo stimulus to ventilation is produced after the spinal cord transection, and if the neural pathway is the only one mediating exercise stimulus to the central ventilation regulatory apparatus, the dog with spinal cord transection during induced exercise should behave "exactly" as our neural dog. The fact remains that after spinal cord transection, several abnormal adventitious stimuli to ventilation happened (such as hypotension, acidosis, pain, etc.) and as the authors discussed, these abnormal happenings made the conclusion of a humoral pathway or any pathway hazardous.

Godfrey: One of the problems of the many experiments we have heard, particularly the ones with hyperventilation in them, is that the subjects are actually breathing at the time and that sort of complicates the picture. Some time ago we were quite interested in looking at the control of breathing using breath-holding. In these experiments you're not being interfered with by the respiration itself. What you're looking for is a stimulus to start breathing. You can show, as everyone knows, that breath holding is controlled by chemical-mechanical factors, much in the same way as conventional respiratory physiology regards ventilation. If you breath-hold and some stimulus to breathing arises and you can't hold your breath any longer, then you take a breath and you can then go on breath-holding again. So presumably respiration removes some respiratory stimulus. What we then thought was that if you breathe a lot we perhaps ought to be able to remove much of the stimulus. In these experiments we found no difference between one breath or 5 breaths or many breaths on the duration of the subsequent breath holding time. If voluntary hyperventilation was going to produce a respiratory stimulus we would have predicted a shortening of breath holding time. We had no effect on it. If voluntary hyperventilation or any other kind of hyperventilation was relieving some stimulus, we would prolong breath holding time, but we did not. I know that it's breath holding and not breathing. I wonder if anybody might comment on that

Eldridge: Well, I think that all you may have shown is the sensation that causes you to quit holding your breath is different from that which stimulates breathing in a normal way.

Godfrey: Well, you can't accept that completely. A breath holding time vs. PCO_2 response curve is very similar in slope to a ventilation PCO_2 response curve.

Eldridge: That shows that they are associated but it doesn't prove them causal. I mean they would be expected to go together, wouldn't they, since they're all time based, but that doesn't prove that one causes the other one.

Godfrey: It is not a time base phenomenon. You can plot a curve of PCO_2 at start of breath hold against breath holding time and you get a very straight line.

Eldridge: But the amount of CO_2 generated during that period is going to be time function, isn't it.

Godfrey: At the quitting time of that breath hold, if you take a breath of CO_2 which pushes your PCO_2 up even higher, you can breath hold again. So the movement of the chest wall or the movement of the respiratory system is removing some respiratory stimulus in that situation.

Kampine: When you do the kinds of animals experiments where you change pulmonary CO_2 by breathing CO_2 or by changing the venous load of CO_2, or by altering the venous load of CO_2 by interfering with oxidative metabolism with drugs, you might be altering mechano-receptor afferent drive also, simply by altering the environment in which these mechano-receptors exist. If there are receptors of some sort in the lung and we know that changes in CO_2 do change the elastic properties of the airways, is this not something that some-one must look at in terms of changing drive to respiration?

Wasserman: You've done some of these studies of diverting blood away from the pulmonary circulation to the systemic circulation. Guz (Bartoli et al., J. Physiol., 240:91-104, 1974) found a markedly reduced ventilation associated with it. I think that he ascribes this reduction to the decrease in lung PCO_2. I believe that there are pulmonary CO_2 chemoreceptors but I'm not sure they're inhibitory or excitatory or that both types exist. Dr. Filley thinks that there are excitatory CO_2 chemoreceptors and I think there is good evidence for it. On the other hand, Guz's observations (Cross, B.A. et al., Clin. Sci. and Molecular Med., 50:439-454, 1976) of a steeper CO_2 response when the airways are anesthetized suggest the presence of CO_2 inhibitory receptors. You're asking me a question that I think, from your own work, you probably know the answer better than I.

Kampine: I wish I did. I think that what we need are some record-ings from something that is a chemoreceptor and distinctly not a stretch receptor or so-called irritant receptor.

Fishman: I agree that first you have to find the chemoreceptor.

Kampine: They've found them in birds. I guess it all depends on whether we want to find out whether we are more or less like birds.

Sampson: I'd like to comment on this last point. You run into some problems when you consider the effects of CO_2 on pulmonary stretch receptors. I refer to some experiments that the Drs. Coleridge have done over the past few months looking at the effects of changes in

PCO_2 on pulmonary stretch receptors. In a divided lung preparation, if the pulmonary artery is occluded and arterial PCO_2 is maintained constant and the PCO_2 in one lung is dropped to zero, the rate of discharge arising from pulmonary stretch receptors in that lung is increased both in the inspiratory phase and in the expiratory phase. It's as though CO_2 exerts some sort of control on the ability of pulmonary stretch receptors to discharge normally. This is not secondary to change in airways resistance as far as I can recall, and so there is a critical level of CO_2 and it has to be above zero.

Fishman: These are very complicated experiments.

Sampson: Yes, but they speak to the point that Karl just mentioned regarding Guz's experiments where they had their dogs on cardio-pulmonary bypass (Bartoli, A. et al., J. Physiol., 240:91-109, 1974). They dropped the CO_2 to zero and their rate of ventilation was slowed tremendously and then they added CO_2 back to normal or above and ventilation returned to normal. That data is quite different from the case they were trying to make in regard to some type of CO_2 receptor in the lungs that responded to CO_2. I don't think there has been any evidence that's been presented from any laboratory on the basis of neuro-physiological recordings that there is a CO_2 receptor in the lung. That CO_2 may play some role in controlling the ability of mechano-receptors to respond normally may be a different story. Within the normal physiologic range of CO_2 there appears to be nothing dramatic going on.

Kampine: I do not exclude the possibility that stretch receptor afferents could be altered in their discharge by a change in the environment in which they exist simply by changing intra-pulmonary CO_2.

Fishman: How did you do this experiment?

Kampine: The experiment is simply to maintain $PaCO_2$ constant on a pump by-pass. First you must demonstrate that the animal is responsive to carotid sinus stimulation or carotid occlusion and so on. Then, with a constant arterial PCO_2, pH and PO_2 one introduces systematic changes in intra-pulmonary CO_2. We see an increase in respiratory frequency, as measured by phrenic nerve output, which is eliminated by vagotomy. One may not have to postulate an alien CO_2 receptor, because it may simply be a change in a mechano-receptor or other type of receptor already described which is driving respiration. We must have recordings from something that responds to CO_2, only to CO_2, and not to mechanical stimuli.

Fishman: In these experiments, how do you take into account the fact that you might be depleting the pulmonary blood volume which contributes to the distensibility characteristics and stretch of the lung?

Kampine: Well, one can do an experiment where you perfuse the systemic circulation and the lung independently. These are difficult experiments to do. Dr. Coon has devised a method where you perfuse one lobe or one side, which is much easier to do. The other one is technically much more difficult.

Fishman: These have been done but to the best of my knowledge, they have not clarified very much along the lines that we are now considering.

Kampine: I don't think that that is the real issue. We have not excluded the possibility that there is something other than a specific CO_2 receptor which responds to changes in PCO_2 to a perfused lung.

Weiser: Concerning the control of exercise hyperpnea, is it wholly neural or wholly chemical, or is control a combination of neural and chemical mechanisms?

Eldridge: Well, I think that Dr. Wasserman's work about the linkage of CO_2 flow to fine control of the ventilatory level during exercise cannot be faulted. There is some linkage between CO_2 and ventilation during exercise. That is not the same thing as saying that this is the sole explanation for the ventilation during exercise. In fact, I visualize the significant part of the increase in ventilation during exercise as being neural in origin whether from some metabolic receptor in the periphery or from other kinds of receptors of a mechanical nature. This is augmented by the process that I'm talking about, and has a fine chemical control superimposed upon it.

Part III
Control of Airway Calibre

12

Control of Airway Calibre: Introduction

John P. Kampine

This review brings up to date several important aspects of the regulation of airway calibre. The subject matter relates principally to the roles of the autonomic nervous system, vagal reflexes, altered gas tension, certain pharmacological agonists, and mechanical and physical factors in the regulation of airway smooth muscle. In addition, it is important to note that a great many non-autonomic humoral substances have been implicated as having physiological and pathophysiological roles in the regulation of airway calibre.

A. Innervation of Major Airways

The sympathetic innervation of larger and intermediate sized airways derives from the intermediolateral cell column of the spinal cord from T_1 to T_5. These preganglionic fibers have synaptic junctions in the ganglia of the thoracic sympathetic chain or in one of the cervical ganglia; and the postganglionic fibers innervate smooth muscle of blood vessels and airways down to the terminal bronchioles but excluding the alveolar ducts. The effect of sympathetic efferent nerve stimulation on airway calibre and lung mechanics has been studied less than the effect of pulmonary vagal efferent stimulation, but generally is thought to cause relaxation of bronchial smooth muscle and a reduction in resistance to airflow. The demonstration of bronchodilator action of pulmonary sympathetic nerve stimulation has depended upon the establishment of some resting tone in airway smooth muscle. In the presence of bronchoconstriction established through the administration of the anticholinesterase eserine or a parasympathomimetic agent such as carbachol, stimulation of the sympathetic nerves produces relaxation of bronchial smooth muscle (9, 24).

The parasympathetic efferent innervation accounts for approximately 90% of the efferent pulmonary innervation and is derived from the dorsal motor nucleus of vagus nerve in the floor of the 4th ventricle. The preganglionic fibers are closely intermingled with sympathetic fibers in the chest and form plexuses in the hilar areas where many parasympathetic ganglion cells are located. Postganglionic fibers arise from these hilar ganglion cells or, more distally, in the peribronchial tissue and bronchial smooth muscle and innervate larger, intermediate, and smaller airways. Functionally, the parasympathetic fibers do not innervate the terminal

179

bronchioles or alveolar ducts (23). Stimulation of pulmonary vagal efferent fibers in most mammalian species produces an increase in resistance to airflow attributed to bronchoconstriction. This bronchoconstriction has been demonstrated in quick-frozen lungs and in radiographic examination of lungs after tantulum powder insufflation to extend to airways of 0.5 mm diameter in the cat and dog with maximum changes in airways with resting diameters of 1.0 to 2.0 mm (4, 13, 14).

The bronchoconstriction, increased resistance to airflow, decreased anatomical dead space and decrease in airway calibre produced by vagal stimulation are blocked by muscarinic blocking agents such as atropine and potentiated by the anticholinesterase eserine. Resting tone in bronchial smooth muscle is thought to be partially due to tonic activity of sympathetic and parasympathetic efferent fibers. Atropine usually can be demonstrated to produce a decrease in airway resistance, and a low level of parasympathetic tone seems to dominate (23).

B. Reflex Regulation

Asphyxia, hypercapnia, and hypoxemia have been shown to produce bronchoconstriction in mammals. Asphyxia and hypercapnia cause an increase in airway resistance through a centrally mediated increase in vagal nerve activity, as reviewed by Widdicombe (23). Bronchoconstriction secondary to hypoxemia has been an inconsistent finding, although reported to be vagally mediated and partially reversed by carotid body denervation (8, 15).

Numerous reflexes arising from upper airways, lung and vascular sources may produce increased resistance to airflow. Mechanical and irritant receptors in the nasal mucosa have been shown to produce bronchoconstriction when stimulated mechanically (22) or when subjected to local irritant effects of cigarette smoke, chloroform, and other irritants (12). These reflexes from nasal and nasopharyngeal mucosal receptors are eliminated by olfactory, trigeminal, and glossopharyngeal denervation or atropine.

Stimulation of the cut central end of the superior or inferior laryngeal nerves produces an increase in lung resistance (23), and mechanical stimulation of the epiglottis and larynx may produce a reflex increase in laryngeal and lower airway resistance (18, 22) which can be blocked by atropine and is thought to be activated through mucosal receptors.

Both upper airway and lung irritant receptors have been implicated in reflex bronchoconstriction in man and animals. In the upper airway, stimulation of cough receptors elicits reflex bronchoconstriction even when the cough is prevented; and stimulation of more distant pulmonary irritant receptors with sulfur dioxide, ammonia, and ether vapor can produce tracheal constriction and bronchoconstriction. Lung inflation has been shown to decrease airway

resistance in animals associated with a decrease in vagal afferent
nerve activity. Although not firmly established, it appears that a
lung inflation reflex bronchodilator response may be initiated in
cats by the Hering-Breuer inflation reflex (23).

Reflexes arising from receptors located in extrapulmonary tissue
may produce changes in airway resistance. A bronchoconstrictor
response to pulmonary artery embolism has been shown to be blocked
by vagotomy or atropine in dogs, indicating the reflex nature of
the response (11). In animals, stimulation of Hering's nerve has
been shown to produce both an increase or a decrease in airway
calibre. Attempts to separate the baroreceptor afferents from
carotid body afferent nerves indicate that stimulation of baroreceptor afferents acts as a stimulus to bronchoconstriction (10),
while carotid body stimulation produces a bronchodilator response
(1). Local axon reflexes have been implicated as a partial
explanation for the bronchoconstrictor response to histamine or
nicotine applied to pleural surfaces of the same lung and the
opposite lung. The bronchoconstrictor response persists after
acute denervation but is abolished by atropine or local administration of lidocaine.

C. Autonomic Airway Receptors (Response to Pharmacologic
    Stimulation)

Cholinergic receptors in parasympathetic, neuro-effector junctions
of airways respond to injection of acetylcholine or its longer
acting analogs by producing airway constriction. These receptors
are blocked by atropine and are believed to constitute the most
important functional group of airway receptors. It has been
reported that, after administration of atropine, acetylcholine
may cause an increase in airway diameter. This mechanism, presumed
to involve release of catecholamines at sympathetic post-ganglionic
nerve endings, does not play a major role in regulation of tracheobronchial smooth muscle (1).

Adrenergic receptors in the airways are predominantly beta, and
the bronchodilator effects of sympathetic nerve stimulation or in
response to administration of epinephrine, isoproterenol, and
norepinephrine are blocked by beta adrenergic blocking agents
such as propranolol. More recently, a distinction has been made
between cardiac and airway beta receptors on the basis of beta-1
receptor blocking agents such as practolol, which will selectively
block the cardiac effects of isoproterenol, and beta-2 receptor
blocking agents such as butoxamine, which will selectively block
the bronchodilator effects of isoproterenol. Under certain conditions in man and animals after blockade of beta receptors, the
administration of epinephrine causes bronchoconstriction which is
reversed by alpha adrenergic blocking agents (1). The increase
in airway resistance in asthmatic individuals after beta adrenergic
blocking agents is not a reflection of unopposed alpha receptor-
mediated increased sympathetic activity (24). In these patients,

a multitude of hormonal, emotional, and tissue factors, such as histamine, kinins, and slow reacting substance, may produce bronchoconstriction. Increased vagally mediated bronchomotor tone (blocked by atropine) as well as increased bronchomotor tone due to systemic hypoxemia, hypercapnia, and stimulation of irritant receptors and other types of pulmonary receptors, may also be involved in the increased airway resistance.

D. Non-Autonomic Receptors

Other receptors have been invoked to explain the direct and indirect effects of a number of humoral agents which have been demonstrated to cause changes in airway diameter in animals and in man. Histamine, serotonin, slow reacting substance, and a number of other substances such as bradykinins can produce bronchoconstriction. The role of purines and related compounds, such as adenosine and adenosine triphosphate, as tissue mediators of bronchoconstriction remains to be determined. It has been proposed that these compounds and the drug theophylline, which produces bronchodilation, combine in the airways with purinergic receptors (3). The prostaglandin E series have been demonstrated to produce bronchodilator responses in animals, while the prostaglandin $F_{2\alpha}$ is a potent bronchoconstrictor substance. While the physiologic role of some of the tissue substances which produce bronchodilator responses, such as prostaglandin E, are unknown, it has been speculated that the release of such substances in the lung may serve an adaptive role during hyperventilation to counteract the local bronchoconstrictor effect of hypocapnia (19). Histamine seems to have complex actions leading to bronchoconstriction. The reflex and direct effects of histamine on medium and small sized airways are complex, and the role of histamine in releasing other substances from lung tissue has not been well documented. Presumably, the changes in membrane permeability produced by histamine may lead to release of other bronchoactive substances as well as increased entry of calcium ions or release of calcium ions to bronchial smooth muscle, resulting in enhanced airway smooth muscle constriction.

E. Agents Which Have a Direct Effect on Airway Smooth Muscle

The local effects of alterations of P_{CO_2}, P_{O_2}, and pH have been studied during pulmonary artery occlusion, hyper- and hypocapnia, and hypoxia in experimental animals and in man (17, 20, 21). Evidence from studies in the intact (7) and isolated (16) lungs of animals indicates that the local effects of increased P_{CO_2} or decreased pH are to increase airway calibre and decrease airway resistance. It has been suggested that the local effects of altered P_{CO_2} and pH may play a role in the regulation of ventilation distribution in response to altered distribution of perfusion. At the present time, these effects are presumed to be direct effects on airway smooth muscle. Although a direct bronchoconstrictor effect of local hypoxia has been reported in the cat and dog (21), the magnitude of the response is less than that observed during hypocapnia or alkalosis.

The response of airway smooth muscle to potent inhalational anesthetics, such as diethyl ether, methoxyflurane, enflurane, and halothane, in experimental animals and in man is a dilator response which is primarily a direct non-specific effect (1, 22). Diethyl ether, in addition to its direct dilator action on airway smooth muscle, has been postulated to increase airway calibre either through a beta adrenergic stimulating action or through release of epinephrine or norepinephrine. Cyclopropane has been shown to increase airway resistance in animals and in man (5). Thiopental and morphine sulfate have been reported to cause bronchoconstriction in animals and in man (1). The effect of thiopental, however, is not well documented in man; and morphine has been postulated to act through the mechanism of histamine release (24).

A great many physiologic and pharmacologic mechanisms acting either on airway smooth muscle or through reflex activation of vagally mediated changes in airway resistance may interact in pathophysiologic states with local factors to produce altered regulation of airway resistance. Although many studies of individual mechanisms have been carried out, the relative importance of many of these mechanisms in physiologic regulation remains to be determined.

REFERENCES

1. Aviado, D.M. Anesthesiology 42:68-80, 1975.

2. Blumberg, M.Z. N. Engl. J. Med. 288:50, 1973.

3. Burnstock, G. Pharmacol. Rev. 24:509-581, 1972.

4. Cabezas, G.A., P.D. Graf, and J.A. Nadel. J. Appl. Physiol. 31:651-655, 1971.

5. Colgan, F.J. Anesthesiology 26:778-785, 1965.

6. Coon, R.L., and J.P. Kampine. Anesthesiology 43:635-641, 1975.

7. Coon, R.L., C.C. Rattenborg, and J.P. Kampine. J. Appl. Physiol. 39:580-589, 1975.

8. Daly, M. DeB., C.J. Lambertson, and A. Schweitzer. J. Physiol., London 119:202-314, 1953.

9. Daly, M. DeB., and L.E. Mount. J. Physiol., London 113:43-62, 1951.

10. Daly, M. DeB., and A. Schweitzer. J. Physiol., London 116:35-58, 1952.

11. Jesser, J.H., and G. DeTakats. Surgery 12:541-552, 1942.

12. Kratschmer, F. S.B. Akad. Wiss. Wien 62:147-170, 1870.

13. Nadel, J.A. Ann. N.Y. Acad. Sci. 221:99-102, 1974.

14. Nadel, J.A., G.A. Cabezas, and J.H.M. Austin. Invest. Radiol. 6:9-17, 1971.

15. Nadel, J.A., and J.G. Widdicombe. J. Physiol., London 163: 13-33, 1962.

16. Nisell, O. Acta Physiol. Scand. 23:352-360, 1951.

17. Patterson, R.W., S.F. Sullivan, J.R. Malm, and F.O. Bowman. J. Thorac. Cardiovasc. Surg. 58:209-216, 1969.

18. Rex, M.A.E. Brit. J. Anaesth. 42:891-899, 1970.

19. Said, S.I., S. Kitamura, T. Yoshida, J. Preskitt, and L.D. Holden. Ann. N.Y. Acad. Sci. 221:103-114, 1974.

20. Severinghaus, J.W., E.W. Swenson, T.N. Finley, M.T. Lategola, and J. Williams. J. Appl. Physiol. 16:53-60, 1961.

21. Tisi, G.M., W.G. Wolfe, R.J. Fallat, and J.A. Nadel. J. Appl. Physiol. 28:570-573, 1970.

22. Tomori, Z., and J.G. Widdicombe. J. Physiol., London 200: 25-49, 1969.

23. Widdicombe, J.G. Physiol. Rev. 43:1-37, 1963.

24. Widdicombe, J.G., and G.M. Sterling. Arch. Intern. Med. 126: 311-327, 1970.

13

Role of CO$_2$ & O$_2$ Tension

Robert L. Coon & John P. Kampine

Widdicombe (38), in a section of a 1963 review concerning the effects of pH and P$_{CO_2}$ on tracheobronchial smooth muscle, made the following conclusion:

"These reservations are not intended to imply scepticism, but to encourage other research on a problem of great physiological interest; its solution could be the basis of a mechanism controlling the ventilation of pulmonary units in response to their gas contents. A similar mechanism may control the circulation in separate parts of the pulmonary vascular bed, and the two could act together as an intrinsic system modifying ventilation/perfusion ratios in units of the lung."

Thirteen years later these conclusions are still valid. Although a number of articles have been published describing various aspects of the problem, the mechanisms of action and the physiological significance of local control by H$^+$, CO$_2$, and O$_2$ of ventilation/perfusion ratios in lung units continue to be areas of research in which definitive answers remain to be ascertained.

Work in our laboratory has been directed toward one aspect of the problem, the direct effect of CO$_2$, H$^+$, and O$_2$ on peripheral airway smooth muscle. As indicated in the reference to Widdicombe's review, this is certainly not an original idea. In 1912, Trendelenburg (34) demonstrated that NaOH produced contraction and HCl relaxation of tracheal rings suspended in a smooth muscle bath. Macht and Ting (11) made a similar observation with respect to NaOH; but, in their preparation, HCl caused a contraction. In addition, both 20% CO$_2$ in O$_2$ and NaHCO$_3$ produced contraction of the tracheal muscle. Wick (37) confirmed the constrictor effect of CO$_2$; but, in his preparation, prolonged exposure to CO$_2$ produced relaxation.

In experiments previously described, muscle strips were used. These were usually taken from the larger bronchi. Sollmann and Gilbert (27) used a more unique smooth muscle bath preparation. They attempted to demonstrate the effects of drugs on bronchiolar smooth muscle by microscopic observation of excised lung tissue from the rabbit, guinea pig, puppy, cat or human. The excised

185

lungs were filled through the trachea with 10% gelatin in Ringer's
solution. The lungs were then excised and placed in cold Ringer's
solution in a refrigerator. When hard, the lobe was sliced to give
0.1 to 0.3 mm thick slices. Sections of these slices were placed
in a Petri dish in warm Ringer's solution. Because of the thinness
of the slices, no aeration was required. Changes in broncheolar
lumen were followed with camera lucida drawings. The drawings were
transferred to a second paper and the area of the bronchial lumen
cut out, weighed, and calculated as a percentage of the original
lumen. Reactions in the bronchioles showed greater percentage
changes in lumen size than the small bronchi, but the qualitative
response was the same. No reactions were obtained in the infundi-
buli and alveoli. Ciliary motion could be observed to be very
active in these preparations and did not appear to be affected by
autonomic drugs. Rhythmic bronchiolar contractions which were
observed could usually be stopped with atropine. The rhythmic contractions were similar to those seen in the intestine: a rapid 10
to 30 per minute superficial, pendular contraction and a stronger,
slower, 3 per minute to 1 in 10 minutes, peristaltic-type contraction. A number of drugs of physiological significance were studied.
Mecholyl, physostigmine, and pilocarpine caused constriction which
was blocked partially by atropine, but more effectively by epinephrine. Atropine in itself caused dilation in the untreated preparation. Decreasing pH to 6.0 by the addition of acetic acid
caused relaxation in both constricted and normal bronchioles.
Carbon dioxide, bubbled through the solution, caused a slight
relaxation of the bronchioles. One species variation was observed.
The guinea pig was found to be unsuitable for the study because the
bronchioles contracted shut when the gelatin was melted, and this
contraction was unaffected by normal dilator drugs. This was
thought to be caused by the fact that the elastic tissue of the
guinea pig is a continuous sheet, whereas, the rabbit, for example,
has a loose meshwork of elastic tissue.

Thornton (31) also used a unique approach to the study of the
effects of various stimuli on isolated bronchi. In this preparation, the lungs, excised from sacrificed animals, were suspended
by a cannula in the trachea. The cannula was attached to a side
arm at the bottom of a U-tube. One side of the U-tube was attached
to a Mariotte bottle which was filled with a physiological solution
and elevated to about 90 cm above the cannula to the lung. The
other side of the U-tube was connected to a water manometer. Solution flowed from the Mariotte bottle through a heating coil and
out through scarifications in the lung. If solution flowed freely
through the lung, there was little pressure recorded by the manometer. When contractions occurred, the pressure rose; and, if
complete occlusion occurred, the pressure would approach the level
of the Mariotte bottle. A similar set-up was used to perfuse the
pulmonary circulation. Cats, rabbits, rats, and guinea pigs were
used. The guinea pig was the most satisfactory, and results
reported were from this animal. The preparation reacted to histamine, pilocarpine, and vagal stimulation with constriction and was

dilated by adrenaline and by atropine when constricted with pilocarpine or vagal stimulation. The more important observation with
regard to this review was that, when the pH of the solution perfusing the tracheobronchial tree was increased to 7.8, an increase
in the tracheobronchial resistance occurred. When the pH was
changed to 7.0, dilation occurred. Also, dilute alkali (NaOH)
constricted and dilute acid (lactic acid) dilated the tracheobronchial tree when injected into the media perfusing it.

Stephens et al. (28) studied the effects of O_2, CO_2, and pH
on 1.0 cm longitudinal sections of left lower lobe bronchus. The
sections were suspended in a modified Krebs-Ringer's solution with
the force transducer perpendicular to the intact bronchial ring.
Hypoxia, hypoxic and hypercapnic acidosis, and hypocapnic alkalosis
caused a slight but significant increase in resting tension. Hypercapnic acidosis and metabolic acidosis caused no change in resting
tension, whereas, compensated hypercapnia caused a small but significant decrease in resting tension.

With some reservations, it may be concluded from the literature that acid relaxes contracted bronchial smooth muscle, and
alkalosis may cause the bronchial smooth muscle to contract. The
degree of contraction demonstrated with alkalosis is variable and
appears to depend on the preparation used. Furthermore, smooth
muscle bath preparations yield qualitative results but do not
indicate the quantitative effects on physiological variables in
the intact animal.

Numerous studies in the intact animal have also indicated a
local effect of H^+ and CO_2 on airway smooth muscle. Graubner and
Wick (6) observed that, on the death of a dog, there was an apparent bronchospasm. Wick (36), in a follow-up article, demonstrated
that 85% of the bronchospasm could be blocked by administration of
3.5% CO_2, and 90% was blocked with 6% CO_2 in the inspired gas mixture. Since this was a postmortem effect, it was considered to be
independent of central control. Atropine was given to insure that
the effect was not on the vagal nerve endings. Lohr (10), using
the isolated cat lung, and Venrath et al. (35), using the dog, also
implicated hypocapnia as the cause of the bronchoconstriction
following pulmonary hypoperfusion. A more complete study was conducted by Severinghaus et al. (26), again using the dog. A
bronchospirometer tube was introduced, and blood flow to one lung
was stopped by unilateral occlusion of the left or right pulmonary
artery. Temporary unilateral pulmonary artery occlusion increased
resistance and decreased compliance, functional residual capacity,
and the anatomical dead space on the occluded side. Samanek and
Aviado (24), using a pump-perfused isolated left lower lobe of the
dog preparation, demonstrated by chronic sympathetic and parasympathetic denervations that the response is locally mediated by a
non-neurogenic mechanism. A local effect of CO_2 on airway smooth
muscle during hypoperfusion of the lung has also been demonstrated
in the human (19, 30).

The airway constriction produced by hypoperfusion and the resultant decrease in alveolar PCO_2 has been ascribed a number of different etiologies. Tiefensee (32) demonstrated that $NaHCO_3$ infusion produced a decrease in lung capacity in the denervated cat lung, but the amount of decreased lung capacity correlated better to the amount of total fluid infused than to the quantity of $NaHCO_3$ infused. Hyperventilation without gross changes in pulmonary blood flow produced increased pulmonary or airway resistance in humans (5, 17, 20, 29). However, the response was partially blocked by atropine (17, 29). Nisell (18), using isolated pump perfused cat lungs, did not observe a dilator effect of CO_2 unless the lungs were preconstricted with a constrictor agent. Tisi et al. (33) demonstrated that the constrictor effect of pure O_2 reverses the constrictor effect of pulmonary artery occlusion. Thus, an interrelationship between the effect of temporary pulmonary artery occlusion, the resultant decrease in alveolar PCO_2 and increase in pulmonary resistance, and oxygen were suggested. Hypoxia by itself appears to have little effect on airway smooth muscle (38).

The purpose of our work in this area was threefold: 1) to better define the alveolar PCO_2-pulmonary resistance and lung compliance relationships, 2) to investigate the mechanism of action of alveolar PCO_2 on pulmonary mechanics, and 3) to demonstrate possible interactions between local and central control of airway smooth muscle.

Our studies have been carried out using the isolated left lower lobe (LLL) of lungs of dogs anesthetized with sodium pentobarbital. The lobe was ventilated separately from the remaining lobes of the lung by a tube-within-a-tube system. The lobe was either autoperfused or pump perfused. In the pump perfused preparation, blood which was pumped into the lobar artery flowed through the lobe into a reservoir and was recirculated back through the lobe. Systemic pressure, LLL airway pressure, LLL pulmonary artery pressure, and main airway pressure were monitored by Statham pressure transducers and recorded by a Grass model 5 polygraph. LLL pulmonary artery pressure was monitored from a T in the perfusion cannula, and LLL airway pressure was monitored from a catheter placed such that the tip of the catheter was in the LLL bronchus. End-expired CO_2 was monitored by a Beckman IR CO_2 analyzer and was also recorded on the Grass model 5 polygraph. Blood gas and pH determinations were made using a Radiometer blood gas and pH analyzer.

The initial problem encountered was devising a method of studying pulmonary mechanics. This was particularly difficult in this study since it was supposed that the resistance changes occur in the respiratory bronchioles and alveolar ducts where gas flow is either very slow or, as during normal ventilation, occurs primarily by diffusion (26). If resistance is to be measured in these areas, flow must be increased sufficiently to produce a measurable pressure drop. The method which we now use in our

studies is a modification of the square flow, constant volume
technique of Rattenborg and Holaday (22). As the name implies,
the method depends on the generation of a square flow pulse in
which flow increases suddenly from zero to a pre-set flow and
remains constant during the druation of the pulse, at which time
it drops suddenly to zero. When flow is initiated (Fig. 13.1),

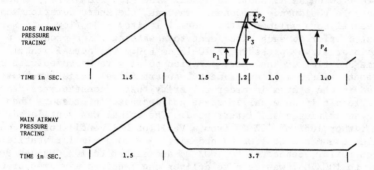

Fig. 13.1. Schematic of main and lobar airway pressure
tracings with expiration of the short duration pulse
delayed for 1 sec.

airway pressure increases abruptly (P_1) in response to the resistance beyond the point of pressure measurement and then, because of
the combined effects of resistance and dynamic compliance, increases
more gradually as the lung is inflated (4). When flow is interrupted and expiration is delayed, airway pressure drops rapidly,
then decreases exponentially to a nearly stable pressure. The rapid
drop in pressure (P_2) results from the rapid decrease in the resistance component of the pressure tracing when flow suddenly drops to
zero. The non-resistive component of pressure (P_3) observed immediately after the interruption of flow results from the dynamic
compliance of the lung, and the pressure observed after the system
has stabilized (P_4) is a measure of the static compliance. The
difference between dynamic and static compliance results from stress
relaxation and from redistribution of air within the lung which
occurs when expiration is delayed (7). Resistance was calculated
both when flow was initiated and when flow was interrupted (or
stopped) by the formulas $P_1/\dot{V}$ = initial resistance, and $P_2/\dot{V}$ = stop
flow resistance, respectively. Two compliance measurements were
calculated using the formulas V/P_3 = dynamic compliance and V/P_4 =
static compliance.

The ventilator used to impose the square flow wave inflations on the LLL was a modification of a ventilator originally designed to ventilate the right and left lungs simultaneously with square flow wave inflations during bronchospirometry (21). This ventilator was used to ventilate the LLL and the animal with simultaneous square flow inflations but was modified so that, during the apneic period of the animal, only the LLL underwent a high flow rate, square flow pulse of short duration. The high flow rate yielded a measurable resistance component, whereas, the short duration kept the ventilatory volumes within normal limits. The flow rate was adjusted prior to each experiment to a setting which produced a peak lobar airway pressure of 10-15 cm H_2O. The actual ventilatory volume and flow of the short duration pulse were measured with a spirometer after each experiment. An artificial resistance was tested in the system in order to verify that a constant resistance would result in an equal increase and decrease in pressure when flow was initiated and interrupted. The animal was ventilated with either 100% or 40% O_2 from a Veriflor MR1 ventilator O_2 controller connected to 100% O_2 and air. A second similar ventilator O_2 controller, connected to 100% O_2 and either to 10% CO_2 and 90% O_2 or to 100% N_2, was used to deliver the required mixtures of CO_2 and O_2 or N_2 and O_2 to the lobe.

Figure 13.2 demonstrates the increase in pulmonary resistance and decrease in dynamic compliance produced by decreasing alveolar PCO_2 and, in turn, increasing pulmonary venous pH during recirculation of blood through the lobe (3). The changes in initial resistance were similar but usually greater in magnitude than the changes in stop flow resistance. The changes in static compliance were similar to the changes in dynamic compliance but were smaller in magnitude.

Alternating sodium bicarbonate and lactic acid infusion while alveolar PCO_2 was maintained below 5 mm Hg (Fig. 13.3) demonstrated the dependence of the hypocapnic response on the acid-base status of the blood perfusing the respiratory airways (4). The increase in resistance and decrease in compliance observed at a pulmonary venous pH of 7.64 was comparable to that observed after lobar pulmonary artery occlusion in the autoperfused preparation. Varying degrees of hypoxia did not significantly affect bronchomotor tone, nor was the bronchoconstriction following lobar pulmonary artery occlusion affected by the hypoxia. The CO_2 effect on airway smooth muscle was not affected by beta receptor blockade.

Vagal stimulation (Fig. 13.4) superimposed on a stepwise increase in pulmonary venous pH from 7.32 to 7.62 resulted in an increase in resistance which paralleled the increase in resistance when pulmonary venous pH alone was increased (4). Compliance was not significantly affected by vagal stimulation at any level of pulmonary venous pH. The resistance increase caused by vagal nerve stimulation appeared to be additive to the increase in resistance caused by increasing pulmonary venous pH.

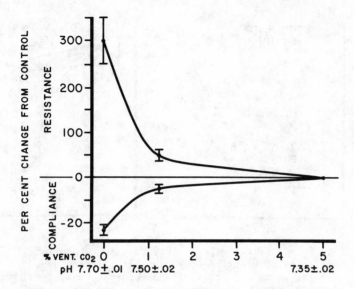

Fig. 13.2. Effects on resistance and dynamic compliance of altering inspired CO_2. Vertical bars represent ± 1 SEM, n = 25. Lobar venous pH is also shown.

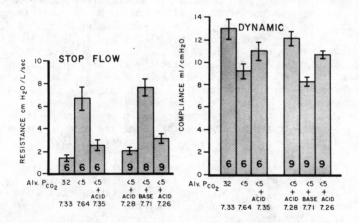

Fig. 13.3. Effect on pulmonary resistance and lung compliance of first decreasing alveolar PCO_2 to less than 5 mm Hg and then of alternate sodium bicarbonate and lactic acid infusion.

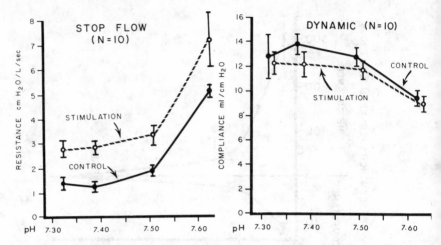

Fig. 13.4. Effect of pulmonary resistance and lung compliance of superimposing vagal stimulation upon response which occurred when pulmonary venous blood pH was increased by decreasing CO_2 concentration in gas ventilating lobe. Brackets represent 1 SEM.

This additive type of response may have been produced by the parasympathetic and chemical stimulation of airway smooth muscle acting on the same end organ by different mechanisms, or it may have been produced by parasympathetic stimulation acting on airway smooth muscle of airways other than (and probably in series with) the airways which were affected by the altered pulmonary venous pH. Vagal stimulation does not constrict the terminal bronchioles and alveolar ducts (14). The additive resistance response of vagal stimulation to the constrictive effect of increased pulmonary venous pH without a concomitant decrease in compliance is probably a further reflection of the separate influence of the vagus nerve on the larger airways as opposed to the mediation of peripheral lung constriction through the pulmonary arteries (15).

Because the airway constriction produced by pulmonary artery occlusion was reduced by ventilation with a gas containing CO_2, Severinghaus et al. (26) proposed that the constricted airways are those into which CO_2 diffuses directly and which are not perfused by the bronchial arteries. The respiratory bronchioles and the alveolar ducts have the ability to constrict. Constriction of the alveolar duct by histamine has been dramatically demonstrated in microscopic section of rapid frozen lung tissue (16). Furthermore, the additive effect on airway resistance of vagal nerve stimulation superimposed on the constrictor effect of increasing perfusate pH suggests that the H^+-induced constriction occurs in the respiratory bronchioles and alveolar ducts. Although the

indirect evidence indicates the location of the local constrictor
effect of increasing perfusate pH, no direct evidence exists which
verifies this indirect evidence. Also, is the pH effect restricted
to the respiratory airways? During hyperventilation, the conductive
airways are also affected by the increased systemic arterial pH of
blood perfusing the airways through the bronchial arteries. Is
there a difference in response to H^+ between the conducting and
respiratory airways?

Woolcock et al. (40) demonstrated that, when the vagi were
stimulated, as was done in the present experiment, but using chloralose anesthesia, the peripheral airways (less than 3 mm in diameter)
were protected from constriction by sympathetic tone. Le Blanc and
De Lind van Wyngaarden (9) stimulated the stellate ganglia and
observed greater dilation when air was breathed than when CO_2 was
breathed. This observation was not confirmed by the studies of
Nisell (18) in which stellate ganglion stimulation was ineffective.
The ability of sympathetic activity to block locally mediated changes
in airway resistance would enhance the physiological role of the
pulmonary sympathetic nerves to the airways.

More pertinent to this discussion, though, is the question of
the physiological significance of local control of airway resistance and lung compliance. The theoretical value of a local system
of regulation of ventilation and perfusion has been discussed by a
number of authors (8, 23, 24, 36, 38). During total pulmonary
artery occlusion, ventilation is shifted away from the occluded
side (1, 26); while, in the perfused lung, hypocapnia-induced constriction produces an increase in shunt flow (13). These studies
demonstrate that, in fact, ventilation can be shifted away from
over-ventilated (with respect to CO_2) lung units. Recently, Sealy
and Seaber (25) reported that CO_2 acts as a dilator of collateral
channels in the lung; although these authors felt that this may be
an important role of the effect of CO_2 on airway smooth muscle, the
physiological significance of collateral ventilation is unknown (12).
Furthermore, whether or not the local control mechanism of altering
ventilation to match perfusion is significant in normal respiration
or exercise, or if it only functions in a pathological system,
remains to be ascertained.

Widdicombe (39) demonstrated that the activity of the pulmonary
stretch receptors was increased by bronchoconstriction caused by
inhalation of histamine aerosol. This was particularly true when a
decrease in compliance accompanied an increase in resistance. A
similar situation probably exists when the respiratory airways are
constricted by hypocapnia. In this way, if hypocapnia caused by
hyperventilation constricted respiratory airways, the activity of
the stretch receptors would be increased and the hyperventilation
reflexly inhibited through the Hering-Breuer reflex. Bartoli et
al. (2) described a reflex increase in breathing frequency when
lungs of dogs on cardiopulmonary bypass were ventilated with CO_2
in the ventilatory gas mixture. These authors did not observe

changes in pulmonary mechanics when CO_2 was varied in their
preparation. Either the preparation was insensitive to CO_2 or
their methods were incapable of showing the changes in pulmonary
mechanics. Additional research will be required to solve this
problem.

Hence, the conclusions which can be extracted from this
discussion sound like the introductory quote from Widdicombe (38):

"These reservations are not intended to imply scepticism,
but to encourage research in a problem of great physiological interest. . . ."

REFERENCES

1. Allgood, R.J., W.G. Wolfe, P.A. Ebert, and D.C. Sabiston, Jr.
    Am. J. Physiol. 214:772-775, 1968.

2. Bartoli, A., B.A. Cross, A. Guz, S.K. Jain, M.I.M. Noble, and
    D.W. Trenchard. J. Physiol., London 240:91-109, 1974.

3. Coon, R.L., and J.P. Kampine. Anesthesiology 43:635-641,
    1975.

4. Coon, R.L., C.C. Rattenborg, and J.P. Kampine. J. Appl.
    Physiol. 39:580-589, 1975.

5. Don, H.F., and J.G. Robson. Anesthesiology 26:168-178, 1965.

6. Graubner, W., und H. Wick. Arch. Int. Pharmcodyn. 84:337-
    348, 1950.

7. Hughes, R., A.J. May, and J.G. Widdicombe. J. Physiol.,
    London 146:85-97, 1959.

8. Laros, C.D. Respiration 28:120-136, 1971.

9. Le Blanc, E., and C. De Lind van Wyngaarden. Pflüger's Arch.
    des Physiol. 204:601-612, 1924.

10. Lohr, H. Klin. Wochschr. 2:2278-2279, 1923.

11. Macht, D.I., and G.C. Ting. J. Pharmacol. Exp. Ther. 18:373-
    398, 1921.

12. Macklem, P.T. Physiol. Rev. 51:368-436, 1971.

13. Monkcom, W., and R.W. Patterson. J. Thorac. Cardiovasc. Surg.
    63:577-584, 1972.

14. Nadel, J.A. Ann. NY Acad. Sci. 221:99-102, 1974.

15. Nadel, J.A. Med. Thorac. 22:231-242, 1965.

16. Nadel, J.A., H.J.H. Colebatch, and C.R. Olsen. J. Appl. Physiol. 19:387-394, 1964.

17. Newhouse, M.T., M.R. Becklake, P.T. Macklem, and M. McGregor. J. Appl. Physiol. 19:745-749, 1964.

18. Nisell, O. Acta Physiol. Scand. 21(Suppl. 73):5-62, 1950.

19. Patterson, R.W., S.F. Sullivan, J.R. Malm, F.O. Bowman, Jr., and E.M. Papper. Circulation 35:212-216, 1966.

20. Pirnay, F., J. Damoiseau, and J.M. Petit. Int. A. Angew. Physiol. 20:420-426, 1964.

21. Rattenborg, C.C., J.R. Benfield, S.L. Nigro, O. Gago, and W.E. Adams. Physiologist 5:199, 1962.

22. Rattenborg, C.C., and D.A. Holaday. Acta Anaesth. Scand. 23:211-223, 1967.

23. Rattenborg, C.C., and D.A. Holaday. Clin. Anesth. 1:23-40, 1967.

24. Samanek, M., and D.M. Aviado. J. Appl. Physiol. 22:719-730, 1967.

25. Sealy, W.C., and A.V. Seaber. J. Thorac. Cardiovasc. Surg. 69:533-538, 1975.

26. Severinghaus, J.W., E.W. Swenson, T.N. Finley, M.T. Lategola, and J. Williams. J. Appl. Physiol. 16:53-60, 1961.

27. Sollmann, T., and A.J. Gilberg. J. Pharmacol. Exp. Ther. 61:272-285, 1937.

28. Stephens, N.L., J.L. Meyers, and R.M. Cherniack. J. Appl. Physiol. 25:376-383, 1968.

29. Sterling, G.M. Clin. Sci. 34:277-285, 1968.

30. Swenson, E.W., T.N. Finley, and S.V. Guzman. J. Clin. Invest. 40:838-835, 1961.

31. Thornton, J.W. Q. J. Exp. Physiol. 21:305-314, 1932.

32. Tiefensee, K. Arch. Exp. Pathol. Pharmakol. 139:139-153, 1929.

33. Tisi, G.M., W.G. Wolfe, R.J. Fallat, and J.A. Nadel. J. Appl. Physiol. 28:570-573, 1970.

34. Trendelenburg, P. Arch. Exp. Pathol. Pharmakol. 69:79–107,
     1912.

35. Venrath, H., R. Rotthoff, H. Valentin, and W. Bolt. Beitr.
     Klin. Tuberk. 107:291–294, 1952.

36. Wick, H. Arch. Int. Pharmcodyn. 88:461–472, 1952.

37. Wick, H. Arch. Int. Pharmcodyn. 88:450–457, 1952.

38. Widdicombe, J.G. Physiol. Rev. 43:1–37, 1963.

39. Widdicombe, J.G. J. Physiol., London 159:436–450, 1961.

40. Woolcock, A.J., P.T. Macklem, J.C. Hogg, and N.J. Wilson.
     J. Appl. Physiol. 26:814–818, 1969.

DISCUSSION

McFadden: Does collateral ventilation affect calculations of the
resistance or compliance in your preparation?

Coon: I am sure that collateral ventilation exists in our preparation. We did not measure it.

14

Properties of Rapidly Adapting Vagal Receptors in Intrapulmonary Airways[1]

S. R. Sampson, E. H. Vidruk[2] & H. L. Hahn[3]

The lungs contain two types of vagal sensory receptor that
have been implicated in the reflex control of airway diameter.
These are: 1) slowly adapting pulmonary stretch receptors, which
reflexly appear to cause bronchodilatation, and 2) rapidly
adapting ("irritant") receptors, whose stimulation has been
associated with reflex bronchoconstriction (17). The properties
(adequate stimulus, conduction velocities of the afferent fibers,
patterns of electrical activity, and responses to certain drugs) of
pulmonary stretch receptors, despite having different thresholds
for activation, have been clearly described (12), probably because
they are easy to study, their activity dominating electrical recordings obtained from most bundles dissected from the vagus nerve.
Moreover, since the time Widdicombe and Nadel (18) reported that
transection of the thoracic vagus nerves abolished tracheal dilata-
tion induced by maintained inflation of the lungs, the role of pulmonary stretch receptors in reflex relaxation of the airways has
generated little, if any, controversy.

The situation pertaining to the intrapulmonary rapidly adapting
receptors, however, is not so straightforward. First recorded by
Knowlton and Larrabee (5) in the cat and later by Paintal (10) and
Armstrong and Luck (1) in this species, impulses from these receptors have since been obtained from vagal afferent fibers in a number
of other mammals including rabbit (4,7,8), guinea pig (6) and most
recently dog (9,13). The available data indicate that there is
considerable species variation with regard to the properties of
these receptors, so much so in fact, that even the selection of
an appropriate name for them has been difficult. Thus, terms
such as "rapidly adapting" (5,16), "deflation" (6), "expiration"
(7) and "irritant" (8,11) have all been used. The last term
was originally offered by Paintal (11), who stated that the
"natural stimulus for these endings...appears to be local

1. Supported by Pulmonary SCOR Grant HL-14201 from the National
   Heart and Lung Institute.
2. Supported by Fellowship HL-00448 from the National Heart and
   Lung Institute.
3. Supported in part by a North Senior Fellowship in Pulmonary
   Disease and by a Fulbright Travel Grant.

mechanical irritation...", and has been adopted by most other investigators. The enthusiasm for this term is based on the presumption that these sensory receptors are stimulated by a number of
irritant substances such as ether vapor, ammonia vapor and cigarette
smoke (see 17). As pointed out by Sampson and Vidruk (13), however,
current evidence does not fully substantiate the implication that
all "irritant" receptors are excited by all irritant substances.
We have elected to retain the older term - "rapidly adapting" - in
the naming of these receptors, because this adequately describes
the basic criterion used for the identification of this category of
receptor in neurophysiological studies, i.e., rapidly adapting responses to maintained hyperinflation and deflation of the lungs
(see 12).

It has been stated that intrapulmonary rapidly adapting receptors reflexly cause bronchoconstriction (see 12,17), as activity
arising from these sensory endings is increased by histamine (1,8,
13) and anaphylaxis (8), which themselves cause bronchoconstriction.
A major unresolved issue, however, is whether increased receptor
activity reflexly initiates bronchoconstriction or only intensifies
that produced by these conditions. Similarly, it is not known
whether excitation of rapidly adapting receptors is a cause or an
effect of bronchoconstriction. Hence, the precise role of these
receptors in the mediation of this effect is difficult to ascer-
tain.

Some of the uncertainty regarding the functional significance
of intrapulmonary rapidly adapting receptors may in part be due to
the extrapolation of data obtained from one species (e.g., rabbit)
to explain observations made in another (e.g., dog), an approach
which is seldom valid. The current investigation was prompted by
the need to characterize rapidly adapting receptors in the lungs of
dogs, the species used by our colleagues, Drs. J.A. Nadel and W.M.
Gold, in their studies on the role of the vagus nerves in the
control of ventilation and airway tone.

METHODS

The methods used in this study are those described in detail
by Sampson and Vidruk (13); only a brief description will be given
here. Adult mongrel dogs, 8-28 kg body weight and unspecified as
to sex, were initially anesthetized with sodium pentobarbital
(35 mg/kg, i.v.) and subsequently maintained with an i.v. mixture
of chloralose (25 mg/kg) and urethane (125 mg/kg). They were
paralyzed with i.v. gallamine triethiodide (1-3 mg/kg) and ventilated artificially. Appropriate cannulae were inserted into the
trachea below the larynx, into the pulmonary artery (via the right
external jugular vein), and into the femoral vein and artery for
injections of drugs and recording of arterial pressure, respectively. A midline thoracotomy was done while the dogs were artificially ventilated with tidal volumes (V_t) of 20-30 ml/kg, and the expiratory line of the respirator was placed under 3-5 cm H_2O to prevent
the lungs from collapsing. End-expiratory PCO_2, measured with a

Beckman LB-1 intra-red analyzer, and transpulmonary pressure
(P_{TP}), measured with a Statham differential pressure transducer
attached to the endotracheal cannula, were recorded on a Grass
polygraph. Deep body temperature was maintained between 34 and
$38^{\circ}C$ with an infra-red heat lamp or a heating pad.

Small strands were dissected from the otherwise intact left
vagus nerve, and afferent activity was recorded with fine platinum
electrodes, amplified and displayed on an oscilloscope. The vertical signal output from this oscilloscope was fed to an audiomonitor,
pulse-height selector and ratemeter, and to a second oscilloscope
from which photographic records were made on moving film. The
output from the ratemeter was also recorded on the polygraph.

Single or few afferent fibers were identified as arising from
rapidly adapting receptors by their responses to hyperinflation
of the lungs with a large plexiglass syringe. If the response
was rapidly adapting (Fig. 14.1A-C, arrows 1 and 2), the location
of the receptor ending was determined by gentle probing of the
left lung, a manoeuver which provokes activity in the fiber when
the receptive field is stimulated (Fig. 14.1A, B, arrows 3,4 and
5). Determination of the pulmonary origin of rapidly adapting
receptors is important because similar patterns of discharge may
arise from receptor endings located in the esophagus or pulmonary
artery (13). Upon identification of the type and location of the
receptors, they were studied further for their responses to chemical substances such as ammonia and ether vapors, and cigarette
smoke (administered via the inspiratory line of the respirator) and
histamine (delivered as an aerosol generated from 0.1-5% solutions
by a Devilbis 35A ultrasonic nebulizer).

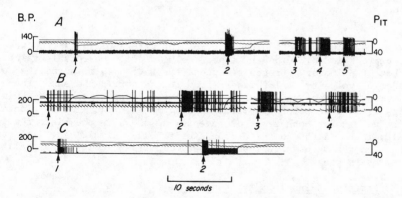

Fig. 14.1 Responses of intrapulmonary rapidly adapting receptors
to hyperinflation (arrows 1 and 2) and direct mechanical stimulation (arrows 3,4 and 5) of the lungs. Recordings from 3 different
preparations are shown in A, B and C. P_{IT}=intratracheal pressure
(cm H_2O),BP=arterial pressure (mmHg). From Sampson & Vidruk (13).

RESULTS

Characterization and conduction velocity.

We have now examined properties of over 100 units identified as rapidly adapting receptors (adaptation index greater than 70%; 17) arising from intrapulmonary airways. All receptors had patterns of responses to constant volume hyperinflation of the lungs encompassed by those illustrated in Fig. 14.1 A-C.

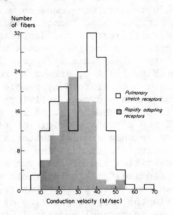

Fig. 14.2. Histogram showing the distribution of conduction velocities measured in afferent fibers arising from 101 rapidly adapting receptors (shaded area) and 167 pulmonary stretch receptors (clear area).

The mean conduction velocity of the afferent fibers from these receptors is 28.2+0.8 S.E. m/sec (n=101). To compare this value with that of pulmonary stretch receptors, we have also measured the conduction velocity of 167 fibers from the latter in the same group of dogs. The mean conduction velocity for afferent fibers from pulmonary stretch receptors is 32.2+0.8 S.E. m/sec. The distribution of the values for both types of receptor is shown in the histogram in Fig. 14.2. Although there is a statistically significant difference between the mean values, the degree of overlap among individual values is great.

Effects of inhaled "irritant" substances and histamine.

Intrapulmonary rapidly adapting receptors in species other than dog have been called "irritant" receptors because they are reported to be strongly stimulated by chemical irritants such as ammonia vapor, ether vapor and cigarette smoke (see 17). We, therefore, examined the effects of these substances on the spontaneous activity from rapidly adapting receptors in canine lung to determine if

they are sensitive to chemical irritants. We also investigated
the effects of histamine aerosol on these receptors, because it
has been proposed that the vagally-mediated reflex component of
histamine-induced bronchoconstriction is due to stimulation of
intrapulmonary rapidly adapting receptors (2,3).

In our initial study, we found that the irritant chemicals did
not consistently stimulate all intrapulmonary rapidly adapting
receptors. Indeed, only 1 receptor was stimulated by ammonia,
ether and cigarette smoke, only 2 by ammonia and smoke, and the
remainder of those few of the total population that were excited
by these substances were affected by only one or other of them (13).
These findings led us to question whether the term "irritant" is
an appropriate name for these receptors.

The most consistent chemical stimulant of intrapulmonary receptors in our studies was histamine, which given as an aerosol to
the lungs, caused a significant increase in rate of activity in
over 80% of the receptors. An example of this effect of histamine
on 2 receptors (recorded from the same nerve strand) is shown in
Fig. 14.3. Regardless of the magnitude of the increase in discharge produced by histamine, ranging from as low as 0.1 to as high
as 12.8 imp/sec, there was a tendency for the receptors to discharge
maximally during inflation. When a prominent effect occurred,
however, the units discharged throughout the respiratory cycle. An
increase in intratracheal pressure either preceded or coincided with
the increase in receptor activity, and both effects were reversed by
stepwise hyperinflation of the lungs produced by occluding the expiratory line through 2-3 respiratory cycles.

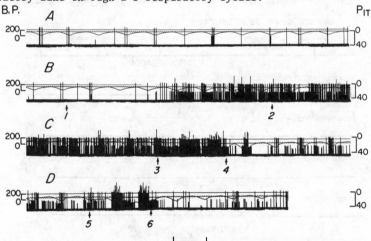

Fig. 14.3. Continuous film records of responses of 2 intrapulmonary
rapidly adapting receptors to an aerosol of histamine (0.1% solution),
given during the time between arrows 1 and 2 in B. At arrows 3 and
4, and again at 5 and 6, the lungs were hyperinflated. Calibrations
as in Fig. 14.1 From Sampson and Vidruk (13).

Mechanism of stimulation by histamine,

There are several questions that arise regarding the histamine-
induced increase in activity of rapidly adapting intrapulmonary receptors. Among them are: 1) Is this effect only secondary to changes
produced by histamine in total lung mechanics or is it due to direct
effects in the vicinity of the receptor? 2) If histamine causes
effects in the vicinity of the receptor, does it stimulate the receptors directly or does it do so indirectly by causing local contraction of airway smooth muscle? To answer the first question, we
have performed experiments with the use of a fiberoptic bronchoscope both to determine the location of the receptor ending and to
apply histamine directly to the vicinity of the nerve ending (14).
      Our procedure is as follows. We first dissect off an afferent
fiber from a rapidly adapting receptor, and determine the lobe in
which it is located by gentle palpation of the external surface of
the lungs. Then, after testing the effects of histamine aerosol to
the whole lungs, we explore the various bronchi in the appropriate
lobe with a small catheter attached to the bronchoscope. When the
region of the receptor is touched gently with the tip of the
catheter, a burst of action potentials is recorded in the afferent
fiber (Fig. 14.4A). Confirmation that the receptor is located in

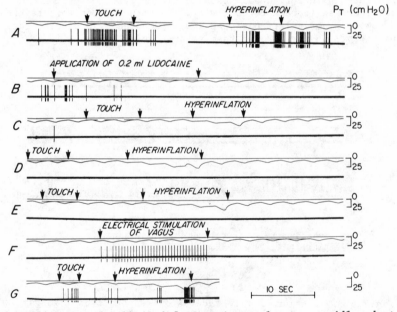

Fig. 14.4. Records obtained from an intrapulmonary rapidly adapting
receptor during study with the fiberoptic bronchoscope. Mechanical
stimulation with tip of the catheter shown in A. B-G are continuous
film records and show effects of small amount of lidocaine (1%
solution) applied to receptor area.

the specific region touched by the catheter tip, and not in a neighboring bronchus being mechanically deformed, is provided by the blocking effects of a small amount of local anesthetic applied to the region which provokes the most intense discharge (Fig. 14.4 B-G). Such local anesthesia reversibly blocks the responses to both touch and hyperinflation of the lungs.

We have currently examined the effects of histamine aerosol, given by both local and general delivery (for 1 min), on the activity of 39 rapidly adapting receptors. An example of the response of one of these receptors to local administration of an aerosol of 1% histamine is shown in Fig. 14.5. Of the 39 units tested, 23 were stimulated by both local and general delivery of histamine, 6 by general delivery only, and 5 by local delivery only. The remaining 5 receptors were not stimulated by histamine given by either means. Typically, receptor activity began to increase during application of histamine, sometimes within 10-15 sec of the onset of administration. The pattern of activity was not related to any phase of respiration, as the ventilator was turned off during administration of histamine to prevent it from being distributed throughout the lungs.

Responses to aerosols of histamine, in concentrations of 0.1-2%, could be obtained repeatedly from these receptors. Fig. 14.6 shows the first and last of a series of 6 responses to an aerosol of 2% histamine given at 20 min intervals. These findings demonstrate

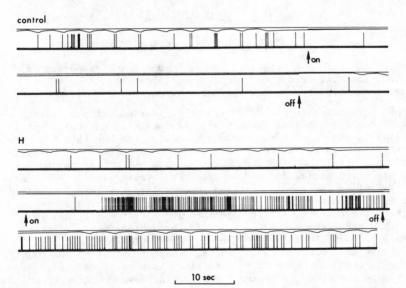

Fig. 14.5. Effects of locally-applied histamine on activity of a rapidly adapting receptor. An aerosol of control buffer solution was applied in the upper two records, and an aerosol of histamine in the lower 3 records, at the times indicated between the arrows.

that the histamine-induced increase in activity of rapidly adapting
receptors occurs as a result of direct effects in the vicinity of
the sensory endings and is not secondary to changes in total lung
mechanics.

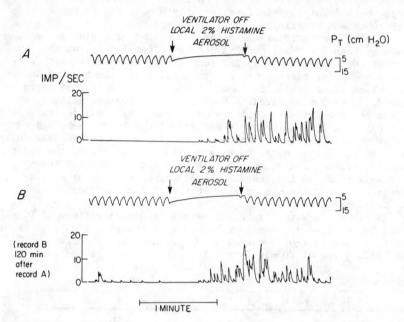

Fig. 14.6. First (A) and last (B) of 6 successive responses of a
rapidly adapting receptor to locally applied histamine. Lower
trace in each record is the ratemeter recording of nerve activity.

We have attempted to determine whether stimulation of intrapulmonary rapidly adapting receptors by histamine is due solely to its
ability to constrict airway smooth muscle,or whether this bronchoconstrictor may act directly on the sensory receptors to increase
their discharge. One approach we have used is to compare the
effects of histamine and ACh on receptor activity (15). ACh, given
as aerosol to the lungs, caused a greater increase in P_{TP} than did
equimolar concentrations of histamine (Table 14.1). Therefore, we
reasoned that if the ability of histamine to stimulate rapidly
adapting receptors was due only to its bronchoconstrictor action,
then bronchoconstriction produced by ACh should be almost as
effective as histamine in increasing receptor activity. We found,
however, that when both drugs were given as aerosol to the lungs,
histamine consistently caused a greater increase in activity of
these receptors than did ACh (Fig. 14.7).

Table 14.1. Effects of ACh and histamine on transpulmonary pressure
(P_{TP}). Each drug was given as aerosol to the whole
lung (n=32 experiments).

	ACh (3.25–32.5 mM)	Histamine (3.25–32.5 mM)
Increase in P_{TP}	11.2	8.1
S.D.	±7.9	±5.9
P	< 0.01	

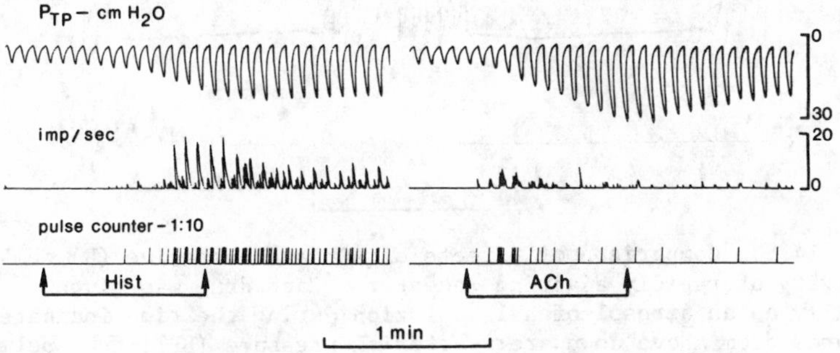

Fig. 14.7. Comparisons of effects of histamine and ACh on activity
of rapidly adapting receptors. Each drug was given as aerosol to
the lungs during the time indicated. Records from above downward
are transpulmonary pressure (P_{TP}), analogue output of rate meter
(imp/sec) and digital output of rate meter (1 vertical bar for 10
nerve impulses).

We also compared the effects of ACh with those of histamine on
receptor activity, when each drug was given locally via a catheter in the fiberoptic bronchoscope in order to provide equal concentrations of each drug in the vicinity of the receptor. In this
series of experiments, we first determined the minimum concentration
of histamine to stimulate the receptor, and then tested the effects
of an equimolar concentration of ACh. The sequence was repeated a
minimum of 3 times, responses to the tests with each drug averaged,
and the results obtained with histamine and ACh compared. An example of effects of the locally-applied drugs is shown in Fig. 14.8,
and the results obtained on a total of 12 receptors are summarized in
Table 14.2. Locally-applied histamine caused a significant increase
in rate of discharge in each of the 12 units, whereas ACh (and buffer solution tested on 7 receptors) did not. Both histamine and ACh,
however, produced noticeable airway constriction in the vicinity of
the receptor visible through the fiberoptic bronchoscope. The lack
of effect of ACh on receptor activity when applied locally, therefore, indicates that local constriction of airway smooth muscle is
not sufficient to stimulate intrapulmonary rapidly adapting receptors.

Hence, histamine appears to stimulate the sensory endings directly; local smooth muscle contraction may further intensify this effect.

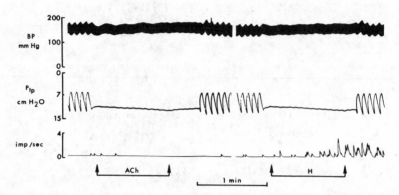

Fig. 14.8. Comparison of effects of ACh and histamine (H) on activity of rapidly adapting receptor. Each drug was given locally as an aerosol of a 1% solution during the time indicated. Records from above down are: arterial pressure (BP); transpulmonary pressure (P_{TP}); rate meter recording of nerve activity (imp/sec).

Table 14.2. Effects of locally-applied aerosols of histamine and acetylcholine on intrapulmonary rapidly adapting receptors. The concentrations of histamine and ACh ranged from 3.25–16.25 mM.

	Histamine	ACh	Buffer
Increase in discharge (imp/sec)	3.2	0.4	0.3
S.E.	± 0.4	± 0.2	± 0.1
P	< 0.001	N.S.	N.S.
n	12	12	7

SUMMARY

Intrapulmonary rapidly adapting receptors in dogs are innervated by afferent fibers whose mean conduction velocity is only slightly less than that of fibers arising from slowly adapting pulmonary stretch receptors. The distributions of individual values of conduction velocity indicate that the afferent fibers from the two types of receptor do not differ significantly with respect to their diameter.

Irritant chemicals, such as vapors of ammonia and ether and cigarette smoke, are relatively ineffective as stimulants of rapidly adapting receptors. Hence, the term "irritant receptor" may be inappropriate for these receptors in canine lungs.

Aerosols of histamine administered to the lungs cause a significant increase in the rate of discharge from the majority of rapidly adapting receptors. This stimulant effect of histamine also occurs when it is given as an aerosol locally via a catheter in a fiberoptic bronchoscope, indicating that the excitation of rapidly adapting receptors by histamine is not secondary to changes in total lung mechanics. In contrast, local application of acetylcholine, which causes greater bronchoconstriction than histamine on an equimolar basis, does not increase activity from these receptors, indicating that they are not stimulated by local smooth muscle contraction alone. We conclude that histamine acts directly on intrapulmonary rapidly adapting receptors to increase their activity, and this effect is intensified by histamine-induced contraction of airway smooth muscle.

REFERENCES

1. Armstrong, D.J., and J.C. Luck. Respir. Physiol. 27:47-60, 1974.
2. DeKock, M.A., J.A. Nadel, S. Zwi, H.J.H. Colebatch, and C.R. Olsen. J. Appl. Physiol. 21:185-194, 1966.
3. Gold, W.M., G.-F. Kessler, and D.Y.C. Yu. J. Appl. Physiol. 33:719-725, 1972.
4. Homberger, A.C. Helv. Physiol. Pharmacol. Acta 26:97-118, 1968.
5. Knowlton, G.C. and M.G. Larrabee. Am. J. Physiol. 147:100-114, 1946.
6. Koller, E.A. Helv. Physiol. Pharmacol. Acta 26:153-170, 1968.
7. Luck, J.C. J. Physiol. (London) 211:63-71, 1970.
8. Mills, J.E., H. Sellick, and J.G. Widdicombe. J. Physiol. (London) 203:337-357, 1969.
9. Mortola, J., G. Sant'Ambrogio, and M.G. Clement. Respir. Physiol. 24:107-114, 1975.
10. Paintal, A.S. J. Physiol. (London) 121:341-359, 1953.
11. Paintal, A.S. Ergeb. Physiol. 52:74-156, 1963.
12. Paintal, A.S. Physiol. Rev. 53:159-227, 1973.
13. Sampson, S.R., and E.H. Vidruk. Respir. Physiol. 25:9-22, 1975.
14. Vidruk, E., H.L. Hahn, J.A. Nadel, and S.R. Sampson. Physiologist 18:432, 1975.
15. Vidruk, E.H., H.L. Hahn, J.A. Nadel, and S.R. Sampson. Federation Proc. 35:841, 1976.

16. Widdicombe, J.G. J. Physiol. (London) 123:71-104, 1954.
17. Widdicombe, J.G. In: MTP International Review of Science
        Physiology Series One, Vol. 2, Respiratory Physiology,
        edited by J.G. Widdicombe. Baltimore, Md.: University Park
        Press, 1974, Chapt. 10, pp. 273-301.
18. Widdicombe, J.G., and J.A. Nadel. J. Appl. Physiol. 18:681-
        686, 1963.

DISCUSSION

Edelman: Do you know the distribution of these receptors?
Slowly adapting receptors occur in the trachea. Are there rapidly
adapting receptors in the trachea too? Is there any implication
to the differences in the distribution of the slow and rapidly
adapting receptors?

Sampson: Rapidly adapting receptors are present in the trachea
but the ones we are primarily interested in are present in the
intrapulmonary airways 2-4mm in diameter. They are probably present
in smaller airways but our methods do not assess these.

Adkinson: Have you information on antagonism of the effect of
histamine by either H_1 or H_2 antihistamines?

Sampson: I am reluctant to answer that question due to the preliminary nature of our experiments. The H_2 antagonist, metiamide,
blocked the histamine stimulation in a few preparations.

Remmers: In view of the fact that they are stimulated by bronchial
contraction, why did acetylcholine not stimulate these receptors?

Sampson: We were surprised at the results of these experiments
and pleased that the secondary effects of histamine could be
abolished. When aerosol acetycholine is administered to the whole
lung rapidly adapting fibers fire, probably as a result of a
secondary mechanical phenomenon.

Claremont: Do you think that these or similar receptors are in the
vascular system, since aerosol antihistamines do not block the
bronchial constriction that follows arterial occlusion?

Sampson: We don't know where all these receptors are. Some lie in
airways, and could well be subepithelial. But the definitive
anatomical and histological work has yet to be done with degenerative
and comparative morphologic studies.

Godfrey: Have you looked at other agonists or antagonists such as
isoproterenol, SRS-A or prostaglandins? You discussed the afferent
half of the reflex. What is the efferent half? These are rather
like Head's paradoxical reflex.

Sampson: I believe the mechanism proposed for the paradoxical reflex of Head is that over stimulation shuts off the discharge from the receptors. However, this proposal is still conjectural. The efferent half of the reflex is vagal since airway constriction is abolished with either cooling of the vagus or pretreatment with atropine. We find that we can reduce but not abolish the rapidly adapting receptor's traffic with isoproterenol aerosol. With extremely large non-physiologic doses of isoproterenol (1mg/kg) intravenously or by aerosol we did abolish the traffic from the receptor.

15

Role of Biochemicals Endogenous to the Lung[1,2]

N. Franklin Adkinson, Jr.[3]

Control of airway caliber is complex and multi-dimensional, reflecting its biological importance for adaptation and survival. Figure 15.1 illustrates schematically four groups of mechanisms which are capable of initiating chains of events which ultimately can affect the caliber of airways in the respiratory tree. First, autonomic innervation of the lung provides for neural control mechanisms. Not only is resting bronchial tone maintained in this way, but reflex arcs provide for constant monitoring of the physical and chemical environment in the lung. Supratentorial controls such as psychological stimuli can also exert an influence through these pathways. The chemical environment such as the state of oxygenation or acid-base balance may also initiate physiological events which result in alteration of airway diameter. The same is true for physical and mechanical factors, as is amply documented by the entire proceedings of this symposium. Finally, immunologic mechanisms of a variety of types may initiate the synthesis and release of chemicals which have direct effects on respiratory smooth muscle.

Such a grouping of mechanisms is somewhat arbitrary and probably incomplete. Furthermore, the scheme tends to obscure the very complex interactions among these pathways, and the existence of elaborate feedback control mechanisms which impinge upon them. For the purposes of this presentation, I will leave to others the discussion of these higher-order regulatory mechanisms in order to focus upon the final common pathways for the control of airway diameter. By this I mean the endogenous biochemicals which ultimately carry the message of contraction or relaxation to airway smooth muscle.

Table 15.1 lists those native chemicals which are thought to possess the capacity to induce relaxation or contraction by direct stimulation of bronchial smooth muscle. This list is almost certainly incomplete, especially with regard to rapidly expanding

[1]Publication No. 233 from The O'Neill Research Laboratories, The Good Samaritan Hospital, Baltimore, Maryland 21239.
[2]Supported by Grant No. AI 11936 from The National Institutes of Health.
[3]Recipient, Allergic Diseases Academic Award No. AI 71026 from The National Institute of Allergy and Infectious Diseases.

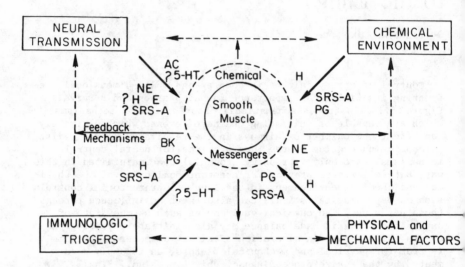

Fig. 15.1.   Mechanisms for control of airway diameter.

knowledge of the role of small chain fatty acids such as the
prostaglandins and thromboxanes in the control of smooth muscle
function. The role of acetylcholine and the parasympathetic nervous system has been addressed by Dr. Sampson and will not be
discussed further here. The catecholamines have long been recognized as important regulators of airway diameter, not only
physiologically but also in terms of pharmacological intervention.
Respiratory smooth muscle clearly possess a $Beta_2$ adrenergic membrane receptor by which agonists such as norepinephrine can induce
muscular relaxation (49). It has been suggested that the responsiveness of this Beta adrenergic system may be in some manner
defective in states of chronic bronchospasm such as bronchial
asthma (47). The role of alpha adrenergic control of smooth
muscle function is less clear (22) and the subject of much current
research. Epinephrine, the drug of choice for therapy of acute
bronchospasm, exerts both beta and alpha adrenergic effects in

lung smooth muscle and elsewhere. Its endogenous release from the
adrenal medulla may be affected by sympathetic stimulation or by
circulating histamine (40, 53).

Serotonin (5-hydroxytryptamine, 5-HT) originates primarily in
the gastrointestinal tract and in circulating platelets in man.
Recently, interest has been aroused in the discovery of serotonin-
containing neuroepithelial bodies in the lung where they appear
to be concentrated at sites of airway bifurcation (37). These
structures appear to be innervated by autonomic nerves. Nothing
is yet known of their physiological role, but it is conceivable
that serotonin will emerge as a neurotransmitter in the lung.
Serotonin is capable of producing contraction of bronchial smooth
muscle (18, 21). It may be speculated that the neuroepithelial
bodies might help to modulate airway diameter at crucial sites of
airway bifurcation. Platelet-derived serotonin may also play a
role in pathological settings in which platelet aggregation, coagulation, or hemorrhage occurs in the lung. There is currently
little evidence to support this view, however.

Bradykinin is a vasoactive nonapeptide which is split off from
a plasma $alpha_2$ globulin precursor (kininogen) by the enzyme
kallikrein. A number of kallikreins have been described. A
kallikrein may be generated in plasma by activation of one of the
Hageman factor- (clotting factor XII) dependent pathways; these
pathways include coagulation, fibrinolysis and activation of the
complement cascade, chiefly through the alternate or properdin
(C3 proactivator) pathway (9). By any of these complex pathways,
involving either immunologic or nonspecific stimuli, bradykinin
may be generated in plasma and presumably in interstitial spaces.
In addition, tissue mast cells and circulating basophils contain
a kallikrein enzyme which is preformed in these cells and released upon appropriate biological stimulation (41, 57). The
physiologic and pathologic roles of bradykinin in man remains to
be established. In human bronchial muscle preparations, bradykinin produces weak and variable contractions compared with
histamine (5, 43). This contractile response is blocked by non-
steroidal anti-inflammatory drugs such as aspirin and meclo-
fenamate (10, 13), an observation which has led some to attribute
the effect of bradykinin on smooth muscle to stimulation of
prostaglandin synthesis. Recently this view has been supported
by direct experimental evidence showing that bradykinin does
directly stimulate prostaglandin synthesis probably by initiating
arachidonic acid release (31).

The remainder of this review will be directed toward a discussion in some depth of the remaining three classes of bronchoactive substances. Histamine and slow reacting substance of
anaphylaxis (SRS-A) were the first known and are the best studied
chemical mediators of immediate hypersensitivity reactions.
Recent evidence suggests that these substances may be liberated
by non-immunologic mechanisms as well (25, 34, 36), opening up

Table 15.1. Endogenous Chemicals with Direct Bronchial Smooth Muscle Activity

Biochemical	Principal Sources	Lung Receptors	Bronchial Activity
Acetylcholine (AC)	Parasympathetic nerves	AC	Contraction
Catecholamines — norepinephrine (NE)	Sympathetic nerves	$\beta_2$adrenergic ($?\alpha$-adrenergic)	Relaxation
— epinephrine (E)	Adrenal medulla	$\beta_2$adrenergic ($?\alpha$-adrenergic)	Relaxation
Serotonin (5-HT)	Neuroepithelial bodies (NEB) Platelets (blood)	?	Contraction
Bradykinin (BK)	Serum kininogen	?	Contraction (variable)
Histamine (H)	Mast cell granules Basophilic leukocytes (blood)	H_1(muscle) ? irritant receptors	Contraction
Slow-reacting substance of anaphylaxis (SRS-A)	Mast cell generated Leukocytes (tissue and blood)	?	Prolonged Contraction
Prostaglandins (PG) and Thromboxanes (Tx)	Most (?all) nucleated cells	PGE PGF ?Endoperoxides ?Tx	Relaxation Contraction Contraction ?

the possibility of a more general physiological function in addition to their well established pathological role. Finally, we are confronted with an ever-expanding number of prostanoic acid derivatives which have profound smooth muscle activity and appear likely to be important in the modulation of airway function. Currently the prostaglandins, their endoperoxide precursors and their thromboxane derivatives appear to exert a general regulatory function in the control of membrane-associated events in a large variety of tissue. This discussion will focus upon recent developments in prostaglandin and thromboxane research which have implications for pulmonary physiology.

Histamine in the Lung

Histamine (B-imidazolylethylamine) is a granule-associated chemical found in tissue mast cells and in basophilic granulocytes. It is formed from L-histidine by the enzyme histidine decarboxylase. Metabolism is by oxidation or methylation and the lung is known to be a rich source for such enzymes. However, unlike serotonin and bradykinin, histamine does not disappear from the circulation during its passage through the lungs (20). Within lung tissue, the richest source of histamine is mast cells which are situated in the perivascular connective tissue. However, there may be some non-mast cell histamine, the nascent or non-mast cell pool being defined as the histamine content which resists the action of drug 48/80, a substance capable of releasing histamine from mast cells (32). The role of non-mast cell associated histamine in the lungs is not known. On the other hand, mast cell histamine is susceptible to release by immunologic events which trigger mast cell degranulation. Mast cells possess Fc receptors for IgE antibody; when these are occupied by antibody and united with specific antigen, a series of biochemical events culminating in mediator release is initiated (1). Split fragments of complement components C3 and C5, known as C3a and C5a anaphylatoxins, are also capable of initiating mediator release through a somewhat different mechanism (52).

Non-immunologic release of mast cell histamine is also possible. Though there are some discrepancies which may be species related, several investigators have provided evidence that alveolar hypoxia may result in pulmonary mast cell degranulation (3, 28, 29). More recently, prostaglandins have been implicated in the bronchospasm resulting from alveolar hypoxia (50). Finally, lung mast cells have been shown to possess cholinergic receptors which are capable of potentiating mediator release (33). This has led to speculation that lung mast cells may be directly innervated by cholinergic nerves. Further study of this intriguing possibility is required.

When injected intravenously or into the airways by aerosol, histamine produces a profound bronchoconstrictor response leading to marked increase in airway resistance with concomitant reduction in compliance (19a). Some, but not all, of these effects can be

blocked by vagotomy of the experimental animal, or pretreatment of
human or animal subjects with atropine (7, 19b). To this extent,
the histamine-induced bronchial constriction may be dependent upon
vagal reflexes initiated by afferent nerves from so-called "irritant" receptors in the pulmonary tree. This effect is supplemented by histamine's direct stimulation of bronchial smooth
muscle (16). In addition, histamine produces increased vascular
permeability predominantly at the level of pulmonary venules (17).

In most but not all animals, the effect of histamine on vascular and bronchial smooth muscle can be largely antagonized by
the classical antihistamines such as mepyramine. Histamine receptors on lung smooth muscle are thus predominantly of the H_1
subtype. Why H_1 antihistamines have proven to be of such little
clinical value in the treatment of bronchospastic states such as
asthma remains unexplained (11). Peripheral leukocytes and presumably mast cells possess histamine receptors of the H_2 subtype
defined by the specific antagonism of a new group of antihistamines of which burimamide and metiamide are the prototypes (6).
This mast cell histamine H2 receptor is linked to the adenylate
cyclase system. Stimulation of the receptor thus increases
intracellular levels of cyclic AMP. It is now clearly established
that agents which increase cyclic AMP inhibit the immunological
release of mediators from mast cells and basophilic leukocytes
(39b, 46). Thus, the mast cell H2 receptor may subserve the
function of feed-back inhibition for the release of vasoactive
and chemotactic substances from lung mast cells. Little is known
of the interaction of histamine with pulmonary "irritant" receptors, presumably on afferent nerve endings.

Slow Reacting Substance of Anaphylaxis (SRS-A) in the Lung

SRS-A is a low molecular weight acidic, sulphur-containing
lipid whose exact chemical structure is as yet uncharacterized.
It is detected by bioassay on guinea pig ileum with the effects of
histamine and cholinergic agents blocked by the use of an H_1 anti-
histamine and atropine. Disrupted mast cells and basophilic
leukocytes contain minimal amounts of SRS-A, suggesting that unlike
histamine, it is not largely preformed. Instead it is generated
from a precursor after cellular activation, usually initiated by
antigen-antibody union. The biochemical pathways leading to the
release of SRS-A are quite distinct from those demonstrated for
histamine (1). SRS-A can be inactivated by an arylsulfatase B of
the type found in human eosinophils (56). Heretofore, SRS-A has
been exclusively identified with anaphylactic or IgE mechanisms
involving tissue mast cells or peripheral blood basophilic leukocytes. However, a mechanism involving IgG_a and complement has
been employed to obtain SRS-A from rat peritoneal neutrophils
(44). Finally, the calcium ionophore A23187, a nonspecific membrane activator, is capable of initiating the generation of SRS
from peritoneal cells other than mast cells (2) and from granulocytes other than basophils (12). It now seems possible that SRS

will be shown to have a more general pathologic and possibly
physiologic role apart from its contribution to anaphylactic
responses.

When injected into skin, SRS-A appears to produce increased
vascular permeability (8). Of greater importance is the slow
sustained contraction of smooth muscle produced by SRS-A. Compared with histamine, the action of SRS-A is both delayed in onset
and protracted in duration. When SRS-A is inhaled as an aerosol,
it produces bronchoconstriction in man (30). When injected intravenously into guinea pigs, a marked decrease occurs in pulmonary
compliance together with an increase in pulmonary resistance.
These changes are independent of cholinergic mechanisms (19b).
The structure of SRS-A has not yet been elucidated and there are
no known specific pharmacologic antagonists. Thus, the nature of
SRS receptors on smooth muscle and possibly other cell types
remains to be defined.

The pharmacological control of immunologically mediated release
of SRS-A is similar in many respects to that of the preformed
mediators such as histamine (45). Substances which act through
adenylate cyclase to increase intracellular levels of cyclic AMP
inhibit SRS-A release. These include beta adrenergic drugs, PGE,
and histamine - each through a distinct receptor. The release
process may be potentiated by cholinergic agonists such as
carbacol, alpha adrenergic agonists such as phenylephine and
possibly by low levels of PGF. Cholinergic, alpha adrenergic,
and PGF receptors may be present on lung mast cells, but they
appear to be absent on human basophils (39a).

Prostaglandins (PGs) and Thromboxanes (Txs) in the Lung

The prostaglandins are a series of C20 hydroxy-fatty acids
derived principally from arachidonic acid. Phospholipases and
other lipolytic enzymes generate the arachidonic acid precursor
which is then converted to prostaglandins by prostaglandin
synthetase, a group of microsomal enzymes. Virtually every
mammalian tissue studied with the exception of erythrocytes
possesses the capacity for prostaglandin synthesis.

The current view of the principal biosynthetic pathways in the
lung may be summarized as follows (26) (Fig. 15.2). The cyclo-
oxygenase converts arachidonic acid to endoperoxide intermediates
(PGG_2 and PGH_2) which have half-life of only four to five minutes
in aqueous solution. They possess potent bronchoconstrictor
activity, estimated at 5 to 10 times that of $PGF_{2\alpha}$ (27). The
endoperoxides are rapidly converted to the primary prostaglandins
PGE, a bronchodilator, and PGF, a bronchoconstrictor. These forms
are stable in aqueous solution, but are rapidly metabolized in
vivo to relatively inactive derivatives by prostaglandin dehydro-
genase enzymes. Recent work from Samuelson and his colleagues
in Sweden have suggested that in the lung, as was shown for human

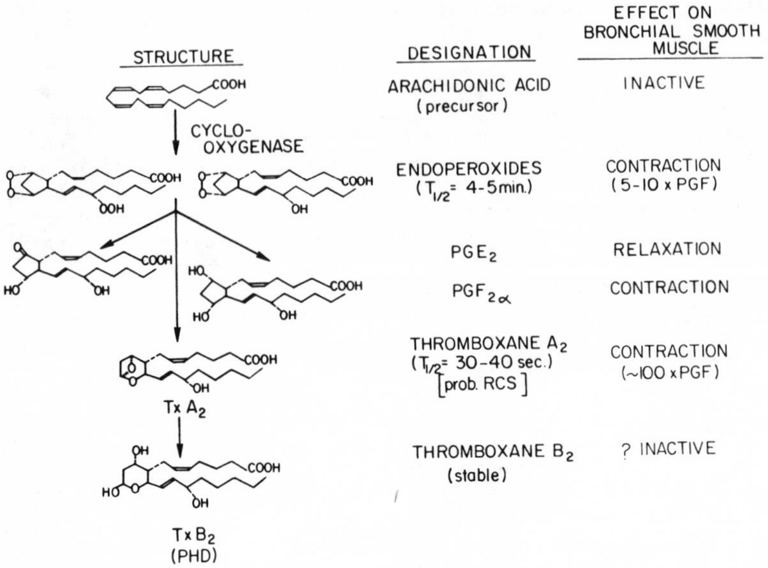

STRUCTURE	DESIGNATION	EFFECT ON BRONCHIAL SMOOTH MUSCLE
COOH	ARACHIDONIC ACID (precursor)	INACTIVE
↓ CYCLO-OXYGENASE		
COOH OOH COOH OH	ENDOPEROXIDES ($T_{1/2}$= 4-5min.)	CONTRACTION (5-10 x PGF)
COOH HO COOH	PGE$_2$	RELAXATION
HO OH HO OH	PGF$_{2\alpha}$	CONTRACTION
COOH OH Tx A$_2$	THROMBOXANE A$_2$ ($T_{1/2}$= 30-40 sec.) [prob. RCS]	CONTRACTION (~100 xPGF)
OH COOH HO OH Tx B$_2$ (PHD)	THROMBOXANE B$_2$ (stable)	? INACTIVE

Fig. 15.2. Principal prostaglandin and thromboxane pathways in lung tissue.

platelets, the primary pathway is not to PGE and PGF but to the thromboxanes (51). Thromboxane A$_2$ is also short lived in aqueous solutions with a half-life of 30 to 40 seconds. Its half-life and biological properties suggest that it may be the elusive rabbit aorta contracting substance (RCS) released from lungs undergoing anaphylactic shock. The smooth muscle contracting potency of thromboxane A$_2$ is estimated to be 10 to 100 fold greater than PGF (26). Its importance in anaphylaxis and in chronic bronchospastic states such as asthma remains to be determined. Thromboxane A$_2$ is rapidly metabolized to thromboxane B$_2$, a stable derivative whose biological function is currently obscure. The non-steroidal anti-inflammatory drugs such as aspirin, indomethacin, and the fenamates are known to block the prostaglandin synthetase enzyme system (55). These drugs have been very useful in studies of the physiological role of the prostaglandins.

Prostaglandins and their metabolites, once formed, are released without being stored. A wide variety of stimuli are capable of inducing prostaglandin synthesis and release. These include gentle stroking of whole lung, mechanical irritation of respiratory mucosa, pulmonary embolization with small particles, and hyperinflation of the lung. The contraction of smooth muscle itself by histamine or other substances appears to stimulate prostaglandin production (24). The smooth muscle constriction response to bradykinin has also been attributed to prostaglandin production, principally on the grounds that it is antagonized by pretreatment with indomethacin (14). Anaphylactic shock of sensitized lungs in experimental animals also results in the production of both PGE and PGF (48). More recently, endoperoxides and thromboxanes have also been found in effluents from lungs undergoing anaphylactic reactions (27). The prostaglandin production is believed by most investigators to be a secondary result of the release of mast cell mediators such as histamine and SRS-A. This belief stems from the fact that sodium cromolyn, a drug which blocks histamine and SRS-A release from sensitized mast cells, also blocks the production of prostaglandins following antigenic challenge of sensitized pulmonary tissue (15).

The fact that both smooth muscle relaxing (PGE) and constricting (all other) prostanoates can result from the same synthetic enzyme system creates, on one hand, the potential for a finely balanced regulatory system and, on the other hand, an immense complexity which has just begun to be unraveled. For example, it is now thought that isomerases and reductases control production of PGE versus PGF, and even the interconversion of PGE to PGF (38). How these enzyme systems may operate to favor the production of muscle-relaxing end products rather than muscle-constricting ones awaits exploration.

In the lung, PGE acts to relax both bronchial and vascular smooth muscle, though these effects are variable and difficult to reproduce in some species. $PGF_{2\alpha}$ has a consistent bronchoconstrictor effect upon isolated bronchial muscle and increases pulmonary vascular resistance when injected into the pulmonary artery. No true pharmacological antagonists for the prostaglandins currently exist. It has been inferred from studies of a PGE cell membrane receptor on lipocytes and a PGF receptor on corpus luteum cells that the effect of prostaglandins on smooth muscles, mast cells, and leukocytes are mediated by specific membrane receptors. There is increasing evidence that PGE may provide a cyclic AMP dependent feed-back inhibition of mediator release from lung mast cells (4). The origin of this PGE may well be the contracting smooth muscle itself.

As mentioned previously, the non-steroidal anti-inflammatory drugs block the synthesis of prostaglandins, their endoperoxides, and thromboxanes. Early work by Vane and associates suggested that corticosteroids had no effect on prostaglandin synthesis (23, 55). However, several investigators have recently confirmed that hydrocortisone and other steroids do inhibit prostaglandin production in some systems (35, 54), probably by interference with the activity of phospholipases in generating the required precursor, arachidonic acid. In view of the diverse biological activity of the prostaglandins and derivatives, it is surprising that almost complete suppression of endogenous production can be

achieved with aspirin or indomethacin without serious physiological consequences. This has been taken by some as evidence against
a major role for prostaglandins in the control of airway caliber
in disease processes such as bronchial asthma. One alternative
explanation is that prostaglandins may be important extracellular
messengers in the micro-environment and exert their regulatory
control at the level of what might be called "fine tuning."

Summary

This presentation has focused upon three groups of endogenous
biochemicals which are likely to exert some measure of control
over airway caliber. They are representative of that list of
chemicals which convey the final chemical message to respiratory
smooth muscle, either to contract or to relax. The interactions
of the multiple stimuli which may initiate the signal are extra-
ordinarily complex; they comprise the domain of classical
pulmonary physiology. In the end, however, it is the molecular
physiology of these chemical mediators which must be understood
if we wish to intervene intelligently to modify therapeutically
pathological processes in the lung.

REFERENCES

1. Austen, K.F. In: Asthma - Physiology, Immunopharmacology
    and Treatment, edited by K.F. Austen and L.M. Lichtenstein.
    New York: Academic Press, 1973, p. 111.
2. Back, M.K., and J.R. Brashler. J. Immunol. 113:2040-2044,
    1974.
3. Barer, G.R., and J.R. McCurrie. J. Exp. Physiol. 54:156,
    1969.
4. Barrett-Bee, K.J., and C.R. Greer. Prostaglandins 10:589-
    598, 1975.
5. Bhoola, K.D., H.O.J. Collier, M. Schachter, and P.G. Shorley.
    Brit. J. Pharmacol. 19:190-197, 1962.
6. Black, J.W., W.A.M. Duncan, C.J. Durant, C.R. Ganellin, and
    E.M. Parsons. Nature 236:385-390, 1972.
7. Bouhuys, A., R. Jonsson, S. Lichtneckerts, S.E. Lindell, C.
    Lundgren, G. Lundin, and T.F. Pingquist. Clin. Sci. 19:
    79, 1960.
8. Brocklehurst, W.E. In: Clinical Aspects of Immunology,
    edited by P.F.H. Gell and R.R.A. Coombs. Oxford: Blackwell,
    1968, p. 611.
9. Colman, R.W. N. Engl. J. Med. 291:509-514, 1974.
10. Collier, H.O.J. Adv. Drug. Res. 5:95-107, 1970.
11. Collier, H.O.J., G.W.L. James, and P.J. Piper. Brit. J. J.
    Pharmacol. 34:76, 1968.
12. Conroy, M.C., R.P. Orange, and L.M. Lichtenstein. J. Immunol.
    (in press), 1976.
13. Crocker, A.D., and S.P. Willavoys. J. Pharm. Pharmac. 28:78,
    1976.

14. Crocker, A.D., and S.P. Willavoys. J Pharm. Pharmac. 28: 78, 1976.

15. Dawson, W., and R. Tomlinson. Brit. J. Pharmacol. 52:107P, 1974

16. DeKock, M.A., J.A. Nadel, S. Zwi, H.J.H. Colebatch, and C.R. Olsen. J. Appl. Physiol. 21:185, 1966.

17. Douglas, W.W. In: Pharmacological Basis of Therapeutics, edited by L.S. Goodman and A. Gilman. 5th ed. New York: MacMillan, 1975, pp. 590-629.

18. Drakonites, A.B., and M.D. Gershon. Brit. J. Pharmacol. 33:480, 1968.

19a. Drazen, J.M., and K.F. Austen. J. Clin. Invest. 53:1679, 1974.

19b. Drazen, J.M., and K.F. Austen. J. Appl. Physiol. 38:834, 1975.

20. Eiseman, B., L. Bryant, and I. Waltuch. J. Thorac. Cardiovasc. Surg. 48:798, 1965.

21. Fleisch, J.H., H.M. Maling, and B.B. Brodie. Amer. J. Physiol. 218:596, 1970.

22. Fleisch, J.H., K.M. Kent, and T. Cooper. In: Asthma - Physiology, Immunopharmacology and Treatment, edited by K.F. Austen and L.M. Lichtenstein. New York: Academic Press, 1973, p. 149.

23. Flower, R.J., R. Gryglewski, K. Herbaczynska-Cedro, and J. R. Vane. Nature (New Biol.) 238:104-106, 1972.

24. Grodzinska, L., B. Panczenko, and R.J. Gryglewski. J. Pharm. Pharmac. 27:88-91, 1975.

25. Haas, F., and E.H. Bergofsky. J. Clin. Invest. 51:3154, 1972.

26. Hamberg, M., J. Svensson, and B. Samuelsson. Proc. Natl. Acad. Sci. USA 72:2994, 1975.

27. Hamberg, M., J. Svensson, P. Hedqvist, K. Strandberg, and B. Samuelsson. In: Advances in Prostaglandin and Thromboxane Research, Vol. 1., edited by B. Samuelsson and R. Paoletti. New York: Raven Press, 1976, pp. 495-501.

28. Hauge, A. Circ. Res. 22:371, 1968.

29. Hauge, A., and N.C. Staub. J. Appl. Physiol. 26:693, 1969.

30. Herxheimer, H., and E. Stresemann. J. Physiol. Lond. 158: 38, 1961.

31. Hong, S.L., R. Polsky-Cynkin, and L. Levine. J. Biol. Chem. 251:776-780, 1976.

32. Johnson, H.L. J. Pharmacol. Exp. Ther. 171:88, 1970.

33. Kaliner, M., R.P. Orange, and K.F. Austen. J. Exp. Med. 136:556, 1972.

34. Kaliner, M., R.P. Orange, D.J. LaRaia, and K.F. Austen. J. Allergy Clin. Immunol. 49:88, 1972.

35. Kantrowitz, F., D.R. Robinson., M.D. McGuire, and L. Levine. Nature 258:737-738, 1975.

36. Lasser, E.C., A.J. Walters, and J.H. Lang. Radiology 110: 49:59, 1974.

37. Lauweryns, J.M., M. Cokelaere, and P. Theunynck. Science 180:410-413, 1973.

38. Levine, L. Personal communication, 1976.

39a. Lichtenstein, L.M., E. Gillespie, and H. Bourne. In: The
     Biologic Role of the Immunoglobulin E System, edited by K.
     Ishizaka and D.H. Dayton. Washington, DC: U.S. Govt.
     Printing Office, 1973, pp. 165-180.
39b. Lichtenstein, L.M., and C.S. Henney. In: Progress in
     Immunology II, Vol. 2, edited by L. Brent and J. Holborrow.
     Amsterdam: North-Holland, 1974, p. 73.
40. Maengwyn-Davies, G.D., J.H. Fleisch, and T.P. Pruss. J.
     Pharm. Pharmacol. 24:295, 1972.
41. Mansell, A., C. Dubrawsky, H. Levison, A.C. Bryan, H. Langer,
     C. Collins-Williams, and R.P. Orange. J. Appl. Physiol. 37:
     297, 1974.
42. Needleman, P., S.L. Key, S.E. Denny, P.C. Isakson, and G.R.
     Marshall. Proc. Natl. Acad. Sci. USA 72:2060-2063, 1975.
43. Newball, H.H., and H.R. Keiser. J. Appl. Physiol. 35:552-
     556, 1973.
44. Orange, R.P., M.D. Valentine, and K.F. Austen. J. Exp. Med.
     127:767, 1968.
45. Orange, R.P., D.J. Stechschulte, and K.F. Austen. Fed. Proc.
     28:1710, 1969.
46. Orange, R.P., and K.F. Austen. In: The Biologic Role of
     the Immunoglobulin E System, edited by K. Ishizaka and D.H.
     Dayton. Washington, DC: U.S. Govt. Printing Office, 1973.
     p. 151.
47. Parker, C.W. In: Asthma - Physiology, Immunopharmacology,
     and Treatment, edited by K.F. Austen and L.M. Lichtenstein.
     New York: Academic Press, 1973, p. 185.
48. Piper, P.J., and J.R. Vane. Ann. N.Y. Acad. Sci. 180:363,
     1971.
49. Prosser, C.L. Ann. Rev. Physiol. 36:503, 1974.
50. Said, S.I., T. Yoshida, S. Kitamura, and C. Vreim. Science
     185:1181, 1974.
51. Samuelsson, B. In: Advances in Prostaglandin and Thromboxane
     Research, Vol. 1, edited by B. Samuelsson and R. Paoletti.
     New York: Raven Press, 1976, pp. 1-6.
52. Siraganian, R.P. J. Immunol. (in press), 1976.
53. Staszewska-Barczaki, J., and J.R. Vane. Brit. J. Pharmacol.
     Chemotherp. 25:728, 1965.
54. Tashjian, A.H. jr., E.F. Voelkel, J. McDonough, and L.
     Levine. Nature 258:739-741, 1975.
55. Vane, J.R. Nature New Biol. 231:232-235, 1971.
56. Wasserman, S.I., E.J. Goetzl, and K.F. Austen. J. Immunol.
     114:645, 1975.
57. Webster, M.E., Z. Horakova, M.A. Beaven, H. Takahaski, and
     H.H. Newball. Fed. Proc. 33:761, 1974.

DISCUSSION

Gee: Another factor perhaps should be added to this superb review. There are some bacterial formulated and acylated tripeptides (eg. formye-methionine-leucine-phenylalanine) which act as chemotaxins and are also capable of releasing histamine from basophils and probably also of mobilizing lysosome enzymes from both monocytes and leukocytes.

Adkinson: I would tend to agree. There are a number of other mediators of inflammation which I did not cover principally because they are not known to act directly on bronchi and vessels. These other mediators are important in the overall inflammatory response in the lung and cannot be ignored in the final analysis of the control mechanisms.

Fishman: Could I ask about the release of histamine during anaphylaxis. Is degranulation of mast cells a prerequisite for the release of histamine? Is it possible to release nascent histamine without affecting the release of histamine from mast cells?

Adkinson: No one knows whether there is non-mast cell histamine in the lung or what physiologic role it might play. Total mast cell degranulation of the type that can be observed under the microscope is not necessary for histamine release but a profound anaphylactic reaction will result in almost complete emptying of contents of mast cell granules. Blood basophils appear to be less prone to extrude their granules than mast cells.

Fishman: Can the basophil and the mast cell release histamine without degranulating?

Adkinson: I think it is fair to call the mechanism degranulation. Histamine is stored in the granules but release does not require total extracellular extrusion of all granules. At least for mast cells, mediator release is probably not an "all-or-none" phenomenon.

Cropp: I was very interested to hear about your comment regarding the cholinergic innervation of the mast cell. As you know, many of us believe that a classical mediator must be involved in one way or another in exercise induced asthma since blockade of mediator release by cromolyn can reduce and often prevent this phenomenon. Would you like to elaborate on the evidence for cholinergic innervation of the mast cell?

Adkinson: I wish that I could. There has been too little work in this area. There are clearly cholinergic receptors on mast cells in the lung and the only known source for cholinergic agonists is the nerve end plate; the presumption has been that cholinergic stimulation potentiates the release of mediators. But that is circumstantial evidence and as far as I know, the anatomists have not yet demonstrated cholinergic terminals on mast cells.

Kampine: We know that there are muscarinic receptors in blood
vessels that are not innervated by parasympathetic postganglionic
nerve endings so to find receptors in sites that are not innervated
is not unique. I have another question. How does histamine produce
contraction of airways smooth muscle? Is it a matter of histamine
acting on myofibriles or does histamine affect calcium entry into
airway smooth muscle to produce contraction? Since calcium has
been implicated in excitation-contraction coupling in most other
systems, is there information on the role that calcium plays in
pharmacologic or chemically mediated contraction of airways smooth
muscle?

Adkinson: There has been relatively little work on the biochemistry
of airway smooth muscle contraction, in part because of technical
problems. The extensive investigations of calcium and cyclic
nucleotide fluxes and their relationship to excitation-contraction
coupling in skeletal and cardiac muscle (S.E. Mayer, In: New
Directions in Asthma, American College of Chest Physicians, Park
Ridge, Ill., pp. 71-83, 1975) may not be applicable to bronchial
smooth muscle (S.E. Mayer, op. cit., pp. 129-130). Additional
research aimed directly at airway smooth muscle will be required
in order to answer your very pertinent question, Dr. Kampine.

L. Smith: If prostaglandins are involved in bronchial smooth
muscle control mainly by exerting regulatory fine tuning, then how
could they exert such a powerful effect in aspirin induced asthma?

Adkinson: In my view, we don't yet have enough data to provide
reasonable speculation as to how aspirin provoked bronchospasm
might come about. In susceptible patients bronchospasm is induced
by aspirin and related anti-inflammatory drugs which are structurely
dissimilar but share the common property of inhibiting the synthesis
of prostaglandins. This fact suggests that the prostaglandin
synthesis system may play some role in the pathogenesis of aspirin
induced asthma, but as yet we have too little knowledge of the
prostaglandin synthetase system to construct a reasonable hypothesis.

16

Role of Mechanical Factors in Ventilation Distribution

Björn Bake

During exercise breathing differs from resting conditions in several respects, e.g. increased tidal volume, increased flow rates and perhaps changed breathing pattern. Effects of these factors on distribution of ventilation among lung regions will be discussed. Regional ventilation is studied by externally positioned scintillation counters which are placed in collimators the geometry of which define these lung regions which therefore, do not correspond to anatomical subdivisions of the lungs. Undoubtedly, the distribution of ventilation within a region may be considerably more uneven than between regions, but so far we know less about intraregional than about interregional ventilation distribution.

Increased Tidal Volume

Regional expansion during static or quasi static conditions has been studied particularly by Milic-Emili and coworkers (14,17). At functional residual capacity (FRC) in a normal upright subject apical alveoli are more expanded than basal ones, whereas during a quasi static tidal breath the change of the degree of expansion of apical alveoli is less than in basal ones (Fig. 16.1). These circumstances are considered to be due mainly to the weight and elastic properties of the lung itself (14). Thus, apical lung regions are relatively overexpanded due to the traction exerted by the dependent portion of the lung. The basal regions are correspondingly relatively underexpanded. In addition, the pressure volume relationship of the lung is curvilinear in such a way that the lung gets stiffer the more expanded it is. Therefore, a given change in transpulmonary pressure causes the expansion of apical regions to change less than basal ones.

It is apparent from Figure 16.1 that an increased tidal breath does not change the distribution of ventilation. Peripheral airways normally close at a certain low lung volume (9). However, if airway closure occurs above FRC, it is conceivable that some airways may open only when tidal volume is increased. This situation is most likely to occur in an old subject (13) who smokes (8) and is obese (10), because under these circumstances airways close at high lung volumes and the breathing mid-position is reduced. The importance of these factors in changing ventilation distribtuion during exercise is, however, unknown.

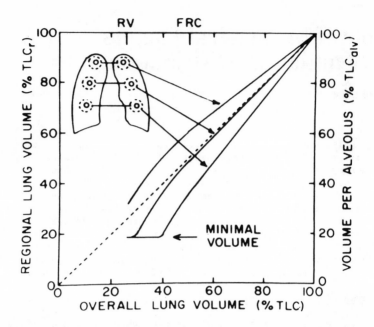

Fig. 16.1 Apical, middle and basal regional lung expansion in relation to overall lung expansion in upright subjects.

Changed Breathing Pattern

Considering various types of exercise it seems likely that the breathing pattern may differ. The breath may be predominantly abdominal or predominantly thoracic and consequently the shape of the thorax-abdomen at any given lung volume may differ. Agostoni and coworkers (1,2) have shown that, e.g. in rabbits, a change of the shape of the thorax can change the distribution of the regional distending pressure. However, in man regional distribution of ventilation seems to be independent of voluntary shape changes (4,5,12) as illustrated in Figure 16.2.

A possible explanation for the discrepancy between results in animals and humans may be the comparatively stiffer thorax in man, not allowing disproportionate change of dimensions (12).

Increased Flow Rate

Regional wash-out rate of a tracer gas has been shown to increase proportionally more in apical regions than in basal ones in seated exercising subjects (7). Otis and collaborators (15) demonstrated that despite equal regional ΔP ventilation dis-

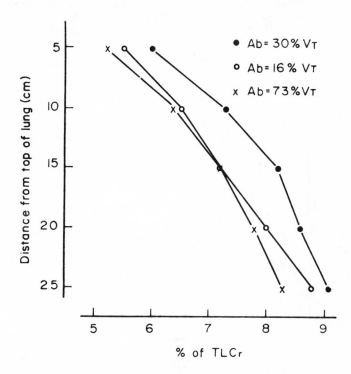

Fig. 16.2 Distribution of a tidal breath (VT) down the lung.
The curves represent mean values from four seated normal subjects.
The abdominal contribution to the tidal volume was voluntarily
varied (Ab = 16% VT; Ab = 30% VT and Ab = 73% VT). The parallel
shift indicates a slightly different size of the average VT's,
whereas the slope of the curves i.e. the ventilation distribution
are unaffected by the breathing process.

tribution among lung regions may change with increasing frequency
of breathing, namely if the regional time constants (i.e. the
products of compliance and resistance) are unequal. Thus, at very
low breathing frequency or at very low flow rate, the regional
elastic properties (i.e. compliances) determine the ventilation
distribution, as has been discussed above. However, at high
breathing frequency or at high flow rates, the resistance of the
airways contributes to determine ventilation distribution. At
FRC in upright position, apical alveoli and presumably also airways
are more expanded than basal ones. Therefore, in apical regions
resistance as well as complicance appears to be less than in basal
regions. With increasing inspiratory flow rate one would there-

fore expect apical regions to receive a proportionately larger
fraction of the inspired air. As illustrated in Figure 16.3,
increase of inspiratory flow makes the regional distribution successively more even (6,16).

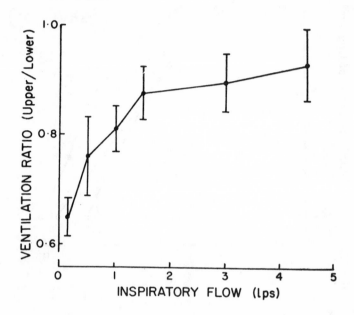

Fig. 16.3 The ratio between upper (apical) and lower (basal)
regional ventilation against inspiratory flow rate in seated
subjects. With increasing flow rates apical and basal ventilation
approach unity.

Contrary to what we would predict the ventilation in apical
regions does not exceed that of basal regions. However, the dead
space may be distributed preferentially to apical regions (11).
One reason for the discrepancy between experimental results and
predictions may be that regional Δ P's are unequal (6). This
hypothesis gains support from measurements in supine position where
there are no differences between apical and basal regions caused
by gravity. The static regional lung volumes were found to be
uneven in the same direction as in upright position (3) and with
increasing inspiratory flow rate apical regional ventilation greatly exceeded that of basal regions (18). Thus it seems likely
that regional Δ P's are unequal, at least under certain conditions. E.g. during swimming it is conceivable that apical ventilation actually exceeds basal, but exercising in upright position
appears only to make ventilation distribution more even.

Summary

Increased tidal volume probably does not change the distribution of ventilation unless airway closure occurs above FRC. Possible changes in the shape of thorax-abdomen associated with breathing during exercise are not predicted to have any effect on regional ventilation distribution. Increased flow rate in upright position makes apical regional ventilation to approach that of basal regions, whereas in supine position ventilation of regions may actually exceed that of basal regions.

REFERENCES

1. Agostoni, E.: Physiol. Rev. 52:57–128, 1972.
2. Agostoni, E. and E. d'Angelo: Respir. Physiol. 12:102–109, 1971.
3. Bake, B., J. Bjure, G. Grimby, J. Milic-Emili, and N.J. Nilsson: Scand. J. Respirat. Dis. 48:189–196, 1967.
4. Bake, B., J. Dempsey and G. Grimby: Amer. Rev. Resp. Dis. in press.
5. Bake, B., A.R. Fugl-Meyer, and G. Grimby: Clin. Sci. 42:117–128, 1972.
6. Bake, B., L. Wood, B. Murphy, P.T. Macklem, and J. Milic-Emili: J. Appl. Physiol. 37:8–17, 1974.
7. Bryan, A.C., L.G. Bentivoglio, F. Beerel, H. MacLeish, A. Zidulka, and D.V. Bates: J. Appl. Physiol. 19:395–402, 1964.
8. Buist, A.S., D.L. Van Fleet, and B.B. Ross: Amer. Rev. Resp. Dis. 107:735–743, 1973.
9. Dollfuss, R.E., J. Milic-Emili, and D.V. Bates: Respiration Physiol. 2:234–246, 1967.
10. Farebrother, M.J.B., G.J.R. McHardy, and J.F. Munroe: Brit. Med. Jour. 10:391–393, 1974.
11. Grant, B.J.B., A. Hazel, H.A. Jones and J.M.B. Hughes: J. Appl Physiol. 37:158–165, 1974.
12. Grassino, A.E., B. Bake, R.R. Martin, and N.R. Anthonisen. J. Appl. Physiol. 39:997–1003, 1975.
13. Leblanc, P., F. Ruff, and J. Milic-Emili: J. Appl. Physiol. 28:448–451, 1970.
14. Milic-Emili, J., J.A.M. Henderson, M.B. Dolovich, D. Trop, and K. Kaneko: J. Appl. Physiol. 21:749–759, 1966.
15. Otis, A.B., C.B. McKerrow, R.A. Bartlett, J. Mean, M.B. McIlroy, N.J. Silverstone, and E.P. Radford: J. Appl. Physiol. 8:427–443, 1956.
16. Robertson, P.W., T. Katsura, and J. Milic-Emili: J. Appl. Physiol. 25:438–443, 1969.
17. Sutherland, P.W., T. Katsura, and J. Milic-Emili: J. Appl. Physiol. 25:566–574, 1968.
18. Sybrecht, G., L. Landau, R. Martin, B. Murphy, L. Engel, J. Milic-Emili, and P.T. Macklen. In press.

DISCUSSION

Kampine: The things that you examined, the change in the breathing
pattern, the change in the lung volumes and the change in the
velocity of flow, would not account for the change in the ventilation during exercise. Could changes in regional blood flow affect
the regional ventilation?

Bake: I think that the main factor changing ventilation distribution during exercise is flow rate or frequency. Hypoventilation
in the bases may cause hypoxic vasoconstriction and not the other
way around.

Dempsey: Bjorn, you showed a similar effect of increasing flow
rate on 133 Xenon distribution in the supine vs. the upright
position. This implies that flow rate affects time constant
distribution which in turn determines the change in Xenon distribution is no longer tenable.

Bake: That is an incomplete description. Otis, et al. (J. Appl.
Physiol. 8:427-443, 1956) could account for the change in compliance with increasing frequency on regional time constant basis
also if Δ P's were everywhere equal. Since then we have tended
not to consider changes in Δ P's because we have not been able to
measure them. However, Δ P's are probably not equal under all
circumstances and small differences may have a large effect on
ventilation distribution.

Kampine: At the plateau part of the curves displaying changes in
flow velocity and the distribution of ventilation, I think that you
were talking about flow velocities that were in the range of 2 to
5 liters per second. These are the kinds of flow velocities that
you do encounter in exercise.

Bake: I can't remember specific measurements on peak flow rates
during exercise, but I think that they would come up in the range
of 3 to 4 liters per second.

Kampine: Are you ever on the plateau area when you are not exercising?

Bake: I think that normally we are operating on the steep part of
that curve. It usually requires exercise to come up to the plateau
of the curve.

Gledhill: We have measured the peak flow rates during exercise and
I would like to respond to the last question. At rest the peak
flow was 0.3 liters per second. During light exercise at a $\dot{V}O_2$
of approximately 1.0 liters per minute peak flow increased to 1.1
liters/sec then at a $\dot{V}O_2$ of approximately 1.5 liters/min and above
the peak flow was in excess of 1.5 liters/sec. This corresponds to
the plateau point on the graph where the apex-base ratio approaches
unity. I believe you said that the apical redistribution of
ventilation seen with increased inspiratory flow rate is due to

the increased alveolar and airway size, and consequent decreased
resistance in the apex. There is recent evidence that differences
in alveolar size exists within a lung slice and I am referring here
to the intraregional differences, not topographical differences.
Can it be expected, therefore, that during exercise the same preferential redistribution of ventilation would occur intraregionally?

Bake: Yes, I would expect that.

Gledhill: And so this would be compatible with an increasing
inhomogeneity within the lung region as opposed to the homogeneity
that you might expect during exercise?

Bake: I wouldn't know about the blood flow though.

Gledhill: Presumably the blood flow is not going to change.

Bake: And assuming that the blood flow is evenly distributed?

Gledhill: Within that region - correct.

Bake: I wouldn't know because if we assume that the distribution
of a slowly inspired breath is compliance determined, then a certain
degree of inhomogeneity may be expected. However, if the airways
within a region are different and the inspired breath during exercise is distributed according to the airways diameter, then intraregional distribution would change. I couldn't tell which inhomogeneity is larger.

Kampine: Aren't we ignoring the fact that the change in the rate
of delivery of acid metabolites during exercise might alter the
caliber of airway smooth muscle and do away with some of the regional
differential that exists ordinarily. Could this be a possible
mechanism for change in the distribution of ventilation during
exercise?

Bake: I do not know. CO_2 tension in airways can affect distribution of ventilation but I do not know if this mechanism is of
any quantitative importance during exercise.

Wasserman: Do you have any data on asthmatics? Since we have to
accomplish a certain amount of ventilation in order to do a given
amount of work, we must affect inspiratory time during exercise.
You showed in normals that the upper-lower distribution of ventilation is very much dependent on inspiratory flow; perhaps,
asthmatics would give a very different picture.

Bake: There are measurements about regional distribution of
ventilation in asthmatics, but not as I am aware of during exercise.
However, the main inhomogeneity is probably intraregional and this
is considered to cause defects in gas exchange. One can't explain
gas exchange in patients on an interregional basis.

Wasserman: Do they have the same time flow pattern?

Bake: I don't know, but I would expect the flow pattern to be different in asthmatics and normal subjects.

Discussion

Kampine: I would like to open the discussion by asking Dr. Coon his views about the primary mechanism of local regulation of airway smooth muscle. We heard some discussion about low PO_2 depravation or hypoxia-hypercarbia and changes in hydrogen ion concentration in the area of smooth muscle as local regulatory features. What is your viewpoint about the primary mechanism or the order in which this regulation occurs?

Coon: I believe from our own studies that the primary regulator is hydrogen ion. Altering the acid-base status of the blood by alternate sodium bicarbonate-lactic acid infusion produced changes in pulmonary mechanics similar to the changes which were observed after acute occlusion of the lobar artery even though alveolar PCO_2 was maintained at less than 5 mmHg.

Sampson: We should keep in mind a couple of other aspects about local changes in hydrogen ion, carbon dioxide and oxygen tension. One of them relates to regulating the sensitivity of afferent nerve endings that could have an important reflex action. Another aspect might relate, not to mediator from mast cells, but to release of acetylcholine from vagal nerve endings. Changes in CO_2 tension or oxygen tension may increase the spontaneous release of neurotransmitter, thereby increasing local smooth muscle tension that could prime sensory receptors in the airways to initiate reflexes. This mechanism might introduce local tone in the muscle that makes the muscle more responsive to other factors that may be released physiologically or pathophysiologically. The variations and permutations are almost endless and should be kept in mind in trying to interpret various findings or in trying to assign a first cause to any particular condition.

Eggleston: I have a question that I hope Dr. Sampson and Dr. Adkinson both will address about the time course of histamine effect on the rapidly adapting receptor. First, why is there a several second delay in onset of effect which doesn't usually apply in a smooth muscle preparation? Second, why does it persist? These receptors rapidly adapt to a stretch stimulus and yet the histamine effect persists for 30 seconds or more unless it is stopped by an abrupt hyperinflation. I wonder specifically whether with abrupt hyperinflation the effect of histamine can be stopped a few seconds after it's applied or whether it must persist at least 30 seconds before the hyperinflation can block it. If there is no hyperinflation, how long does the effect continue?

Sampson: Let me start at the end and work forwards. If we do not hyperinflate the lungs after giving histamine for 30 to 60 seconds the discharge will persist for upwards of 5 to 10 minutes in these receptors. We have never done a precise study of the time course of the effect. It is difficult to control the concentration of histamine at the receptor unlike an _in vitro_ organ bath approach.

233

Even by blowing in an aerosol through a fiberoptic-bronchoscope we
do not know the precise amount that gets there.

The problem of adaptation is a difficult one to discuss. We
refer to rapid adaptation specifically with regards to hyperinflation of the lungs or forced deflation of the lungs. The
mechanisms by which receptors adapt to this stimulus are not fully
understood. One possibility is that mechanical deformation in
the tissues are not transmitted directly to the nerve endings on
a one to one basis. So, for one reason or another, eg. elasticity
or inelasticity of tissue around a nerve ending may limit the
stimulus from being transmitted directly to the receptor ending
for the whole time that we think we are stimulating the receptor
with a maintained hyperinflation. You might have noticed on the
first slide that I showed that when we locate a receptor by
touching an area, the receptor didn't seem to adapt rapidly to
that stimulus. As long as we maintained the touch there was some
stimulation. But, of course, we cannot control how much vibration
we may have on the little cotton tipped applicator we are holding.
We have some additional information from other studies done by a
graduate student, Richard Jaffe, on sensory nerve cells in the
nodose ganglion (Jaffe and Sampson, J. Neurophysiol., 1976, in
press). We recorded intracellularly from the sensory neurons and
passed long depolarizing pulses that were suprathreshold and
caused action potential to be generated. There are different
populations of nerve cells. Some nerve cells discharged only a
single action potential, or two or three, and then were totally
silent throughout the next ten seconds of this maintained super
threshold depolarization. Others responded with a continuous
steady discharge such as you see in slowly adapting stretch
receptors. What I am trying to point out is that the mechanisms
underlying adaptation are not clearly defined. This is particularly
true when we study receptors in the lungs. Let me add that we have
defined them in terms of adaptation induces of Widdicombe (Widdicombe, J.G., J. Physiol. (London) 123:71-104, 1954). Anything
that decreased its firing by 70% or more after one or two seconds
of maintained inflation was classified as rapidly adapting. I am
not so certain as to how meaningful that is.

Remmers: May I make a comment? Together with Dr. Sambrosio, we
have carried out experiments, not unlike yours. We resected the
mucosal site we defined as the receptive field for the irritant
receptor. This eliminated the sensitivity to light touch (and
in a few experiments to local histamine administration), but the
receptor still responded to inflation and deflation with a
rapidly adapting response, suggesting that we may be actually
dealing with two endings or with a bifurcating ending, one superficial in the mucosa and another deep.

Sampson: Many sensory fibers branch quite extensively. We don't
know where they all may go. Some sympathetic afferent fibers have
one ending in the esophagus and another in the pulmonary artery.

But it is also possible that the light touch and histamine sensitivity occur at the generator region of the nerve and the stretch or mechanical deformation at the first node or its equivalent.

Eggleston: Do you feel that the time required for histamine to penetrate to the receptor accounts for the response lag and that the response continues as long as histamine is present? If so, tissue metabolism must be relatively slow.

Sampson: I suppose it penetrates somewhat slowly. I would think it persists. Dr. Kampine raised the question regarding how it constricts smooth muscle; whether it is a calcium dependent phenomenon; I don't know what it does to the nerve endings, I don't know what it does to the tissue around the nerve endings, I don't know what factors it may release that may secondarily excite the ending. There is evidence that cutaneous pain fiber endings are stimulated by histamine, but again, I don't know what the mechanism is.

Fishman: I wonder Dr. Sampson, if I could put to you, and possibly to Dr. Remmers, a question that is puzzling me. You keep calling these inflation, deflation receptors and yet I sense that these are mechanoreceptors. But we provoke the mechanoreceptors with histamine. Do you think these are histaminergic endings or do you believe that the mechanoreceptors are responding non-specifically to histamine? My other question invites your speculation: how do these receptors relate to exercise?

Sampson: You have touched on a very important nerve ending. They are mechanoreceptors, I think. All neurons are not rapidly adapting and are not all sensitive to histamine. About 80% of them are stimulated by histamine. Even application of histamine locally to the other 20% of histamine insensitive receptors was ineffective. So I wouldn't say that they are all histamine sensitive receptors and would agree that they are mechanoreceptors. They are rapidly adapting airway receptors which is the only way we really want to classify them. So I would be happy to call them rapidly adapting mechanoreceptors as a descriptive term to compare them with slowly adapting pulmonary stretch receptors.

How does this all relate to exercise? I don't know yet how these nerve endings relate to overall control of ventilation or of the calibre of the airways. Rapid hyperinflations of the lung increase the activity from these receptors. Perhaps forced rapid inflations of the lungs could increase activity and do something that might be important to exercise. Perhaps local changes in blood gases might do something to these receptors that might be important to exercise. It is important to keep in mind that at the same time we have activity in rapidly adapting receptors we also have increased firing from slowly adapting pulmonary stretch receptors and the more you ventilate the more active they are. I think the clue as to how this all relates to exercise will be

found in how it relates to the control of ventilation and how the
central nervous system decoding processes operate. I think the
central control of respiration is the area in greatest need of
a lot of work and is one of the most difficult areas in neurophysiology, what with the literally thousands and thousands of inputs
that a single respiratory neuron can have.

Kampine: Not to mention the tracheal and laryngeal and other
receptors that are probably activated during exercise as well.
Dr. Yamamoto's approach in thinking about the complexities of
these interactions is correct.

Wasserman: I don't know if Dr. Coon's work addresses the issue
of the exercise or post-exercise bronchoconstriction, but he did
mention that he thought that the bronchoconstriction was primarily
activated by hydrogen ions and I was wondering if Dr. Coon thought
that the hydrogen ion was having a direct effect on the myofibriles
or was it stimulating release of histamine or some other bronchoconstrictor agent or was it acting through some reflex pathway?

Coon: There has been a suggestion that there might be a mediator,
yet the evidence for a mediator is not very strong. In other
smooth muscle areas the pH effect seems to be direct. I did not
give atropine to the preparation I used. Samanek and Aviado
(J. of Appl. Physiol. 22:719-730, 1967) have performed chronic
denervations and demonstrated that an axon reflex is not required
for airway constrictions to occur in response to a reduction in
pulmonary blood flow and the resultant decrease in alveolar PCO_2.

Forster: I would like to ask Dr. Bake how strongly he feels that
the redistribution during exercise is due to the changes in flow
rates?

Bake: I think that the data of Bryan and co-workers (J. Appl.
Physiol. 19:395-402, 1964) can be accounted for almost exclusively
by increased flow rates.

Dempsey: Dr. Bake, do you feel that in a healthy person, breathing
normally at rest or with moderate exercise, the predominate or the
only thing determining distribution of ventilation and airway
calibre, are mechanical and physical factors? Is there a tone to
smooth muscle that is physiologically important?

Bake: The way I look at this is that the basic framework is the
mechanical factors, such as resistance and compliance, and the
driving force to any given region, but upon that, act those
mechanisms which might regulate compliance or resistance. There
is a tone in airways normally, but I don't know its importance.

Kampine: But how does the tone get there? What is it dependent upon? If there is some tonic level of parasympathetic activity in the control of airway calibre there has to be something putting it there.

Cropp: Perhaps I look at this problem too naively; however, I feel that there is a fundamental need for vascular as well as airway tone. The purpose of the lung is gas exchange in the most efficient way possible, and that depends on matching of ventilation with perfusion. While the tone in the airways as well as in the pulmonary circulation may normally not be very high, it probably serves to maintain good ventilation-perfusion matching. Whenever we disturb this matching by disease, the effects are maldistribution or mismatching of ventilation and perfusion because tone is too high in either the vascular or bronchial tree. Abnormal ventilation-perfusion relations can be brought about by pulmonary vasoconstriction in response to hypoxia, or by bronchoconstriction in consequence to airway irritation as a lack of perfusion. Smooth muscle tone in pulmonary arterioles and bronchioles is aimed to maintain ventilation-perfusion matching at an optimum.

Dr. Kampine, I was surprised that you said that there was no innervation of terminal respiratory bronchiolar and alveolar ducts.

Kampine: No functional innervation.

Cropp: We must accept, however, that there is innervation. This was recently reviewed by Murray (Murray, J.F., The Normal Lung, W.B. Saunders Comp., Philadelphia, 1976), and the physiological evidence suggests that there is both sympathetic and parasympathetic innervation down to alveolar ducts.

Kampine: The studies by Nadel and Widdicombe fail to disclose a functional innervation. I think the nerves are there, but the role they play remains to be determined.

Godfrey: Dr. Bake, I was fascinated by the fact that when those subjects lay horizontally the effect of inspiratory flow rate on maldistribution was exaggerated. It occurred to me that what you are showing is due to the inertia of the abdominal contents - back to the "sloshing guts" again. In the horizontal position this might be more exaggerated so that, in fact, with a fast inspiratory rate you may not be able to expand the lower part of the thorax as rapidly as the upper part because of the inertia of the abdominal contents. I wondered what you thought about that?

Bake: Firstly, those data are not mine. The study was done by Sybrechl et al. in Montreal (to be published). As to the mechanism, I can only speculate. If inertia of the abdomen were the cause, I would expect that breathing more or less with the abdomen and diaphragm would have an influence on ventilation distribution, whereas we have shown that it did not within the range we studied. I would not expect inability to move the diaphragm down at a sufficient speed to have any effect on the apex to base distribution.

Godfrey: But I don't believe you have actually looked at the rib cage versus abdomen with speed of inspiration.

Bake: No, we haven't.

Godfrey: That is critical - perhaps Dr. Goldman might be able to say something about it.

Goldman: I don't have any data of my own, but I believe that Dr. Bake's co-workers in Montreal have begun to look at that. The suggestion made by Dr. Bake and re-enforced by Jerry Dempsey makes one tend to think that an explanation based on time constant distribution doesn't give one the whole answer. One alternative explanation might be local change in transpulmonary pressure being different in different areas. I think the recent evidence from Montreal (and I have only heard it described in a casual discussion) supports that possibility after looking at the separate volume displacements of rib cage and abdomen.

Dempsey: What is the normal physiologic function of bronchial smooth muscle? Certainly the mechanical factors and the tone are probably both important. Dr. Cropp gave a lot of nice examples, all of them in diseased lungs or breathing hypoxic gases or noxious agents. During change in posture, talking, exercise and other activities is the smooth muscle playing a role that can't be handled by the mechanical and physical factors determining calibre and distribution?

Kampine: Can you design an experiment to eliminate smooth muscle activity?

Dempsey: That is a good question John, I would like you to answer it.

Kampine: I don't think you can because after removal and reimplantation of a lung which covers all neural pathways, the smooth muscles still have hypersensitivity to humoral factors.

Cropp: I think that the experiment has been done. Severinghaus occluded a pulmonary artery many years ago and the ventilation in that part of the lung was almost down to zero - at least it became very low (Severinghaus, J.W., E.W. Swenson, T.N. Finley, M.T. Lategola and J. Williams, J. Appl. Physiol. 16:53, 1961).

Kampine: He is asking about physiologic regulation, I think.

Cropp: My point is that physiological regulation is there to
provide us with a mechanism to withstand insults. We are not living
in an environment totally without insults and, therefore, we have
to have reserve mechanisms to adjust our physiology to adverse
situations.

Sampson: Do we come back to Barcroft's locomotive in trying to
answer this type of question?

Reed: Dr. Sampson or Dr. Adkinson do either the nervous system
or these chemical mediators act sufficiently locally to control
regional areas of the lungs? For example, will stimulation of a
rapidly adapting receptor in an airway constrict just that airway
or does it affect the rest of the lung as well?

Sampson: I would imagine that it would affect the rest of the
lung if one could do that type of experiment. The closest thing
that comes to it perhaps are the divided lung studies of Gold and
associates (Gold, W.M., G.F. Kessler and D.Y.C. Yu, J. Appl.
Physiol. 33:719-725, 1972) who gave antigen to one lung and produced reflex bronchoconstriction in the opposite lung. I can't
imagine that the local control is so finely tuned to be able to
govern what goes on in an individual airway.

Kampine: Widdicombe's review indicates that histamine applied to
pleural surface of one lung can cause bronchoconstriction which
is reflexly mediated in the opposite lung. The reflex requires
an intact vagus and is abolished by atropine so that I think there
is good evidence that local application of humoral substances have
an effect, not only in that particular area but can have widespread
influences.

Adkinson: I would like to comment about the converse of that
situation. That there is also the possibility of relatively
regional effects of some of the mediators. Some of the mediators
when infused either into the pulmonary circulation or given by
aerosol will have differential effects on smooth muscle at various
levels of the respiratory tree. Bradykinin (and perhaps that means
prostaglandins) tends to have very peripheral effects down to the
level of the alveolar duct. I would like to comment on the converse of that situation; namely, that there is also the possibility
for restriction of the activity of some mediators to certain regions
of the respiratory tree. For example, Drazen and Austen (J. Clin.
Invest. 53:1679-1685, 1974) have shown that in the guinea pig intravenous SRS-A preferentially affects peripheral airway diameter when
compared with histamine and $PGF_{2\alpha}$. Newball and Keiser (J. Appl.
Physiol. 35:552-556, 1973) have provided evidence that in man
Bradykinin may act principally at the level of the alveolar duct.
Histamine, on the other hand, produces constriction of both large
and small airways. There appear to exist, therefore, differential
regional effects for various chemical mediators in the lung.

These observations suggest the potential for regional restriction
of airway responses to some stimuli, whereas histamine tends to
have a broader effect constricting central or peripheral airways
depending upon the route of administration. Slow reacting
substance of anaphylaxis again acts more peripherally. So,
there is the opportunity for these humoral mediators to have
differential effects presumably on the basis of relative receptor
specificity of smooth muscle in various portions of the lung.

Wasserman: I just want to add a function of the smooth muscle in
the airways besides that for optimization of gas exchange that
Dr. Cropp mentioned. It is probably also very important in the
clearance of foreign materials by increasing the velocity of air
flow secondary to airway narrowing. Essentially, it assists the
cough mechanism.

Part IV
Exercise-Induced Bronchospasm

17

Exercise-Induced Bronchospasm: Introduction

E. R. McFadden, Jr.

Because bronchial asthma is such a common disorder, one would think that it would be possible to describe its pathophysiology and immunobiology with great precision. Unfortunately, despite the large amount of work that has been accomplished this is not yet the case. Many aspects of this disease continue to remain poorly understood particularly that of the phenomena of exercise-induced bronchospasm. The attraction in investigating this aspect of asthma is that it is a way of producing acute exacerbations of this disease without having to resort to pharmacologic or immunologic interventions that introduce the question of the relationship of the evoked response to that which occurs spontaneously. Consequently it would appear to be an ideal system in which to study the pathophysiology of asthma in general. Unfortunately its utility remains compromised because of the many unresolved issues that surround it.

One of the earlier reports that physical exertion could alter pulmonary function in asthmatic patients in the absence of other exogenous factors such as infection, or exposure to antigens, or irritants, was made by Herxheimer in 1946 (15). At that time he postulated that the cause was due to lactic acid stimulating excess ventilation which resulted in a decrease in carbon dioxide stores and hypocapnia and that the latter was the stimulus for bronchoconstriction. Subsequently post-exercise asthma has been studied by many investigators, and a considerable number of alternative explanations have been proposed. A brief review of the literature reveals that increased minute ventilation with stimulation of mechanoreceptors (6,13,28,31,36), hypocapnia (15,9,10,36,39), abnormalities of oxygen transport (3,18), lactic acidosis (6,10,29,38), various metabolic imbalances (4,12) and release of humoral factors (23) have all been incriminated as being the mechanism responsible for this phenomenon.

In addition to the above controversies, or perhaps as a result of them, there has been conflicting evidence put forth regarding the efficacy of various drugs in preventing the occurrence of exercise-induced asthma. Attempts to block its onset with disodium cromoglycate have been reported as being uniformly successful (8,20, 24), partially successful (25,27,39), successful in only some patients (16,32) and unsuccessful (33). Likewise, isoproterenol has been found to be efficacious in some instances but not in others (7,17,20,35) and varying protection has been found with salbutamol

(20,25), atropine (6,10,17,23,31,36), corticosteroids (23) and carbon dioxide (1,6,9,10,13,28,36,38). Some of the possible reasons for this confusion have to do with the following interrelated factors. Until relatively recently, detailed investigations of the extent and types of changes that occurred in pulmonary mechanics were not available, and most studies predefined what a response would be by stating that there had to be a 10 to 25% fall in some index of forced exhalation. Application of these criteria gave rise to the speculation that exercise was a unique stimulus that caused airway narrowing in only selected individuals. However as more data became available it became apparent that not all aspects of lung function need to change at the same rate during either remission or induction of asthma (5,22,21) and more authorities now feel that exercise may just be one of many non-antigenic provocations that will trigger acute exacerbations in the general asthmatic population. Although the precise incidence is still unknown, data are available that indicate that if multiple aspects of lung function are examined, exercise appears to be a general stimulus that produces some alteration in lung function in all asthmatics if the physical task being performed is sufficiently stressful (14,37).

The second source of variation has to do with the fact that the stimulus response relationship has not yet been precisely defined, and because of this multiple exercise tasks have been employed to date. The types of provocation used have included ascending and descending stairs (10,23), running or walking along corridors (2, 11,28), treadmill running (3,9,14,38), treadmill walking at constant speed and incline (9,32,33,35), cycling on an ergometer (3, 4,6,10,12,18,30, 36-38) and swimming (11). Very few investigations have compared different methods, but from the available data it appears that running evokes responses more frequently and of greater severity than does cycling or swimming (2,11). In addition considerable emphasis has been laid on the fact that the duration of exercise should last for 8 to 10 minutes. The reasons for the above differences are unknown, but because of this great heterogeneity of stimuli, one can not be certain that the conclusions drawn from any given investigation necessarily apply to all patients with this problem.

The final factor, and perhaps the most important of all, is that the literature is unclear as to the reproducibility of post-exercise asthma. The work of McNeil and colleagues (23) and Chan-Yeung et al. (6) suggest that in some patients repeated exercise on the same day lessens the response, but the data of others are at variance with this (10,18,26,27,30). Obviously if it were true that the response progressively decreased over the course of a day, it would be quite difficult to place any meaningful interpretation on the results of successively performed studies, particularly if they were being performed to test the effects of various therapeutic interventions.

The papers contained in this section have bearing on one or more of the above issues. It is hoped that they will bring into focus

newer insights that will allow for a better understanding of this
perplexing problem.

REFERENCES

1. Allen, T.W., W. Addington, T. Rosendal, and D.W. Cugell. Amer.
   Rev. Resp. Dis. 107:816-821, 1973.
2. Anderson, S.D., N.W. Connolly and S. Godfrey. Thorax 26:396-
   401, 1971.
3. Anderson, S.D., M. Silverman, and S.R. Walker. Thorax 27:
   718-725, 1972.
4. Barboriak, J.J., A.J. Sosman, J.N. Fink, M.G. Maksud, L.H.
   McConnell, and L.H. Hamilton. Clin. Allergy 3:83-89, 1973.
5. Cade, J.F., A.J. Woolcock, A.S. Rebuck, and M.C.F. Pain. Clin.
   Sci. 40:381-391, 1971.
6. Chan-Yeung, M.M.W., M.N. Vyas, and S. Grzybowski. Amer. Rev.
   Resp. Dis. 104:915-923, 1971.
7. Crompton, G.K. Thorax 23:165-167, 1968.
8. Davies, S.E. Brit. Med. J. 3:593-594, 1968.
9. Ferguson, A., W. Addington, and E.A. Gaensler. Ann. Int. Med.
   71:1063-1072, 1969.
10. Fisher, H.K., P. Holton, R.St.J. Buxton, and J.A. Nadel. Amer.
    Rev. Resp. Dis. 101:885-896, 1970.
11. Fitch, K.D., and A.R. Morton. Brit. Med. J. 4:577-581, 1971.
12. Griffiths, J., F.Y. Leung, S. Gryzbowski, and M.M.W. Chan-
    Yeung. Chest 62:527-533, 1972.
13. Hafez, F.F., and G.K. Crompton. Brit. J. Dis. Chest 62:41-45
    1968.
14. Haynes, R.L., R.H. Ingram, Jr., and E.R. McFadden, Jr. Amer.
    Rev. Resp. Dis. Submitted for publication.
15. Herxheimer, H. Lancet 1:83-87, 1946.
16. Jones, R.S. and M.I. Blackhall. Arch. Dis. Child 45:49-53,
    1970.
17. Jones, R.S., M.J. Wharton, and M.H. Busted. Arch. Dis. Child
    38:539-545, 1963.
18. Katz, R.M., B.J. Whipp, E.M. Heimlich, and K. Wasserman. J.
    Allergy 47:148-158, 1971.
19. Kjellman, B. Scand. J. Resp. Dis. 50:41-51, 1969.
20. McCarthy, O.R. Brit. J. Dis. Chest 66:133-140, 1972.
21. McFadden, E.R., Jr., R. Kiser, and W.J. deGroot. N. Eng. J.
    Med. 288:221-225, 1973.
22. McFadden, E.R., Jr., and H.A. Lyons. J. Appl. Physiol. 27:
    452-459, 1969.
23. McNeil, R.S., J.R. Nairn, J.S. Millar, and C.G. Ingram. Quart
    J. Med. 35:55-67, 1966.
24. Muittari, A., and K-E. Kepus. Brit. Med. J. 4:170, 1969.
25. Palmer, K.N.V. and J.S. Legge. Lancet 2:219, 1969.
26. Pierson, W.E., C.W. Bierman, and S.J. Stamm. J. Allergy 4:
    136-144, 1969.

27. Poppius, H., A. Muittari, K.E. Kreus, O. Korhonen and A.
     Viljanen. Brit. Med. J. 4:337-339, 1970.
28. Rebuck, A.S. and J. Read. Lancet 1:429-431, 1968.
29. Seaton, A., G. Davies, D. Gaziano, and R.O. Hughes. Brit.
     Med. J. 3:556-558, 1969.
30. Silverman, M. and S.D. Anderson. Arch. Dis. Child 47:882-
     889, 1972.
31. Simonsson, B.G., B.E. Skoogh and B. Ekstrom-Jodal. Thorax
     27:169-180, 1972.
32. Sly, R.M. Ann. Allergy 29:362-366, 1971.
33. Sly, R.M. Ann. Allergy 28:299-306, 1970.
34. Sly, R.M. Ann. Allergy 28:1-16, 1970.
35. Sly, R.M., E.M. Heimlich, R.J. Busser and L. Strick. Ann.
     Allergy 25:324-327, 1967.
36. Stanescu, D.C. and D.B. Teculescu. Respiration 27:377-383,
     1970.
37. Strauss, R.H., R.L. Haynes, R.H. Ingram, Jr. and E.R.
     McFadden, Jr. J. Appl. Physiol. Submitted for publication.
38. Vassallo, C.L., J.B.L. Gee and B.M. Domm. Amer. Rev. Resp.
     Dis. 105:42-49, 1972.
39. Ward, F.G., S. Gomes, R.S. McNeil. Brit. Med. J. 2:176-
     177, 1969.

18

Clinical Variables
of Exercise-Induced Bronchospasm

Simon Godfrey

Effort intolerance or shortness of breath on exertion is
common to many types of cardiac and pulmonary disease but the
reaction of the asthmatic to exercise is rather different because
exercise acts as a non-specific trigger mechanism for provoking a
brief attack of asthma. This phenomenon of exercise-induced
asthma (EIA) was documented as early as the 17th century (26), but
has only attracted scientific study in the past few years when it
was realized that EIA could provide clues to mechanisms operating
in clinical asthma. Although EIA is probably a safer term since
the mechanical events leading to airways obstruction are not certain, the speed of its onset and remission make it almost certain
that spasm of bronchial smooth muscle is the major contributory
factor.

It has sometimes been implied that EIA is a disease entity
in its own right and that some patients only become symptomatic
in response to exercise. However, there is a very considerable
body of evidence that true EIA only occurs in asthmatics and careful enquiry or investigation will reveal that the patient currently
or previously has had other episodes of reversible airways obstruction. Although it is tempting to equate EIA with clinical asthma,
especially from the point of view of drug trials, there are some
important differences which will be discussed later.

The physiological mechanisms underlying EIA are considered
more fully elsewhere in this symposium but the basic profile of
changes in lung mechanics are very characteristic and can be
documented quite simply by measurements of peak expiratory flow
(PEFR) as shown in Figure 18.1. Provided the exercise test is of
an appropriate type there is initially some bronchodilation during
the exercise period which is more marked if the resting level of
lung function is reduced (24). Towards the end of a 6-minute test,
PEFR begins to fall but the severe, rapid reduction only occurs
after exercise has ceased so that EIA is really post-exercise
induced asthma. The lowest levels of PEFR are usually reached
about 1 to 3 minutes after exercise in children and a minute or
two later in adults. The attack then starts to wear off spontaneously and PEFR has usually returned to the pre-exercise level by
20 to 30 minutes after exercise. At any stage the attack can be
rapidly aborted by giving an aerosol bronchodilator.

247

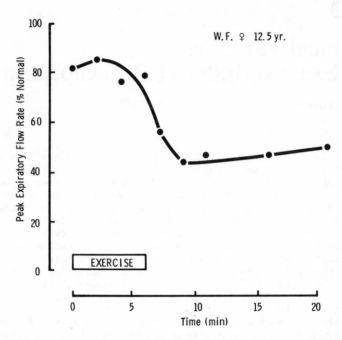

Fig. 18.1. Typical pattern of exercise induced bronchospasm provoked by six minutes of running in an asthmatic child. During
exercise, there is initially a rise in peak expiratory flow rate
(PEFR). This is followed by a fall in peak in PEFR which reaches
its lowest point at the height of the attack of exercise induced
asthma shortly after the stopping of the running and the attack
then begins to wear off spontaneously.

For simple, practical purposes the response to exercise can
be quantitated in terms of the percentage rise in PEFR (or similar
index) during exercise and the percentage fall after exercise
compared with the resting pre-exercise level (11). In any individual the percentage fall remains reasonably independent of the
resting level, but for comparative purposes it is wisest to use
only those tests which commence from similar baseline levels.

Exercise-Induced Bronchial Reactivity in Normal Subjects and Asthmatics

In order to evaluate the bronchial reactivity of asthmatics
to exercise it is necessary to know the reactivity to be expected
from normal subjects and the use of arbitrary criteria such as a
post-exercise fall of 20% is clearly unscientific. Because of the
importance of the nature of the exercise (see later) only those
tests in normal subjects using highly asthmagenic exercise can be

used for determining normal ranges and such data are relatively
scarce. We recently reviewed the available information (1) and it
appeared that the post-exercise fall in normal subjects was between
8 and 14%. Using highly standardized treadmill exercise in normal
adults and children we obtained the values shown in Table 18.1.
In an extensive study of school children who were not only themselves healthy but were also not closely related to asthmatics,
Burr et al. (5) found that 92% of them had a post-exercise fall in
PEFR of less than 10% and 98% had a fall of less than 15%. In
fact many normal subjects do not have any fall in PEFR after exercise. If, after a technically adequate test, the subject has a
fall in PEFR greater than 10% it is probable that he is a current
or recent asthmatic and if the fall is over 15% it is almost
certain.

While a sufficient post-exercise fall in PEFR is diagnostic
of asthma, it is not certain that the absence of such a fall pre-
cludes asthma. There have been few systematic studies of the
incidence of EIA in known asthmatics especially in adults who
rarely take enough exercise to provoke significant bronchospasm.
Those who have studied adults have generally found them just as
labile as children (Fitch, personal communication, 1976). More
information is available about children and the inability to
demonstrate EIA has been suggested as a reason for reconsidering
the diagnosis (13). In a series of 107 clinically asthmatic
children tested in my department, we found that 89% had a post-
exercise fall greater than 10%. When the 11% of non-responders
were retested, the overall incidence of abnormal tests rose to
91%. In a further small proportion the percentage fall was just
in the normal range but the total lability (percentage rise during
exercise plus percentage fall after exercise) was abnormal.
Admittedly the children attending our clinic tend to be drawn from
the more troublesome end of the spectrum of asthma but this high
incidence was seen almost as often amongst our milder bronchodilator-controlled children (83%) as amongst our severe steroid-
dependent group (93%). It must be stressed that this high
incidence can only be expected following a highly asthmagenic
type of exercise and lesser stresses will inevitably produce a
lower incidence of abnormal results.

EIA occurs in asthmatics and not in entirely healthy subjects
but abnormal total bronchial lability has been found in various
other groups of subjects. Any condition such as chronic bronchitis
or cystic fibrosis in which there is bronchial inflammation might
be expected to result in increased bronchial tone and hence to have
an element of reversibility. Exercise tests in such patients
have indeed shown increased bronchial lability which consists
mostly of bronchodilation during exercise and with very little
post-exercise bronchoconstriction (6,25). The contrast between
the pattern of lability in asthmatic children and those with
cystic fibrosis can be seen in Figure 18.2.

Of more theoretical interest was the finding that adults who
had asthma in childhood but were no longer symptomatic still
manifested increased bronchial lability (5), as did healthy ex-

	% Rise in PEFR During Exercise ± SEM	% Fall in PEFR After Exercise ± SEM	Number of Subjects
Treadmill			
Children	8.2 ± 0.7	3.5 ± 0.7	60
Adults	6.6 ± 0.9	3.2 ± 0.5	22
Cycling			
Children	11.6 ± 4.1	1.0 ± 3.0	9
Adults	8.2 ± 1.5	3.1 ± 0.8	8

Table 18.1. Changes in peak expiratory flow rate in healthy adults and children during and after treadmill and cyclogometer exercise (from the data of Anderson et al., Brit. J. Dis. Chest. 69:1-39, 1975).

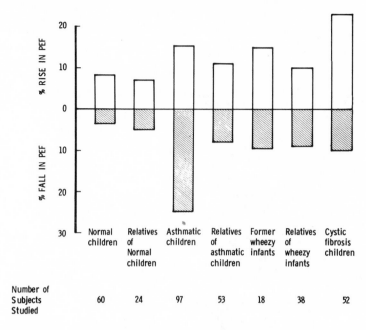

Fig. 18.2. Pattern of bronchial lability in response to exercise in various groups of subjects studied by the author and other investigators. The bronchodilation during exercise is shown as the percentage rise in peak expiratory flow rate (PEF) above the line and the exercise induced asthma is shown as the percent fall in PEF below the line. Only the asthmatic subjects developed severe post exercise bronchoconstriction (from Godfrey, S., Exercise testing in Children, W.B. Saunders, London, 1974).

wheezy babies (16). Increased lability has also been found amongst healthy close relatives of asthmatic children and wheezy babies (17,18). Once again, the pattern of lability in these relatives of wheezy children was predominantly bronchodilation during exercise with little post-exercise constriction (Fig. 18.2). True EIA has only been seen in current or recently active asthmatics. The evidence suggests that increased bronchial lability rather than clinical asthma is inherited and we have found increased lability even in clinically healthy monozygotic twins of asthmatic patients (19). Wheezy babies seem to come from similar stock to asthmatic children and since only a small proportion of the babies go on to become asthmatic children (4). It is probable that some environmental effect (e.g. viral infection) converts the pattern of bronchial lability to the dominant bronchoconstriction seen in active asthma.

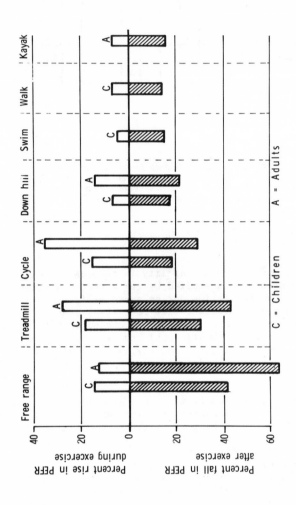

Fig. 18.3. Response of asthmatic subjects to different types of exercise of similar relative severity. The format is similar to that used in the previous illustration. The data has been collected from various published studies (from Fitch K.D. and Godfrey, S., J. Amer. Med. Assoc. in Press, 1976).

Response to Different Types and Patterns of Exercise

Sir John Floyer (10) reported that different types of exercise
caused different amounts of EIA, but for many years it was generally assumed that this was because the severity of exercise was
also different. However, a review of published data about
exercise testing strongly suggested that EIA was more severe and
more frequently demonstrable after running than after other types
of exercise (1). Formal studies have now been carried out comparing different types of exercise of similar physiological
intensity (2,8) and the results of a number of such investigations
are summarized in Figure 18.3. It can be seen that free range
running was the most potent stimulus and on average resulted in
some 47% fall in PEFR after exercise. Treadmill running was a
little less potent, causing a 33% fall in this series and cycling
was even less asthmagenic resulting in a 25% fall. Swimming,
kayak paddling and walking, even when strenuous enough to require
the same oxygen consumption as running, caused very little asthma
resulting in only a 13-15% fall. The implications of these
observations are important not just in terms of physiology and
the results to be expected from exercise tests, but also for the
everyday life of the asthmatic and especially for children. It
means that the asthmatic is unlikely to be able to compete with
his peers in running events unless he take prophylactic medication, but should do reasonably well in swimming. We have recently
reviewed the subject of the athlete with asthma (9) and noted that
several Olympic gold medals have been won by asthmatics, but all in
swimming events. Until this year doping regulations forbade all
potent sympathomimetic drugs which are the most effective in sup-
pressing EIA leaving only Cromolyn sodium which is less effective
(12), but it is understood that the Olympic authorities now permit
the use of the selective beta adrenergic agent, Salbutamol.
    The severity of EIA depends not only on the type of exercise
but also on the duration, power output, steady or progressive
nature of the test and the interval between serial exercise tests.
Clinical experience has shown that brief exercise or intermittent
exercise, even if quite severe, may be quite well tolerated while
more persistent exercise lasting 6 to 8 minutes usually provokes
troublesome EIA. Paradoxically, even longer exercise lasting 15
to 20 minutes or more is often well tolerated and the asthmatic
finds he is able to "run through" his asthma. Formal studies were
carried out to document these observations in the author's laboratory (22) by having groups of children run for different times
at a constant work level or for 6 minutes at different work levels.
The results are summarized in Figures 18.4 and 18.5. It can be
seen that the severity of EIA (post-exercise percentage fall)
increased with the duration of the preceding exercise period up
to about 6 to 8 minutes. With longer tests the mean percentage
fall tended to decrease because some patients failed to develop
EIA after a 12 to 16 minute run even through they had regularly
done so with shorter runs. When the children exercised for 6
minutes at different treadmill gradients, it was found that a

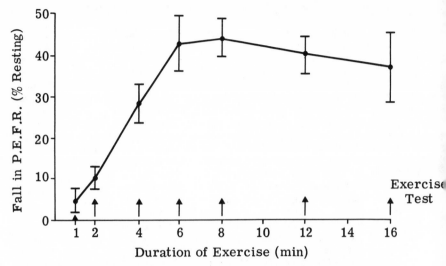

Fig. 18.4.   Effect of duration of exercise on asthma induced by
running at constant speed and slope.   Each point represents the
mean of tests in ten subjects who performed each duration of exercise on a separate occasion (from Godfrey, S., Exercise testing
in children, W.B. Saunders, London, 1974).

maximum amount of EIA was produced when their heart-rates reached
about 180 beats per minute (rather less in adults) and their
oxygen consumption was about 70% of their maximum oxygen uptake.
Later studies have suggested that short, very severe exercise may
produce as much EIA as moderately long, less severe exercise
provided the total oxygen consumed by the subject is about 200
ml/kg in less than 8 minutes.

It is desirable to repeat exercise tests, especially when
studying the effects of drugs (23) but early reports suggested
that once EIA had been provoked a second test had less effect (21).
In these studies the interval between tests was sometimes as short

A popular test for EIA consists of having the patient run up
and down stairs, but downhill running does not provoke much EIA and
so this test is a combination of high and low asthmagenic work so
that the results are unpredictable.   Likewise, the use of progressively increasing work-loads either on a cycle ergometer or a
treadmill results in prolonged tests with the possibility of the
patient exhausting the constrictor mechanism (see below) and in
effect running or riding through his asthma.   Although individual
studies have reported EIA with stair running or progressive exercise, careful comparison of the results show that a smaller proportion of subjects develop EIA and those who do so develop less
than when a single steady level of asthmagenic exercise is used.

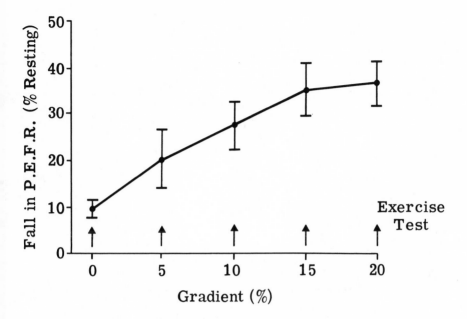

Fig. 18.5.   Effect of gradient on asthma induced by treadmill
running at a constant speed for six minutes.   Each point represents
the mean of tests in nine subjects who performed each gradient on
a separate occasion (from Godfrey, S., Exercise testing in children,
W.B. Saunders, London, 1974).

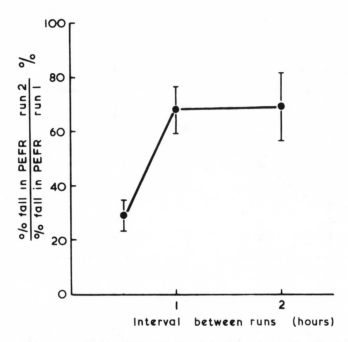

Fig. 18.6. The effect of interval between exercise tests on the
severity of exercise induced asthma. The percentage fall in peak
expiratory flow rate in the second of each pair of tests is
expressed as a fraction of the fall in the first test. The points
represent the mean and SEM for a group of six children who carried
out each pair of tests on different days.

as 45 minutes and our own investigations showed that the mechanism
had usually recovered if 2 hours were left between tests. In order
to demonstrate this more fully we have subsequently carried out
exercise tests after varying intervals in a group of asthmatic
children (7) and the results of these studies are summarized in
Figure 18.6. It can be seen that the severity of EIA in the second
test depended on the time that had elapsed since the first and
that after 1 to 2 hours the first test had only a moderate affect
on the second. The time taken for the mechanism producing EIA to
recover varied somewhat from child to child. When we reduced the
amount of EIA produced in the first test by lowering the workload, then the second test was able to provoke EIA after a
shorter interval.
        These observations could be explained by exercise release of a
stored mediator from mast cells which then caused bronchospasm
either by direct action on bronchial smooth muscle or possibly
by stimulating vagal receptors. The effect of this mediator is

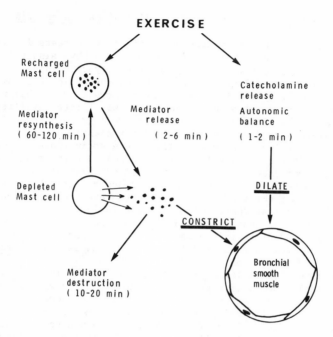

Fig. 18.7. Hypothetical scheme to describe the effect of exercise
on the asthmatic patient. During exercise, there is a balance
between the bronchodilator effect of increased sympathetic drive
and the constrictor effect of mediator released from mast cells.
On stopping exercise the constrictor effect dominates to produce
the exercise induced asthma. The suggested times taken to release,
metabolize and resynthesize mediator are indicated.

antagonized during exercise by the concurrent increase in sympathetic activity (Fig. 18.7) and therefore it only becomes effective
on stopping exercise when sympathetic activity falls off – hence
the post-exercise fall in PEFR. This mediator is also metabolized
quite quickly so that if the subject has "run through" his asthma.
The resynthesis of mediator also takes time and hence a second
test will be less effective during this refractory period. Returning to athletics and sports in general, a low-intensity warm-up
period may well serve to "discharge" the mast cells, so that the
subsequent strenuous exercise is no longer asthmagenic. Likewise
prolonged alternating hard and light exercise (e.g. football)
may be quite well tolerated because the mast cells are never fully
recharged.

The Relation Between Severity of Clinical Asthma and EIA

Because of the diagnostic value of exercise tests in differentiating asthma from other conditions attempts have also been made to relate the severity of EIA to the severity of clinical asthma. Jones (14) proposed 3 groups of asthma on the basis of total bronchial lability and found that these correlated roughly with clinical severity but we have found the use of total lability complicates the picture. When children were grouped according to their maintenance drug requirements after stabilization, we found that post-exercise percentage fall was higher in those on continuous prophylactic therapy (cromolyn sodium) than those who just needed intermittant bronchodilators, and was highest in the steroid-dependent group (1). This work has recently been extended and the results obtained from 116 children are shown in Figure 18.8. It can be seen that there is an increase in lability with increase in severity of asthma as defined by maintenance treatment required and in fact 70% of steroid-dependent children had a post-exercise fall greater than 30% while 74% of mild bronchodilator-controlled children had a fall less than 30%.

We have also followed the pattern of bronchial lability in longitudinal studies of a group of asthmatic children (3) carried out over a 4 to 6 year period. During this time some of the children became clinically more severe and some became less severe and even "grew out" of their asthma and there was no evidence of significant loss of lability so far even in those children growing out of their asthma. We conclude from these studies that while bronchial lability is essential for the development of asthma, environmental factors or altered host responsiveness to them probably determine the clinical pattern.

In the pharmacological field there are some important differences between clinical asthma and EIA. While both clinical attacks and EIA are responsive to bronchodilators and both can largely be prevented by prophylactic use of cromolyn sodium (12), clinical asthma also responds to steroid therapy while EIA rarely does so (20). In this context, as well as in the speed of its onset and remission, EIA resembles acute antigen-induced asthma and it seems quite possible that both antigen and exercise act through the final common pathway of the mast cell. Clinical asthma may involve other mechanisms as well, especially inflammatory reactions, and caution is therefore needed before extrapolating directly from EIA (or antigen challenge) to the clinical situation.

Summary

Exercise results in bronchospasm in asthmatic subjects which is most intense shortly after stopping. The severity of this exercise-induced asthma depends upon the nature of the exercise, running being the most potent stimulus, its duration and intensity.

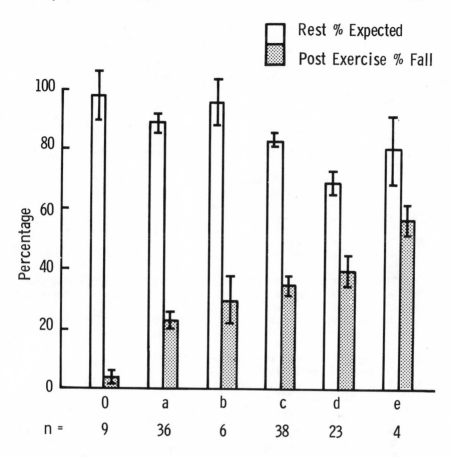

Fig. 18.8. Resting peak expiratory flow rate as percent expected and the severity of exercise induced asthma expressed as the percent fall in peak expiratory flow rate in the various groups of subjects indicated. The heights of the columns show the mean and SEM. Group 0 = children subsequently shown not to have asthma, A = asthmatic children controlled by bronchodilators alone, B = children needing occasional steroids, C = children on continuous prophylaxis with cromolyn sodium, D = children needing continuous aerosol steroid therapy, and E = children on regular oral steroid therapy.

Increased total bronchial lability is found amongst close relatives
of asthmatics but they do not develop the severe post-exercise
constriction. The intensity of exercise-induced asthma reflects
the clinical status of the patient but there are differences
between clinical and exercise-induced attacks.

REFERENCES

1. Anderson, S.D., M. Silverman, and S. Godfrey. Brit. J. Dis.
    Chest. 69:1-39, 1975.
2. Anderson, S.D., N. Connolly, and S. Godfrey. Thorax. 26:396-
    401, 1971.
3. Balfour-Lynn, L., M. Tooley, and S. Godfrey. Longitudinal
    studies of bronchial lability in asthmatic children. In
    preparation, 1976.
4. Boesen, I. Acta Paediatrica, 42:87-96, 1953.
5. Burr, M.L., B.A. Eldridge, and L.K. Borysiewicz. Arch. Dis.
    Childh. 49:923-926, 1974.
6. Day, G., and M.B. Mearns. Arch. Dis. Childh. 48:355-359,
    1973.
7. Edmunds, A.T., M. Tooley, and S. Godfrey. Exercise-induced
    asthma following serial exercise tests in asthmatic children.
    In preparation, 1976.
8. Fitch, K.D., and A.R. Morton. Brit. Med. J. 4:577-581, 1971.
9. Fitch, K.D., and S. Godfrey. J. Amer. Med. Assoc., in press,
    1976.
10. Floyer, Sir John. A Treatise of the Asthma, R. Wilkin &
    W. Innis, London, 1698.
11. Godfrey, S., M. Silverman, and S. Anderson. J. Allergy Clin.
    Immunol. 52:199-209, 1973.
12. Godfrey, S., and P. König. Thorax. 31:137-143, 1976.
13. Jones, R.S., M.J. Wharton, and M.H. Buston. Arch. Dis.
    Childh. 38:539-545, 1963.
14. Jones, R.S. Brit. Med. J. 2:972-975, 1966.
15. Jones, R.H.T., and R.S. Jones. Brit. Med. J. 2:976-978, 1966.
16. König, P., S. Godfrey, and A. Abrahamov. Arch. Dis. Childh.
    47:578-580, 1972.
17. König, P., and S. Godfrey. Arch. Dis. Childh. 48:513-518,
    1973a.
18. König, P., and S. Godfrey. Arch. Dis. Childh. 48:942-946,
    1973b.
19. König, P., and S. Godfrey. J. Allergy Clin. Immunol. 54:280-
    287, 1974.
20. König, P., P. Jaffe, and S. Godfrey. J. Allergy Clin. Immunol.
    54:14-19, 1974.
21. McNeill, R.S., J.R. Nairn, J.S. Millar, and C.G. Ingram.
    Quart. J. Med. 35:55-67, 1966.
22. Silverman, M., and S.D. Anderson. Arch. Dis. Childh. 47:882-
    889, 1972.
23. Silverman, M., P. König, and S. Godfrey. Thorax. 28:574-578,
    1973.

24. Silverman, M. M.D. Thesis, University of Cambridge, England, 1973.
25. Skorecki, K., H. Levison, and D.N. Crozier. Acta Paediat. Scand. 65:39-44, 1976.
26. Willis, T. Pharmaceutice Rationales, Part 2, Dring, Harper & Leigh, London, 1679.

DISCUSSION

Eldridge: Since normal people have some decrease in flow rate after
they exercise, is the difference between normals and asthmatics not
really qualitative, but quantitative? Airway resistance is an in-
verse function of the 4th power of the radius. This means that true
responsiveness of the airway may be the same in the asthmatics as
in the normal but because the asthmatic starts with narrowed airways the response appears greater. This would explain a lot of the
variations from time to time and subject to subject.

Godfrey: You are absolutely right, but I think it is a sematic
question. Why are asthmatics obstructed in the first place?

Eldridge: The time curve of airway resistance with exercise is like
the lactic acid curve with exercise, is it not?

Godfrey: I do not believe that the decrease is due to lactic acid.
With Anderson (Brit. J. Dis. Chest, 63:177, 1969) we compared the
lactic acid level, pH and PCO_2 after running and cycling in a group
of adults of identical size and weight. Hypocapnia, lactic acidosis
and pH were all worse after cycling and the asthma was worse after
running.

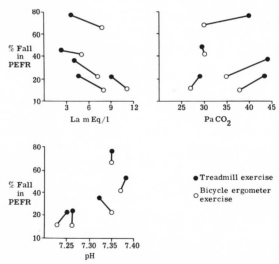

Fig. A. Post-exercise fall in peak expiration flow rate related to
blood lactate, arterial PCO_2 and pH during the cost minute of exercise in 5 asthmatic adults who exercised by running and cycling at
similar metabolic rates. The severity of exercise induced asthma
was greater for running even though the lactate was lower, PCO_2
higher and pH the same.

McFadden: The important point about the resistance-radius relationship not only applies to exercise, but to all forms of bronchial challenge.

Eggleston: The time required for recovery from exercise induced asthma may introduce a problem in interpretation. Many of your asthmatics had not recovered to their baseline pulmonary function before your second exercise stimulus.

Godfrey: This is the same problem of baseline values. About half of the children had returned to their pre-exercise values before the second test. Their response was no different from those who did not. Complete recovery time is two or two and a half hours.

Gee: There are two additional problems with exercise induced asthma. First, the effect of exercise must depend on the initial pre-exercise physiologic status. Apart from the 4th power of the diameter problem, a stimulus is likely to give a different response in a subclinical as opposed to a clinically detectable asthmatic "state". Second, a fall in peak flow is the last event in the development of progressively increasing airway obstruction. Therefore, to use this as a measure of response can be very misleading. Major obstruction may not be detected and the apparent induction of asthma may be really a worsening of pre-existing obstruction.

Godfrey: We do not consider the question of which test to use very important. We are looking for qualitative differences.

Fishman: Why is it called post-exercise asthma when the obstruction may begin during exercise?

Godfrey: We usually call it exercise induced asthma. I think the mediator, whatever it is, starts at the beginning of exercise. The reason asthma doesn't begin until later is that enough mediator has not been produced.

19

Cardiorespiratory Adaptations
of Normal & Asthmatic Children
to Exercise[1]

Gerd J. A. Cropp & Nobuo Tanakawa

Asthma is a disease characterized by chronic or recurrent, reversible airway obstruction and by acute bronchospasm after exercise.
The cardiorespiratory adaptations of asthmatics to exercise have not
been thoroughly investigated; it is also not known whether any
abnormal pulmonary mechanical events during exercise predispose
these patients to post-exertional airway obstruction. We, therefore,
studied the physiological responses of normal and chronically asthmatic children to cycle ergometer work in the hope to answer the
following questions: (1) Does the ability of asthmatics to perform
aerobic work differ from that of normals; (2) How do normal and
asthmatic children differ in their physiological adaptations to
physical exertion; (3) What is the effect of pre-exercies pulmonary
functions in asthmatics on their post-exertional lung functions, and
(4) What is the correlation between unusual physiological adjustments of asthmatics to exercise and the development of exercise-
induced bronchospasm.

METHODS

Thirteen normal children were recruited as a control group for
these studies. None of these children gave histories of allergic
or respiratory diseases, none were smokers and all were moderately
active, although none belonged to competitive athletic teams. The
21 asthmatic children were full-time residents at our treatment
center. They were referred to the laboratory for diagnostic evaluation regarding the presence and severity of exercise-induced
bronchospasm. All patients were taking bronchodilator medications,
and 17 required oral steroids on alternate days or inhaled steroids
two or four times daily for satisfactory control of symptoms. The
time between the last drug administration and exercise was 3 to 5
hours. Patients were tested only when they felt in their usual
state of health and when they had normal air exchange on auscultation. Five patients exhibited localized wheezing on forced
expiration before exercise. Table 19.1 summarizes the anthropometric
data of our study population.

All subjects had spirometric and body plethysmographic pulmonary
function tests before exercise. Spirometric measurements consisted
of vital capacity (VC), forced expiratory volume in one second

(1) This study was supported by NHLI grant #16074-03.

265

TABLE 19.1

STUDY POPULATION

		Normals	Asthmatics	Difference
Number		13	21	
Sex	Male	7	12	
	Female	6	9	
Age (yrs.)	Mean ± SE	12.1 ± 0.69	12.3 ± 0.53	n.s.
	Range	8.4 – 17.1	8.1 – 16.0	
Height (cm)	Mean ± SE	149 ± 4.1	143 ± 2.7	n.s.
	Range	122 – 173	125 – 168	
Weight (kg)	Mean ± SE	43 ± 4.0	39 ± 2.1	n.s.
	Range	23 – 76	24 – 62	

(FEV_1) and maximum mid-expiratory flow rate (MMEF). We assessed the functional residual capacity (FRC) and airway resistance (R_{aw}) in the plethysmograph. The asthmatics were also tested after exercise to evaluate any post-exercise deterioration in lung function. The first post-exertional spirometric examination was performed 4 to 6 minutes after exercise. Subsequent assessments of lung function consisted of plethsmographic measurements followed by spirometric measurements between 6 and 10, 15 and 20 and 25 and 30 minutes after exercise. Residual volumes (RV) were calculated from the FRC and the expiratory reserve volume. Specific airway conductance (SG_{aw}) was determined from R_{aw} and the simultaneously measured thoracic gas volume. Spirometric tests were performed at least twice and only the best effort was counted. Plethysmographic measurements were done 3 to 5 times and the results were averaged. All measurements were adjusted to BTPS conditions and were expressed in % of predicted values to allow for the marked differences in body size of children, or in % of baseline (pre-exercise) values when post-exertional pulmonary functions were reported.

Exercise was performed on a cycle ergometer. After the test had been explained to the subjects, they sat quietly on the ergometer seat for 6 minutes, while breathing on the mouth piece with a nose-clip in place. After the resting period, the children commenced pedaling at a rate between 50 and 60 rpm. The initial and subsequent increments in work rate were adjusted to 0.25 Watts/kg for asthmatics and 0.33 W/kg for normals. Subjects worked at each increment for 3 minutes until they became exhausted. All subjects were encouraged to perform to the best of their ability, however, no efforts were made to reach maximum aerobic work capacity. Throughout exercise we measured the work rates performed (W/kg), the beat-to-beat heart rates (HR), and inspiratory ($\dot{V}_{Insp}$) and expiratory flow rates ($\dot{V}_{Exp}$). During the last minute of each 3-minute work increment, we averaged the above measurements and recorded mixed expired oxygen (FE_{O_2}) and CO_2 concentrations (FE_{CO_2}) at the exit of a gas-mixing chamber and expired volume, using a

mass spectrometer and 120 l gasometer respectively. Taking into
account barometric pressures, water vapor pressures, room and gasometer temperatures, we calculated minute ventilation ($\dot{V}_E$) at BTPS,
and oxygen consumption ($\dot{V}_{O2}$) at STPD. The oxygen pulse
($\dot{V}_{O2} \cdot kg^{-1} \cdot HR^{-1}$) was determined from $\dot{V}_{O2}$ and the HR. Endtidal
pressures of CO_2 (P_{ECO2}) and oxygen (P_{EO2}) were measured in mm Hg
at the mouth piece and averaged during the 30 seconds preceding the
collections of expired gas. The individual analog signals were
relayed to a mini-computer for processing. The derived measurements
were printed out. Individual values were checked for accuracy by
comparing the analog records and the computer print-out.

In order to compare measurements of various physiological
responses in normal and asthmatic children at arbitrarily chosen
values of $\dot{V}_{O2} \cdot kg^{-1}$, we calculated by computer best-fit regression
equations which related physiological adaptive responses of each
subject (independent variable) to $\dot{V}_{O2} \cdot kg^{-1}$ (dependent variable).
Excellent fits were obtained by linear or quadratic regressions for
all relations described in this report (Fig. 19.1). Using the

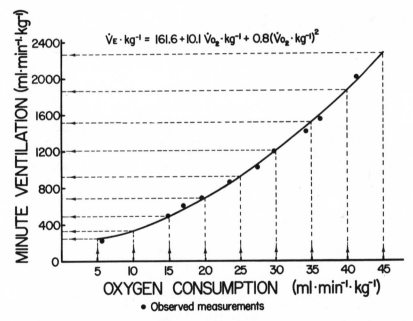

$$\dot{V}_E \cdot kg^{-1} = 161.6 + 10.1\ \dot{V}_{O2} \cdot kg^{-1} + 0.8(\dot{V}_{O2} \cdot kg^{-1})^2$$

MINUTE VENTILATION (ml·min⁻¹·kg⁻¹)

OXYGEN CONSUMPTION (ml·min⁻¹·kg⁻¹)

• Observed measurements

Fig. 19.1: Method used to evaluate a subject's ventilatory adjustments to exercise at oxygen consumptions between 5 and 40
ml·min⁻¹·kg⁻¹, using a computer-derived quadratic regression
equation. This method enabled us to compare ventilatory and other
physiological adaptations to exercise at specific oxygen
consumptions in normal and asthmatic children.

appropriate regression equations for each subject, we calculated
the average physiological responses in normal and asthmatic children
at $\dot{V}_{O_2}$'s of 5, 10, 15, 20, 25, 30, 35 and 40 ml·min^{-1}.kg^{-1} (for
example see Fig. 19.1). The statistical significance of the
differences between the means of physiological responses at each
$\dot{V}_{O_2}$·kg^{-1} in normals and asthmatics was assessed by t-tests.

In order to summarize the overall severity of pulmonary function
abnormalities, as assessed by 5 pulmonary function tests, we
calculated a Pulmonary Function Abnormality Score according to the
criteria given in Table 19.2. Total scores of one or less were
considered to indicate no significant abnormalities, scores between
2 and 5 indicated mild, scores between 6 and 10 moderate and scores
of 11 or higher severe abnormalities.

TABLE 19.2

CRITERIA FOR PULMONARY FUNCTION ABNORMALITY SCORE

	Score=0 (Normal)	Score=1 (Mild)	Score=2 (Moderate)	Score=3 (Marked)
VC	>80*	70-80	60-69	<60
RV	<145	145-215	216-285	>285
FEV$_1$	>80	70-80	60-69	<60
MMEF	>65	50-65	30-49	<30
SG$_{aw}$	>50	35-50	25-34	<25

* all values are % of predicted normal values

The total post-exertional changes, also assessed by 5 different
pulmonary function tests, were expressed by an Exercise-Induced
Asthma Score, using the criteria summarized in Table 19.3. Insig-
nificant exercise-induced asthma (EIA) corresponded to a score of
one or less, mild EIA corresponded to a score of 2 to 5, moderate
EIA to a score of 6 to 10, and severe EIA to a score of 11 or above.

TABLE 19.3

CRITERIA FOR EXERCISE-INDUCED ASTHMA SCORE

	Score=0 (No EIA)	Score=1 (Mild EIA)	Score=2 (Mod. EIA)	Score=3 (Severe EIA)
VC	>80	60-80	40-59	<40
RV	<140	140-200	201-300	>300
FEV$_1$	>75	50-75	25-49	<25
MMEF	>75	50-75	25-49	<25
SG$_{aw}$	>75	50-75	25-49	<25

* all values indicate % of baseline or resting values

The anaerobic threshold (AT) of exercise was defined as the $\dot{V}_{O_2} \cdot kg^{-1}$ above which minute ventilation rose in an accelerated manner with further increases in aerobic work (4). When the AT could not be determined with ease from the plot of $\dot{V}_E$ vs. $\dot{V}_{O_2}$, we evaluated the graphic relation between changes in F_{ECO_2} and/or F_{EO_2} as $\dot{V}_{O_2}$ increased. We have previously shown that the $\dot{V}_{O_2}$ at which F_{ECO_2} reaches a maximum or F_{EO_2} a minimum corresponds to the AT as determined from the relation between $\dot{V}_E$ and $\dot{V}_{O_2}$ (unpublished personal observations). In every case it was possible to establish an AT, and it was expressed in ml $\dot{V}_{O_2} \cdot kg^{-1}$.

RESULTS

Pre-exercise pulmonary function tests were within normal limits for all control subjects. Asthmatics as a group showed mild abnormalities; 6 patients had essentially normal lung functions, 13 showed mild and 2 moderate abnormalities. Severe pulmonary function abnormalities were observed in only two patients who exhibited hyperinflation (RV=292 and 265% of predicted respectively). Following exercise, pulmonary functions deteriorated in generally mild asthmatics, however, there were considerable individual variations; 8 patients developed no significant EIA according to the criteria established in Table 19.3, 4 developed mild, 4 moderate and 5 severe EIA. Table 19.4 summarizes pre- and post exercise pulmonary function test results.

TABLE 19.4

PULMONARY FUNCTION TEST RESULTS IN NORMAL AND ASTHMATIC
CHILDREN BEFORE AND AFTER EXERCISE

| Tests | Pre-Exercise (% Pred.±SE) | | | Post-Exercise (Asthmatics only) | |
	Norm.	Asth.	Diff.	% Baseline±SE	Diff.
VC	106*	115	n.s.	78	p<0.005
	±4.3	±2.8		±4.8	
RV	121	203	p<0.005	171	p<0.005
	±10.1	±12.3		±21.5	
FEV_1	100	96	n.s.	61	p<0.005
	±3.5	±3.3		±5.3	
MMEF	94	67	p<0.005	61	p<0.005
	±6.2	±5.7		±5.3	
SG_{aw}	75	53	p<0.005	62	p<0.005
	±5.0	±4.6		±7.6	
Pul.Fct.	0.5	3.0	p<0.005		
Abn.Sc.	±0.22	±0.50			
EIA Sc.				5.1	p<0.005
				±1.15	

* Means ±S.E.

There was no correlation between results of pre-exercise pulmonary function tests and the development of EIA in our 21 patients. Whether we looked at specific tests of lung function before and after exercise, or at the combined pre- and post exercise scores, no significant correlations were detected (Fig. 19.2).

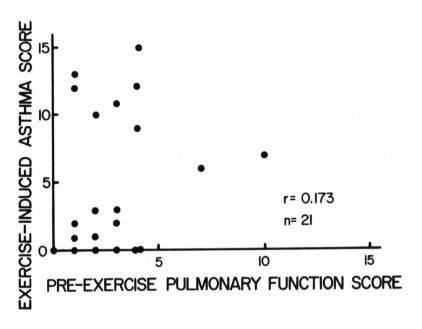

Fig. 19.2: Relation between pre-exercise pulmonary function scores and development of EIA in 21 chronically asthmatic children. Note that there was no significant relation between severity of pre-exercise pulmonary function abnormalities and severity of EIA.

There was no correlation between the maximum heart rates reached by asthmatics and the development of acute bronchospasm after exercise. If we assume that near maximal HR's indicate extreme physical efforts, these observations suggest that marked EIA is just as likely to develop after moderate as after very severe exertion. There were no indications from physical examination or from reports by patients that bronchospasm developed during exercise, and no patient stopped cycling because of respiratory distress at peak work rates.

Table 19.5 shows the average values of selected physiological measurements in normal and asthmatic children at rest and during peak exertion. At rest asthmatics as a group had significantly higher $\dot{V}_E$ and HR's than normal subjects. At the height of exercise normal children were able to work more and achieve higher $\dot{V}_{O2} \cdot kg^{-1}$

TABLE 19.5

MEASUREMENTS OF PHYSIOLOGICAL PARAMETERS AT REST AND AT END
OF EXERCISE IN NORMAL AND ASTHMATIC CHILDREN

Parameter (units)	Rest			End		
	Norm.	Asth.	Diff.	Norm.	Asth.	Diff.
	Mean ±SE	Mean ±SE	p	Mean ±SE	Mean ±SE	p
Work Rate $(W \cdot kg^{-1})$	0	0	n.s.	2.77 ±0.163	1.82 ±0.081	<0.001
Oxy. Cons. $(ml \cdot min^{-1} \cdot kg^{-1})$	5.2 ±0.20	5.9 ±0.26	n.s.	41.4 ±1.62	32.4 ±1.08	<0.001
Heart Rate (per min)	88 ±4.0	103 ±2.5	<0.01	197 ±3.6	184 ±2.6	<0.01
Min. Vent. $(ml \cdot min^{-1} \cdot kg^{-1})$	178 ±10.4	226 ±11.7	<0.01	1608 ±83.7	1322 ±65.7	<0.05
PE_{CO2} (mm Hg)	31 ±0.7	29 ±0.5	n.s.	30 ±0.5	28 ±0.6	n.s.
$\dot{V}_{Insp}/\dot{V}_{Exp}$	1.54 ±0.122	1.66 ±0.081	n.s.	1.11 ±0.030	1.40 ±0.052	<0.001
Anaer. Thresh. $(ml \cdot min^{-1} \cdot kg^{-1})$	26.2 ±1.09	22.4 ±0.95	<0.05			

than asthmatics. Peak HR's and $\dot{V}_E$ were lower in asthmatics than in normal children, however, it should be noted that asthmatics also did less work. In asthmatics an increase of one ml $\dot{V}_{O2} \cdot kg^{-1}$ was associated on the average with a rise in HR of 3.1 bpm (±0.17 SE). This rate of rise in HR was no different from that observed in normal subjects (3.1±0.13 SE). The ratio of $\dot{V}_{Insp}$ to $\dot{V}_{Exp}$ at rest was similar in patient and control groups. At rest, $\dot{V}_{Insp}$ was 1.5 to 1.7 times as high as $\dot{V}_{Exp}$. During exercise $\dot{V}_{Insp}$ rose approximately equally in asthmatics and normals, however, $\dot{V}_{Exp}$ increased less in patients than in control subjects. Consequently the ratio $\dot{V}_{Insp}/\dot{V}_{Exp}$ decreased to near unity in normals, but remained much higher in asthmatics. The AT was significantly lower in asthmatic than in normal children.

Table 19.6 shows the average values for several size-adjusted physiological measurements at low, intermediate and high $\dot{V}_{O2} \cdot kg^{-1}$ in normal and asthmatic children. The significance of differences between normals and asthmatics is also given. The results indicate that at most $\dot{V}_{O2} \cdot kg^{-1}$, asthmatics tended to breathe more, have higher tidal volumes (V_T), have higher endtidal PO_2's and lower PCO_2's than normals. As $\dot{V}_{O2} \cdot kg^{-1}$ increased, asthmatics were also unable to increase their $\dot{V}_{Exp}$ as effectively as control subjects, resulting in the ratio $\dot{V}_{Insp}/\dot{V}_{Exp}$ to fall less in patients than in normals.

The ventilatory adjustments to exercise were described well by

TABLE 19.6

RELATION BETWEEN PHYSIOLOGICAL ADAPTATION AND GRADED EXERCISE
IN NORMAL AND ASTHMATIC CHILDREN

Parameter	Subjects		Oxygen Consumption ($ml \cdot min^{-1} \cdot kg^{-1}$)			
			5	15	25	35
$\dot{V}_E \cdot kg^{-1}$	Norm.	Mean	179	434	784	1231
		±S.E.	9.8	23.1	37.4	45.3
	Asth.	Mean	190	503	926	1375
		±S.E.	13.3	12.6	24.5	45.8
	Diff.	(p)	0.58	<0.008	<0.003	<0.04
$V_T \cdot kg^{-1}$	Norm.	Mean	11.5	17.7	23.3	28.3
		±S.E.	0.81	0.82	0.96	1.13
	Asth.	Mean	12.8	20.3	26.9	34.0
		±S.E.	0.51	0.63	0.76	1.16
	Diff.	(p)	0.16	<0.02	<0.006	<0.003
$\dot{V}_E \cdot \dot{V}_{O_2}^{-1}$	Norm.	Mean	33.1	30.2	30.8	34.9
		±S.E.	1.48	1.35	1.40	1.52
	Asth.	Mean	37.2	34.0	36.7	39.6
		±S.E.	1.30	0.74	1.11	1.31
	Diff.	(p)	0.051	<0.02	<0.003	<0.03
HR	Norm.	Mean	86	115	146	180
		±S.E.	4.2	3.6	4.1	5.5
	Asth.	Mean	99	127	161	182
		±S.E.	2.5	2.6	3.8	2.5
	Diff.	(p)	<0.006	<0.008	<0.02	0.70
$\dot{V}_{O_2} \cdot kg^{-1} \cdot HR^{-1}$	Norm.	Mean	0.09	0.12	0.16	0.20
		±S.E.	0.005	0.004	0.004	0.004
	Asth.	Mean	0.05	0.12	0.16	0.19
		±S.E.	0.002	0.003	0.003	0.005
	Diff.	(p)	<0.001	0.16	0.54	0.13
$\dot{V}_{Insp} \cdot \dot{V}_{Exp}^{-1}$	Norm.	Mean	1.53	1.35	1.21	1.12
		±S.E.	0.101	0.052	0.046	0.045
	Asth.	Mean	1.67	1.53	1.44	1.38
		±S.E.	0.090	0.042	0.049	0.036
	Diff.	(p)	0.32	<0.02	<0.005	<0.0004
P_ECO_2	Norm.	Mean	31	33	33	31
		±S.E.	0.6	0.7	0.7	0.7
	Asth.	Mean	29	30	30	28
		±S.E.	0.5	0.4	0.5	0.7
	Diff.	(p)	<0.02	<0.002	<0.001	<0.006
P_EO_2	Norm.	Mean	76	76	78	81
		±S.E.	0.8	0.7	0.8	1.0
	Asth.	Mean	79	79	81	84
		±S.E.	1.0	0.6	0.8	0.9
	Diff.	(p)	<0.05	<0.008	<0.004	<0.02

linear or quadratic regression equations in normals and asthmatics. In 12 out of 13 normal subjects quadratic regression equations provided optimal fits for the relations between $\dot{V}_E$ and $\dot{V}_{O2}$; in only one subject did a linear regression describe the same relation just as satisfactorily as a quadratic one. In asthmatics the increase in $\dot{V}_E$ was linear in 9 out of 21, and parabolic in 12 out of 21 patients. In all asthmatics, $\dot{V}_E$ at rest and throughout exercise was above the mean for the normal subjects. There were no statistically significantly differences in the ventilatory adjustments to exercise between asthmatics who developed mild or severe EIA and those who had no or mild pulmonary functional abnormalities before exercise.

There was one asthmatic girl who was unable to increase her $\dot{V}_E$ in proportion to energy demands. As a result of this inadequate ventilatory response to exercise, her endtidal P_{CO2} rose 3 mm Hg as $\dot{V}_{O2} \cdot kg^{-1}$ increased (Fig. 19.3). This patient had moderate

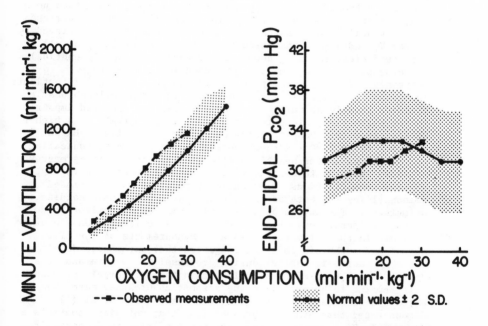

--■--Observed measurements   ▬▬▬ Normal values ± 2 S.D.

Fig. 19.3: Inadequate ventilatory response and rise of endtidal P_{CO2} in response to exercise in an asthmatic child with moderately abnormal pulmonary function tests before test. The patient was, however, in no clinical distress, and remained symptom-free, even during heavy work.

pulmonary function abnormalities prior to cycling (in % of predicted
values: VC=82%, FEV_1=59%, MMEF=30%, SG_{aw}=30% and RV=365%). Despite
these changes she did not complain about respiratory impairment
before or during exercise. Her air exchange on auscultation was
good, and wheezing was noted only during forced expiration. She
developed moderate EIA 3 to 4 minutes after exercise. Since this
patient failed to increase ventilation in proportion to CO_2 production, we consider this type of a ventilatory response to exercise
indicative of relative hypoventilation at work rates above the AT.
Although the ventilatory adjustment to aerobic work was not normal
in this patient, she still breathed more than the average normal
subject at all $\dot{V}_{O_2} \cdot kg^{-1}$ so that there was no pathological degree
of hypercapnia.

DISCUSSION
The results of this investigation show that asthmatic children
without major symptoms of respiratory impairment before exercise
differ from normals in their adaptation to physical exertion. In
general, asthmatic children breathed significantly more than normal
subjects at rest and at all work rates examined. The higher than
normal ventilation in asthmatics at comparable $\dot{V}_{O_2}$ was achieved by
larger V_T and not by increased RR. The increases in $\dot{V}_E$ at all $\dot{V}_{O_2}$'s
were sufficient to bring about significant increases in endtidal
and probably alveolar P_{O_2} and decreases in endtidal $P_{C_{O_2}}$.
    The significantly lower peak powers and peak $\dot{V}_{O_2} \cdot kg^{-1}$ in patients
indicated lower aerobic work capacities in chronically asthmatic
children than in normals. The cardiac reserves appeared impaired
in the asthmatics, since they achieved given $\dot{V}_{O_2} \cdot kg^{-1}$ at a higher
HR than normals. Despite this fact the rate of rise in HR per
unit increase in $\dot{V}_{O_2} \cdot kg^{-1}$ was normal in the patients, indicating
no reductions in the heart's ability to respond to rising energy
demands. We tend to believe that the higher HR at most $\dot{V}_{O_2} \cdot kg^{-1}$
are due to medications these patients received which included
aminophylline and beta-adrenergic agonists, both known cardiac
stimulants. The oxygen pulse was also similar in patients and
normal subjects, suggesting that there was no limitations in oxygen
delivery in the asthmatic children. Measurements of the AT in
normal and asthmatic children suggested that asthmatics developed
metabolic acidosis earlier during progressive exercise and at a
$\dot{V}_{O_2} \cdot kg^{-1}$ of 3.8 $ml \cdot min^{-1} \cdot kg^{-1}$ less than that of normal children.
    It remains to be explained why asthmatics breathed more than
normals at rest and during exercise. Byrne-Quinn et al (1)
demonstrated that athletes breathe less than untrained controls at
comparable $\dot{V}_{O_2}$, however, since the rates of rise in HR per unit
rise in $\dot{V}_{O_2} \cdot kg^{-1}$ were the same in our normal and asthmatic children,
we doubt that differences in physical fitness were responsible for
the asthmatics hyperventilation at all $\dot{V}_{O_2}$'s studied. Our
observations indicate that hyperventilation got progressively more
marked as aerobic work rates increased. For instance, at a $\dot{V}_{O_2}$
of 5 $ml \cdot kg^{-1}$ asthmatics breathed approximately 6% more than normals;

this fraction rose to 16% at a $\dot{V}_{O2}$ of 15 ml·kg^{-1} and to 18% at a $\dot{V}_{O2}$ of 40 ml·kg^{-1}. The difference in the ventilatory equivalent between normals and patients also rose with increasing aerobic work rates. If hyperventilation in asthmatics at rest is a mechanism to compensate for ventilation-perfusion mismatches, maldistribution of inspired air and non-uniform increases in airway resistance, our observations suggest that these abnormalities got worse in asthmatics during exercise. Although there may be a temporary improvement in lung functions early during exercise because of heightened sympathetic tone and bronchodilation (2), we predict from our observations that the (A-a) gradient increases in chronic asthmatics during heavy exercise and that some patients may develop a decrease in arterial P_{O2} and in hemoglobin saturation with oxygen. The high pulmonary ventilation in asthmatics during exercise is an at least partially effective compensatory mechanism aimed to keep alveolar P_{O2} high and P_{CO2} low, thus assuring optimal oxygenation of blood and elimination of CO_2. The excessive ventilatory response of asthmatics to exercise is probably more effective in maintaining CO_2 elimination, arterial P_{CO2} and pH than it is in keeping the arterial P_{O2} and hemoglobin saturation at normal levels.

Asthmatics tended to stop cycle exercise at a lower heart rate than normals. This may have been due in part to an earlier onset of leg fatigue in patients and in part to an increased work of breathing. Although the patients did not complain about respiratory distress at the end of exercise, there may have been a subclinical degree of dyspnea present which influenced the asthmatics to stop pedaling, possibly at a time when the amount of $\dot{V}_{O2}$ devoted to the work of breathing exceeded a critical fraction of the total $\dot{V}_{O2}$.

Comparisons of inspiratory and expiratory flow rates during tidal breathing suggests that asthmatics had significantly more expiratory than inspiratory airway obstruction which became increasingly obvious as flow rates increased during exercise. In normal subjects expiratory flow rates approached and sometimes exceeded inspiratory flow rates, indicating that even at the peak of exertion expiration was unobstructed. In asthmatics we did not see the reduction in the $\dot{V}_{Insp}/\dot{V}_{Exp}$ ratio which was regularly observed in normals with progressive ergometer work. This strongly suggests that in asthmatics expiratory airway obstruction became an increasingly limiting factor as exercise got severe. The high expiratory obstruction in asthmatics probably increased significantly the work of breathing in asthmatics and may have added to a feeling of exhaustion late in exercise.

When expiratory obstruction exceeds tolerable limits, it is likely that asthmatics are unable to ventilate sufficiently to eliminate CO_2 and maintain alveolar P_{CO2} at levels appropriate for heavy exercise. Mild, relative CO_2 retention was noted in one patient who had moderate airway obstruction and marked hyperinflation before exercise. These admittedly preliminary observations suggest that there has to be considerable deterioration in lung function before asthmatics cannot increase their ventilation adequately in response to physical exercise. However, such a limitation exists in childhood asthmatics and may be reached when the FEV_1 is reduced to less than 60%, when the vital capacity is reduced to less than 80%, and when the RV exceeds 350% of predicted values.

This study has confirmed previous observations (2,3) that the development of exercise-induced asthma is not related to pre-exertional abnormalities in lung functions. We were also unable to relate post-exertional deteriorations in lung function in asthmatics to abnormalities in their physiological adjustments to exercise. Any abnormalities in the cardiorespiratory adaptations of asthmatics to work were based on their pre-exertional abnormalities, and exercise aggravated these pre-existing functional aberrations. It is conceivable that exercise-induced functional abnormalities may have contributed to early discontinuation of exertion.

SUMMARY

1. Asthmatic children reached significantly lower aerobic power, $\dot{V}_{O_2} \cdot kg^{-1}$, AT and HR during incrementally increasing cycle ergometer exercise than age-matched normal children. This suggests that asthmatics have reduced cardiovascular and metabolic reserves. Asthmatics had a normal rate of rise in HR per unit increase in $\dot{V}_{O_2} \cdot kg^{-1}$. The low aerobic work capacity of asthmatics may be due, in part, to drug induced increases in HR at all $\dot{V}_{O_2} \cdot kg^{-1}$.

2. Asthmatics breathed more at rest and during exercise than normals, as indicated by higher $\dot{V}_E \cdot kg^{-1}$, lower P_{ECO_2}, higher P_{EO_2} and $\dot{V}_E \cdot \dot{V}_{O_2}^{-1}$ at all $\dot{V}_{O_2} \cdot kg^{-1}$ examined. Increases in ventilation were accomplished by higher V_T and not by higher RR. Hyperventilation before and during exercise served as a partially effective compensatory mechanism to maintain normal elimination of CO_2 and the best possible oxygenation of mixed venous blood.

3. Asthmatics were unable to increase $\dot{V}_{Exp}$ normally during exercise. This indicates significant expiratory obstruction and may contribute to the work of breathing in asthmatics.

4. When pre-exercise pulmonary functions are poor, asthmatics may be unable to increase their ventilation sufficiently to assure adequate elimination of CO_2.

5. We confirmed that abnormalities of pre-exercise lung functions in asthmatics are not correlated with the development of EIA.

6. There was no apparent relation between abnormalities in the physiological adaptations of asthmatics to exercise and the occurrence of post-exertional airway obstruction.

REFERENCES

1. Bryne-Quinn, E., J.V. Weil, I.E. Sodal, G.F. Filley, and R.F. Grover, J. Appl. Physiol. 30: 91-98. 1971.
2. Cropp, G.J.A. Ped. Clin. N. Am. 22: 63-76, 1975.
3. Cropp, G.J.A. Pediatrics 56: 868-879, 1975.
4. Wasserman, K., B.J. Whipp, S.K. Koyal, and W.L. Beaver. J. Appl. Physiol. 35: 236-243, 1973.

DISCUSSION

Sutton: The major differences between your normal and asthmatic
subjects seems to be twofold. (1) The normals were fitter than
asthmatics. (2) The higher $\dot{V}_E$ response to exercise in the asthmatic
patients appears to be a result of increased alveolar ventilation
and not due to increased dead space because ($PetCO_2$ - $PeCO_2$) was
similar in both groups. However, I would be very cautious in im-
plicating increased dead space ventilation. A possible explanation
for this increased alveolar ventilation is an increased ventilatory
sensitivity to hypoxia and/or CO_2.

Cropp: All of 18 asthmatic children had a perfectly normal response
to CO_2 and hypoxia. It is very interesting that the normal child
living at altitude has a perfectly normal ventilatory response to
hypoxia. Only after the age of 25-30 could Weil et al. (J. Clin.
Invest., 50:186, 1971), demonstrate a decrease in the ventilatory
response to hypoxia. Probably it is a matter of a combination of
severity and duration of prolonged hypoxia which eventually leads
to a loss of sensitivity to hypoxia and possibly also to CO_2. But
we cannot demonstrate any such loss in our pediatric patients.

Sutton: Of course, you would need a higher sensitivity to PCO_2
(i.e. higher slope) not a lower sensitivity to explain your exercise findings of a lower $PetCO_2$ in the asthmatics during exercise.

Cropp: That is correct.

Sutton: Your asthmatics had a lower peak $\dot{V}O_2$ than the normals. Is
one of the major differences that your asthamtics had a lower level
of cardiorespiratory fitness?

Cropp: I thought myself that this would be a major difference, but
the fact that the increase of heart rate per unit rise in $\dot{V}O_2$ was
the same in the two groups suggests to me that the cardiovascular
system, while it starts off at a higher set point, possibly because
of drugs, responds to physical stress in the same way in normal and
asthmatic children.

Sutton: But your asthmatics had a lower $\dot{V}O_2$ max than normals regardless of heart rate and as this is the criterion of cardiorespiratory fitness, by definition, your asthmatics were less fit.

Musch: You showed that there was a difference in the response of
the asthmatic to anaerobic thresholds. Your values were in $\dot{V}O_2$ in
ml/Kg. If you take these values in ml/Kg for oxygen consumption as
a percent of maximal oxygen consumption, is there a difference in
response as a percent of max $\dot{V}O_2$ reflecting an abnormal response in
the asthmatic person.

Cropp: If you express it as percent of peak O_2 consumption there
probably is no difference.

Wasserman: The lack of a rapid rise in ventilation after the subject surpasses his anaerobic threshold suggests to me insensitive carotid bodies. Do these patients have a depressed ventilatory response to hypoxia?

Cropp: We have not done that. Almost half of our asthmatics had a linear rise in their ventilation in response to exercise. You might expect that in some of these patients, you may find a significant reduction in response to hypoxia or to CO_2, but we have not found that.

20

Effect of Exercise on Airway Mechanics in Asthma & Observations on Mechanisms[1]

E. R. McFadden, Jr., R. L. Haynes, & R. H. Ingram, Jr.

As indicated in Chapter 17, perhaps no other aspect of asthma
has received more attention in recent years and has resulted in
more controversy than the phenomenon of exercise-induced asthma.
However, as newer and more complete observations have been made,
many areas of previous confusion have become, at least, partially
clarified. Thus, despite the limitations alluded to earlier, sufficient evidence has become available to allow for the development
of a general overview of the effects of exercise on airway mechanics. The purposes of this brief review are to describe the
changes that occur in pulmonary function with physical activity,
provide some observations on mechanism and to develop the concept
that exercise is a non-specific stimulus that can be a useful
non-pharmacologic, non-immunologic technique to provide insights
into the pathophysiology of asthma.

From the standpoint of pulmonary mechanics, there is general
agreement that various forms of strenuous physical exertion result in episodes of bronchoconstriction in asthmatic individuals.
However, there is as yet no general consensus as to how one should
assess the response. Most authors tend to view the latter as an
all or none event with a clear cut end point that can be completely
assessed by measuring some aspect of forced exhalation (1-3,9,11,
18-21,28-31). In most instances, this may be true but it need
not always be so, for there is ample evidence in the literature
that shows that when serial observations are made of multiple aspects of lung function during either resolution or provocation of
acute attacks of asthma, not all parameters will be altered to the
same degree at any point in time, nor will they improve or deteriorate at the same rate (5,22,24). In general, those tests that
are predominantly influenced by large airway events change rapidly
in either direction while those that reflect small airway pathology
tend to change quite slowly. Therefore, the response that one en-
counters may depend upon the size of airways involved, as well as
the extent and/or location of any pre-existing obstruction that
may be present before testing. The significance of this reasoning
is that considerable obstruction could be missed by looking only
at those tests that are influenced predominantly by changes in

1. Supported in part by: Research Career Development Award HL
00013 (E.R.McF.) and grants HL 17873 and HL 17382 from the
National Heart and Lung Institute.

large airways. Thus the choice of endpoints that one measures
becomes extremely important.

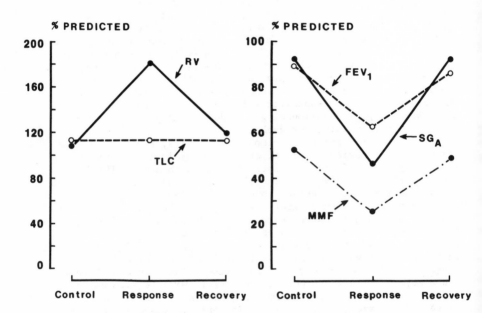

Figure 20.1.   Changes in pulmonary mechanics with exercise. FEV_1
= one second forced expiratory volume; GS_A = specific conductance;
MMF = maximum mid-expiratory flow rate; RV = residual volume; TLC
= total lung capacity.

A typical exercise response is shown in Figure 20.1. These
data were obtained from a 21 year old atopic individual with an
18 year history of asthma who was challenged by running on a treadmill. As can be seen, her pre-challenge lung function was compromised in that both maximum mid-expiratory flow rates (MMF) and
residual volume (RV) were abnormal suggesting small airway obstruction (23). Although this person did not have a history of exercise

induced asthma, the response was quite dramatic in that the one second forced expiratory volume (FEV_1), MMF, and specific conductance (SG_A) all decreased markedly while RV almost doubled. Total lung capacity did not change. Freedman and colleagues (10) have recently evaluated the disturbances that occurred in the pressure-volume and flow inter-relationships of the lungs of asthmatics following exercise and have also found that virtually all aspects of pulmonary mechanics are altered.

Total lung capacity increased significantly in four of their seven patients. In one of these patients the increase in TLC was associated with an increase in static transpulmonary pressure at full inflation, but in the remaining three it was associated with a parallel shift of the pressure-volume curve of the lung without a change in slope. In all of their patients, RV increased and expiratory flow limitation was present. Recent observations from this laboratory have shown similar results. Eight of 12 subjects were found to shift their pressure volume curves, and 20 of 20 significantly and reproducibly increased their RV after exercise (13,14). However only 4 reproducibly increased TLC. Thus it would appear that the mechanical consequences of exercise provocation are no different from those observed with other forms of challenges (27) or with those seen with spontaneously occurring episodes of asthma (12,24,34), and like the other situations there is a great deal of within and between subject variability.

With the data shown in Figure 20.1 and those discussed above there is little question as to endpoints. However, when we began to assess reproducibility of EIA by repeatedly studying a large group of asthmatics, we found that endpoints mattered greatly (13). On each occasion of study we applied the same exercise task and quantitated its consequences by measuring minute ventilation (V_E), oxygen consumption (V_{O2}) and carbon dioxide production (V_{CO2}) both during exercise and recovery. There were no differences between exercise trials as measured by any of the above variables. Prior to and 5 to 10 minutes after exercise we measured spirometric, plethysmographic and lung volume variables. When the response data were analyzed as a function of the pre-exercise state of lung function we found that the same stimulus applied to the same patients at different times evoked a continuum of changes ranging from relatively minor increases in RV to overt attacks of asthma depending upon the pre-existing state of the subject's lungs (Table 20.1).

When lung function was normal before challenge the only significant post-exercise finding was an abnormally large RV. In a second set of studies, the only deviation from normal at baseline was an elevated RV. With this as a pre-existing abnormality, the exercise response was much more dramatic and now all measured parameters changed significantly. However, no additional variables exceeded their predicted ranges. In contrast, when both MMF and RV were abnormal initially (Group 3. Table 20.1), the post-exercise changes were more marked and resembled those seen during a mild attack of asthma with all parameters, except TLC, now becoming abnormal. When initial lung function was compromised suf-

ficiently to reduce the FEV_1 below its lower limit, exercise
brought about changes comparable with moderately severe exacerbations of asthma. These data suggest that it may be an over-
simplification to view the effects of exercise as an "all or none"
event that can be reliably detected by measuring a 10 to 15% fall
in FEV_1 or some other spirometric variable. If the latter reasoning were applied to our data, those individuals in groups 1 and 2
would clearly have been mislabelled.

These observations also offer some insight into the reasons why
the incidence of exercise-induced asthma has been reported to vary
from 13 to 90% (16-18). Our data suggest that in large measure
this inconsistency is the direct result of the manner in which the
response has been assessed, and that the true figure may be 100%
if sufficient exercise stress is applied to any given subject.

As a case in point, we recently had the opportunity of evaluating a world class cross country skier who was suspected of having
exercise-induced asthma. This individual was able to complete 20
minutes of treadmill running at 10 miles per hour at a 20% grade
without developing any measurable alterations in lung function.
However, when the exercise task was readjusted by having him run on
the treadmill as before, but also simultaneously lifting weights
with his arms by a pulley mechanism so as to more closely approximate the work performed during his athletic endeavors, he developed
significant reductions in lung function that could be prevented by
prior administration of disodium cromoglycate. The results of this
study led to a formal investigation of the relative asthmogenicity
of arm versus leg work in asthma (33). Our purpose in undertaking
this endeavor was to determine if the reported variation in severity and frequency of exercise-induced asthma with different forms
of exercise (2,3,9,30) could be attributed to the use of different
muscle groups.

To achieve our ends, we had a group of asthmatics crank an ergo-
cycle with their arms while seated. The external loads applied
were such that exhaustion occurred in about 7 minutes. Pulmonary
function was measured before and after completion of the work load
and gas exchange variables were recorded during the work and recovery periods. After the subjects recovered the exercise was repeated, this time with the subjects seated on the bicycle with
their arms at rest and using their legs to pedal the load. The
work loads, RPM and duration of exercise were held constant for
each individual for both experiments.

The results of this investigation have been presented in detail
elsewhere (33) but in summary, we observed that arm work resulted
in significantly greater minute ventilations ($\dot{V}_E$), heart rates,
arterial hydrogen ion (H^+) concentrations and airway obstruction
and significantly lower arterial carbon dioxide tensions (PaO_2)
than did the identical external leg work. Furthermore, the effects
of lung function were found not to be specific for either muscle
group because when the work load on the legs was increased, the
above differences were eliminated. These observations taken in
combination indicate that the determining factor as to whether an

Table 20.1

Analysis of the Effects of Baseline Lung Function on the Response to Exercise

Baseline Status	No.	RA		SGA		Vmax iso		FEV1*		MMF*		RV*		TLC*	
		B	A	B	A	B	A	B	A	B	A	B	A	B	A
1. Normal Mechanics	6	1.78	1.97	0.19	0.15	5.50	4.29	106.2	94.5	96.8	84.0	103.7	141.2	108.5	115.5
		0.11	0.36	0.02	0.04	0.41	0.97	2.4	8.7	3.5	7.0	4.9	5.6	2.7	3.5
P value		NS		NS		NS		NS		NS		<0.001		<0.005	
% change		11		21		22		11		13		36		8	
2. Abnormal RV	21	1.46	1.90	0.21	0.16	4.55	3.48	100.2	90.2	103.2	90.8	170.0	239.2	113.6	116.5
		0.08	0.13	0.01	0.01	0.19	0.36	1.8	2.3	4.0	5.8	6.6	10.8	3.0	3.4
P value		<0.005		<0.001		<0.01		<0.01		<0.01		<0.02		<0.05	
% change		30		24		24		10		12		41		3	
3. Abnormal RV & MMF	18	1.94	3.32	0.19	0.10	3.55	1.79	90.1	70.4	68.8	43.4	150.2	229.8	108.3	117.9
		0.10	0.25	0.02	0.01	0.18	0.30	1.8	4.4	1.9	4.2	3.7	19.2	2.8	3.3
P value		<0.01		<0.001		<0.001		<0.001		<0.001		<0.001		<0.001	
% change		71		47		50		22		37		53		9	
4. Abnormal FEV1	18	2.94	4.94	0.12	0.06	1.70	0.64	67.2	51.1	40.8	22.4	170.8	282.2	107.8	120.5
		0.28	0.70	0.01	0.01	0.37	0.18	3.2	4.6	3.3	3.4	16.9	34.1	3.3	4.7
P value		<0.005		<0.001		<0.005		<0.001		<0.001		<0.001		<0.005	
% change		68		50		62		24		45		65		12	

Data shown are mean values ± one standard error. No. = the number of studies with the characteristics outlined under Baseline Status; R_A = airway resistance in $cmH_2O/L/sec$; SG_A = specific conductance in $L/sec/cmH_2O/L$; Vmax iso = maximum flow rate at 60% of control TLC in L/sec; FEV_1 =
one second forced expiratory volumes; MMF = maximum mid-expiratory flow rate; RV = residual volume;
TLC = total lung capacity. * indicates per cent of predicted.

283

asthmatic will develop post-exertional bronchospasm appears to be
related to the extent to which the participating muscle groups are
stressed. If the work load is high in relation to the mass of the
exercising muscles an acute exacerbation of asthma will be provoked
However if the relationship is low, airway obstruction will not
occur, at least over relatively short periods of work. These findings, therefore, suggest that if one wished to induce an acute attack of asthma, any exercise task would suffice as long as it was
of sufficient duration, and employed a reasonably large group of
muscles under sufficient load.

Since $\dot{V}_E$ was higher and $PaCO_2$ lower in the most asthmogenic
forms of exercise, and since many investigators feel that these
factors are causally related to the induction of post-exertional
airway obstruction (6-8,15,29,31), it seemed appropriate to systematically investigate the influence of these two variables. To
accomplish this, we utilized a partial rebreathing technique with
an adjustable bias flow that permitted minute and alveolar ventilations to be separated so that a desired target ventilation could
be achieved with end tidal CO_2 tensions ($PetCO_2$) held constant at
any chosen level (25). This system thus allowed for an independent evaluation of the effects of bulk airflow per se as well as a
systematic study of hypocapnia in a dose response fashion. The
data from this series of experiments was then compared to those
obtained during a standardized exercise challenge in a group of
asthmatic subjects whose exercise response was known to be reproducible.

The protocol that was followed consisted of first determining
the effects of treadmill running at 5 miles per hour at 5% grade
for ten minutes. During exercise and recovery $\dot{V}_E$ was recorded at
minute intervals and $PetCO_2$ was monitored continuously at the
mouth. Prior to, and 5-10 minutes after exercise, SG_A, lung volumes and spirometry were measured. On another day, three separate
experiments were performed in each subject with the rebreathing
apparatus. In each, the target ventilations were matched to the
individual $\dot{V}_E$ that the subjects reached during their last minute
of exercise. In the first study $PetCO_2$ was held constant at approximately 40 mmHg so as to evaluate only the effects of bulk airflow on lung function. In the second and third studies, $PetCO_2$
was lowered to approximately 30 and 20 mmHg respectively. Pulmonary mechanics were remeasured before and after each of these maneuvers in a manner identical to the exercise study.

Treadmill running caused every measured variable to worsen ma-
terially. Airway resistance, RV and TLC rose 87, 81, and 8% respectively, while SG_A, FEV_1 and MMF fell 61, 34, and 46%. The
mean $\dot{V}_E$ during the last minute of exercise was 83 liters and the
mean $PetCO_2$ was 28.9 mmHg. Isocapnic hyperpnea and hyperpnea with
a mean $PetCO_2$ of 30.6 mmHg were found to be totally without effect
and did not result in any measurable changes in lung function.
Lowering the $PetCO_2$ to 21.3 mmHg caused R_A to rise and SG_A, FEV_1
and MMF all to fall significantly but only to the same degree as
seen in normals (4,32). In addition, when these effects were com-

pared with those seen during running, it was found that in every index measured, exercise produced the most marked alterations and did so at values of PetCO$_2$ that had no effect when studied in a controlled fashion. Thus it would appear that neither high $\dot{V}_E$ per se nor hypocapnia can be considered as the mechanism underlying the phenomenon of exercise induced asthma.

In summary, the changes that are produced in pulmonary mechanics in asthmatics following exercise do not appear to be different from those observed with other forms of challenges or with those seen during spontaneous episodes of asthma. Some of the factors that determine the response that will occur at a point in time in any given subject after exercise provocation appear to be related in part to the pre-exercise state of lung function, thus suggesting that exercise-induced asthma need not be an all or none event, but rather a continuum of responses profoundly influenced by the pre-challenge state of the airways. Other factors that enter into the amount of obstruction that will develop appear to be related to the task performed and the extent to which the participating muscle groups are stressed. If the work load is high in relation to the mass of the exercising muscles an acute exacerbation of asthma will occur. If the relationship is low the converse appears to be true. Although the precise mechanism underlying exercise-induced asthma is unknown, it appears unlikely that either bulk air movement, or hypocarbia play primary roles.

REFERENCES

1. Allen, T.W., W. Addington, T. Rosendal, and D.W. Cugell. Amer. Rev. Resp. Dis. 107:816-821, 1973.
2. Anderson, S.D., N.M. Connolly, and S. Godfrey. Thorax 26: 396-401, 1971.
3. Anderson, S.D., M. Silverman, and S.R. Walker. Thorax 27: 718-725, 1972.
4. Bradford, J.M., R.H. Ingram, Jr., J.A. Davis, and G.D. Finlay. J. Appl. Physiol. 37:139-144, 1974.
5. Cade, J.F., A.J. Woolcock, A.S. Rebuck, and M.C.F. Pain. Clin. Sci. 40:381-391, 1971.
6. Chan-Yeung, M.M.W., M.N. Vyas, and S. Grzybowski. Amer. Rev. Resp. Dis. 104:915-923, 1971.
7. Crompton, G.K. Thorax 23:165-167, 1968.
8. Fisher, H.K., P. Holton, R.St.J. Buxton, and J.A. Nadel. Amer. Rev. Resp. Dis. 101:885-896, 1970.
9. Fitch, K.D., and A.R. Morton. Brit. Med. J. 4:577-581, 1971.
10. Freedman, S., A.E. Tattersfield, and N.B. Pride. J. Appl. Physiol. 38:974-982, 1975.
11. Godfrey, S., J. Aller. Clin. Immun. 56:1-17, 1975.
12. Gold, W.M., H.S. Kaufman, and J.A. Nadel. J. Appl. Physiol. 23:433-438, 1967.
13. Haynes, R.L., R.H. Ingram, Jr., and E.R. McFadden, Jr. Amer. Rev. Resp. Dis. Submitted for publication.

14. Haynes, R.L., J.J. Wellman, R.H. Ingram, Jr., and E.R.
     McFadden, Jr. J. Appl. Physiol. Submitted for publication.
15. Herxheimer, H. Lancet 1:83-87, 1946.
16. Irnell, L. and S. Smartling. Scand. J. Resp. Dis. 47:103-
     113, 1966.
17. Itkin, I.H., and M. Nacam. J. Allergy 37:253-263, 1966.
18. Jones, R.S. Brit. Med. J. 2:972-975, 1966.
19. Jones, R.S., M.H. Busted and M.J. Wharton. Brit. J. Dis.
     Chest 56:78-86, 1962.
20. Katz, R.M., B.J. Whipp, E.M. Heimlich, and K. Wasserman. J.
     Allergy 47:148-158, 1971.
21. McCarthy, O.R. Brit. J. Dis. Chest 66:133-140, 1972.
22. McFadden, E.R., Jr., R. Kiser, and W.J. deGroot. N. Eng. J.
     Med. 288:221-225, 1973.
23. McFadden, E.R., Jr., and D.A. Linden. Amer. J. Med. 52:725-
     737, 1972.
24. McFadden, E.R., Jr., and H.A. Lyons. J. Appl. Physiol. 27:
     452-459, 1969.
25. McFadden, E.R., Jr., D.R. Stearns, R.H. Ingram, Jr., and D.E.
     Leith. J. Appl. Physiol. Submitted for publication.
26. McNeil, R.S., J.R. Nairn, J.S. Millar, and C.G. Ingram.
     Quart. J. Med. 35:55-67, 1966.
27. Olive, J.T., and R.E. Hyatt. Amer. Rev. Resp. Dis. 106:366-
     376, 1972.
28. Poppius, H., A. Muittari, K-E. Krzus, O. Korhonen, and A.
     Viljanen. Brit. Med. J. 4:337-339, 1970.
29. Rebuck, A.S., and J. Read. Lancet 1:429-431, 1968.
30. Silverman, M., S.D. Anderson, and S.R. Walker. Brit. Med. J.
     1:207-209, 1972.
31. Simonsson, B.G., B-E. Skoogh, and B. Ekstrom-Jodal. Thorax
     27:169-180, 1972.
32. Sterling, G.M. Clin. Sci. 34:277-285, 1968.
33. Strauss, R.H., R.L. Haynes, R.H. Ingram, Jr. and E.R.
     McFadden, Jr. J. Appl. Physiol. Submitted for publication.
34. Woolcock, A.J. and J. Read. Amer. Rev. Resp. Dis. 98:788-
     794, 1968.

DISCUSSION

Godfrey: You have proved that hypocapnia or hyperventilation does not explain exercise bronchospasm. Could lactic acidosis?

McFadden: Critical experiments still need to be done. One would be to infuse lactic acid without exercise and the other would be to block any effect of H+ by bicarbonate during exercise and recovery.

Godfrey: In the study of Anderson (Brit. J. Dis of Chest, 69:1, 1975), exercise on a bicycle ergometer generated higher lactate but less of drop in peak flow than exercise to the same oxygen consumption running on a treadmill. Incidentally, two of these adults had pCO_2 of 44 and 45 after exercise showing that they can underventilate. The lactate is higher on the bicycle.

McFadden: In comparing different types of exercise no matter what endpoint is chosen the work will be different by definition. The exercise in Anderson's study, for example, may have differed in the relative amount of arm and leg work performed though ventilation was similar.

Cropp: We can exhaust the exercise response by repeated exercise if we do the exercise frequently enough and at short enough intervals. I cannot believe that you have less lactate production during and after the second and third exercise than you have after the first.

MdFadden: I am not saying lactate is responsible, please understand. I am just saying that is just a possibility.

Sutton: The question of lactate as a stimulus in exercise induced asthma has yet to be resolved. Have you thought of attempting to differentiate between H+ ion and lactate as possible stimuli? In a recent study (Sutton, et al., Clin. Sci., 50:241–247, 1976) we gave NH_4Cl and on a separate day $NaHCO_3$ and were able to separate H+ ion and lactate during exercise. This method could be used in asthmatic patients during exercise and may help determine if either H+ or lactate is responsible for EIA?

McFadden: Yes, we are very much interested in this work.

Kampine: Remarks about acidosis and calcium ion don't seem to fit with the fact that as hydrogen ion concentration increases calcium ionization becomes more complete and calcium ion concentration also increases.

McFadden: That is correct, but I understood the point to be that lactate binds calcium and pulls it away from the ionized fraction.

Kampine: But still, increasing hydrogen ion concentration will increase the pool of available ionized calcium.

Eggleston: It would be important to know how great a change in pulmonary function was produced both by hyperventilation and exercise when not attached to the servo-system to be able to apply these experiments to mechanisms involved with exercise induced asthma. Did the patients subjected to the servo-system exercise or did they hyperventilate while at rest?

McFadden: They just hyperventilated without exercising. One can induce asthma by hyperventilation on room air to extremes of volume and alveolar CO_2. We did not do that. We allowed our subjects to choose a comfortable ventilatory pattern that avoided volume extremes and then we simply adjusted pCO_2 to various levels.

Gee: What is the effect of repeated short term exercise on lactate production?

McFadden: Recent data in the Journal of Applied Physiology (Karlsson et al., J. Appl. Physiol., 38:763-767, 1975) has demonstrated metabolic changes in non-working muscles during exercise, eg. pyruvate/lactate ratios. I don't know the role of this exercise induced asthma.

Wasserman: Was the arm work done on the cycle ergometer?

McFadden: Yes, the patient was seated in a chair and peddled with the arms.

21

Effect of Drugs on Exercise-Induced Bronchospasm

C. Warren Bierman, William E. Pierson, & Gail G. Shapiro

INTRODUCTION

Bronchospasm induced by exercise (EIB) resembles acute asthma physiologically and pharmacologically but with a shortened time frame from initiation to resolution. In EIB changes are measured in minutes (1), while in acute asthma, changes must be measured in days. A comparison of spirographic changes in exercise induced bronchospasm (EIB), (Fig. 21.1A) and acute asthma (Fig. 21.1B) from a paper by Dr. McFadden (2), indicates these physiological similarities.

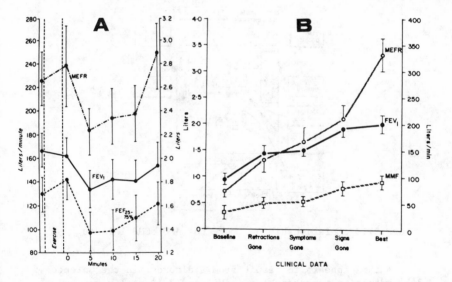

Fig. 21.1 Comparison of airway changes in EIB and acute asthma.

In both conditions, the MEFR response, probably respresenting changes in large airways, returns to normal rapidly and long before the very slow return of the FEF$_{25-75\%}$ or mid-maximal flow (MMF) which reflects changes in smaller airways. The FEV$_1$ response is

somewhere between the two measurements. Other similarities between
acute asthma and EIB include an increase in residual volume and
total lung capacity, a decrease in PaCO2, and a decrease in
specific conductance (3). Like asthma, exercise-induced bronchospasm appears to result from a number of mechanisms and is not a
specific disease state. EIB is an event with great intersubject
variability, though the response of the individual subject tends
to be consistent if baseline pulmonary function before stimulus,
workload, ambient temperature and allergen exposure are constant
(4). As in asthma, it is often family related, though discordance
in response has been demonstrated even in identical twins (5).
It is not caused by, but is frequently intensified by, viral
infections (especially adenovirus, rhinovirus and respiratory
syncytial virus) as well as by exposure to extrinsic airborne
allergens and cold air (6,7). As in asthma, the effectiveness of
any one drug in modifying EIB varies from one patient to another,
and drug therapy must be individualized. The approach to pharmacologic modification of EIB requires an understanding of current
knowledge of the biochemical basis for asthma, noted in Figure
21.2.

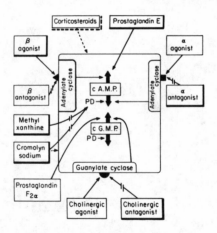

Figure 21.2 Relationship of drugs to cAMP/cGMP balance.

Asthma appears to result from a disorder in the balance of
3'5' adenosine monophosphate (cAMP) and 3'5' cyclic guanosine
monophosphate (cGMP) in three cell types (8). An increase of
cGMP over cAMP in bronchial smooth muscle results in bronchoconstriction, in pulmonary mast cells in the release of mediators
such as histamine, SRS-A and ECF-A and in lymphocytes in production and release of lymphokines.
    Pharmacologic agents useful in asthma appear to act to
increase cAMP over cGMP directly or indirectly (9). Beta

adrenergic stimulators or agonists such as isoproterenol stimulate
adenylate cyclase, an enzyme which converts ATP to cAMP, to
promote bronchodilation. Conversely, the beta adrenergic anatagon-
ist, propranolol, inhibits this effect. Alpha adrenergic agonists
such as norepinephrine inhibit adenylate cyclase production which
results in bronchoconstriction while alpha adrenergic antagonists
such as phentolamine block this effect and promote bronchodilation.
     Theophylline is thought to inhibit a phosphodiesterase which
promotes the breakdown of cAMP though it undoubtedly has other effects on the cAMP/cGMP ratio which have not yet been identified
(such as possible increase in intracellular calcium levels) (10).
Cromolyn sodium, which appears to act only the mast cell and not
on bronchial smooth muscle or lymphocytes may inhibit cAMP phosphodiesterase as well as acting directly on cell membranes to
inhibit release of performed cytoplasmic mediators. Less is
known about pharmacologic modulation of the cAMP system.
Acetylcholine increases cGMP synthesis by stimulating guanylate
cyclase and is blocked by atropine. Prostaglandins appear to
stimulate direct production of cAMP and cGMP independent of
adenylate or guanylate cyclases. Prostaglandin E_1 and E_2
stimulate cAMP to promote bronchodilation while F_2 stimulates
cGMP and is an intense bronchoconstrictor. How adrenocortico-
steroids act in asthma remains controversial. They do not appear
to have direct effects on cAMP/cGMP, but appear to facilitate the
action of beta adrenergic drugs and/or methylxanthine to increase
cAMP.

Beta Adrenergic Agonists

     In an attempt to modify EIB, McNeil (11) administered epi-
nephrine prior to exercise and showed inhibition in an uncontrolled
study. Heimlick (12) showed a response to a combination of ephedrine and theophylline, but again it was an uncontrolled study.
Subsequent work has pointed out the extreme importance of employing a placebo control in EIB studies (13).
     In a controlled study in our laboratory, ephedrine by it-
self had no greater protective value than did the placebo
control, though when administered with theophylline, it did enhance the theophylline effect (1). Subsequent studies have focused on beta adrenergic agents with more specific effects on
bronchial smooth muscle as compared to cardiac muscle.
     Metaproterenol has been effective either when inhaled 10
minutes prior to exercise (14), or when administered orally 2 to
3 hours prior to exercise (15). Terbutaline administered orally
showed a similar but enhanced effect three hours after administration which could still be detected 6 hours later when the metaproterenol effect had disappeared (16). Godfrey showed salbutamol
to be effective when administered by aerosol 10 minutes pre-
exercise or orally two hours prior to exercise (17). Whether
the mechanism of action of beta agonist agents is primarily that
of bronchodilation or inhibition of mediator release or both is
still not clear. Sly and Heimlick, studying metaproterenol,

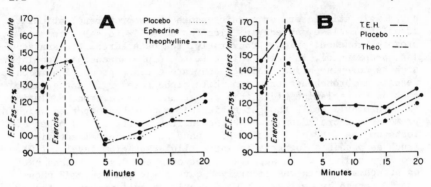

Fig. 21.3 Comparison of Ephedrine, Theophylline and placebo with Theophylline, Ephedrine and Hydroxyzine combined.

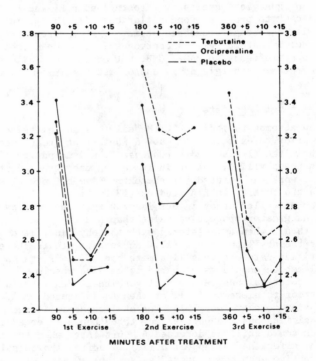

Fig. 21.4 Comparison of exercise response to placebo, Metaproterenol (Ocriprenaline), and Terbutaline 1½ hours, 3 hours and 5 hours after medication (16) (used with authors' permission).

found a dichotomy between bronchodilation and protection from
EIB (18). It is evident that EIB can be modified in most
patients by beta adrenergic drugs, and that pretreatment with
salbutamol or terbutaline orally 2 to 3 hours prior to exercise or
by inhalation 10 minutes prior to exercise offers advantages of
prolonged bronchodilation as well as specific inhibition of EIB
in most patients (19). Beta adrenergic agents appear to reverse
both large and small airway bronchospasm.

Methylxanthines

Theophylline has been shown to be effective in reversing small
and large airway bronchospasm in EIB when administered in an average dosage of 3.5 mg/kg, 1 to 2 hours prior to exercise (Fig. 21.3).
Weinberger administered theophylline in dosages adequate to produce
a serum theophylline concentration of between 10 and 20 µg/ml and
demonstrated appreciable enhancement of its effectiveness (20).
Figure 21.5 showsinhibition of EIB versus plasma theophylline concentrations from a study in progress in our laboratory. As
theophylline serum concentration increases there is inhibition of
EIB up to a level of 10 to 20 µg/ml. Over 20 µg no further benefit
occurred. Dyphyllin, a theophylline analog which is less potent,
more soluble and has a shorter half life, has also been studied
and has some activity in EIB (21). Dyphylline is useful in
patients who are intolerant to theophylline, but the dosage
required is greatly in excess of that recommended in the package
insert (15 mg/kg/dose).

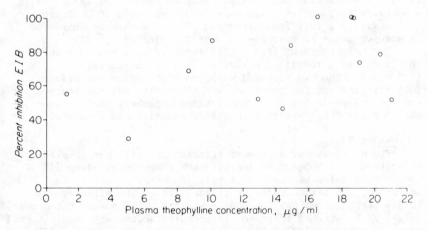

Fig. 21.5 Inhibition of EIB vs Theophylline serum concentrations.

Beta Adrenergic Antagonists

Administration of a beta adrenergic blocking agent has
intensified asthma in allergic subjects (22), though it has little
effect on airways of normal subjects even when they are challenged

with treadmill exercise. Sly et al. (1967)(23) investigated
propranolol in asthmatics. Following I.V. administration they
demonstrated an 18% fall in PEFR pre-exercise but failed to modify
the post exercise response. Both control and experimental groups
had similar bronchospasm after exercise. Irving et al. (24)
demonstrated a rise in both epinephrine and norepinephrine in normal
subjects following exercise in subjects pretreated with beta
adrenergic blockers. Such a study would be of interest in
patients with EIB.

Alpha Adrenergic Receptors
        Controversy persists about whether alpha receptors exist in
the human bronchial tree. Phentolamine, a weak alpha receptor
blocker has been demonstrated to be a weak bronchodilator but
has no influence on EIB even after administration intravenously
in the dosage of 0.1 mg/kg (24). Recently, Patel and co-workers
studied a new agent, thymoxamine (25), a more specific alpha
receptor antagonist. They administered this drug in a 1.5%
aqueous aerosolized solution for a total dosage of 15 mg, 15
minutes pre-exercise. Reduction in EIB dropped from an average
of 35% with placebo to 8% with thymoxamine.

Cholinergic Receptor Modification
        Considerable controversy exists concerning the role of
cholinergic receptors and of their blockade by atropine. Jones
et al. (1963) (26) identified two subjects who appeared to respond
to atropine administered intravenously (0.02-0.03 mg/kg). Sly
was unable to identify a response to 0.1 mg/kg in 10 children
(23). Kiviloog (27) found atropine effective when administered
by aerosol prior to exercise in 5 of 9 subjects with EIB.
        Recently Kershnar et al. (28) reported on a study in which
they compared aerosolized atropine (1 mg) with isoproterenol
(625 μg) and the two combined with cromolyn sodium and placebo.
Both atropine and isoproterenol significantly modified the post
exercise response but when administered together, the two agents
showed a greater response than either administered separately.

Cromolyn Sodium
        The mechanism of action of cromolyn is still not completely
understood. It appears to inhibit cAMP phosphodiesterase in
tissue mast cells as well as stabilizing membranes of these
cells thus inhibiting mediator release (29). Its effectiveness
in EIB as in asthma has been quite variable. Simonsson noted that
only 1 of 6 patients responded to cromolyn sodium when administered
prior to exercise (30). Sly, employing treadmill exercise (31)
and Eggleston (32) employing cycloergometer exercise were able to
show only minimal cromolyn protection post-exercise. By contrast,
Silverman et al. (33) showed that cromolyn produced a highly
significant degree of protection and that in 14 of 31 patients
EIB was completely abolished. Silverman and Godfrey criticised
the Eggleston and Sly studies on the basis that 1) the exercise
stimulus was not sufficient to induce maximal bronchoconstriction

and 2) that the drug was administered too long before exercise
(13). We have recently completed a study which compared free
running, cycloergometer exercise and treadmill exercise when the
drug or placebo were administered within 10 minutes of exercise
to 10 subjects who exhibited significant cycloergometer induced
bronchospasm (Fig. 21.6). In each trial, there was a statistically
significant benefit for cromolyn on large airways (FEV_1) but not
on smaller airways (MMF or $FEF_{25-75\%}$). While there was a quantitative difference between the three forms of exercise, free
running inducing more bronchospasm than other forms of exercise,
there was no difference in drug effect or placebo of the
different forms of exercise (34). Changes in large airways vs.
smaller airways with cromolyn therapy were also noted by Anderson
et al. (35) who measured post exercise airway changes employing
a body plethymograph. Haynes, Ingram and McFadden (36) have
recently demonstrated beneficial effects of cromolyn on EIB
demonstrating that measurements of residual volume (RV), specific
airway conductance and maximum flows at absolute lung volume
between 40 and 60% (Vmax 1SO) are more sensitive indicators of
changes than spirometric changes. All studies of cromolyn show
more marked intersubject variability than of other agents, a
situation paralleling cromolyn effectiveness in control of asthma.

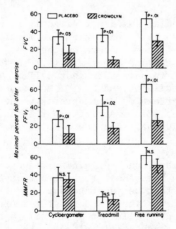

Fig. 21.6 Comparison of effect of pretreatment with Cromolyn
Sodium on FVC, FEV_1 and MMFR with cycloergometer, treadmill and
free running exercise.

Corticosteroids

Even greater variation in patient response has been noted
with corticosteroids. McNeill et al. (11) found that EIB was unchanged by administering 100 mg of hydrocortisone parenterally
to 5 adult asthmatics, 15 minutes prior to exercise. Konig (37)
found improvement in post-exercise bronchoconstriction on
administering or prednisone to 9 asthmatic subjects for one week,

but only 3 of the 9 had a change greater than that which could have
been due to random variation.

A comparison of the exercise response of a group of patients
on chronic prednisone therapy with those receiving placebo did not
show a protective effect, but the patients were not matched for
severity of disease or for responsiveness to exercise prior to
the beginning of steroid therapy.

The administration of betamethasone in a single aerosolized
dosage (37) showed no significant difference over placebo and
even with chronic administration failed to block EIB in 5 of 6
children studied. Frears and coworkers (38) on the other hand
found increased exercise induced bronchoconstriction and exercise
lability when placebo was substituted for betamethasone valerate
aerosol in children who had been receiving it in long term
therapy. Hodgson et al. (39) also found some protection from EIB
on long term administration. Steroids thus appear to have an
effect on exercise induced bronchospasm similar to that found in
asthma where their addition to a standard treatment protocol with
aminophylline and isoproterenol failed to alter airway obstruction
but rather worked tangentially to increase PaO_2 levels probably
by improving pulmonary perfusion/ventilation ratios as well as
response to beta adrenergic agents (40).

Prostaglandins

The prostaglandins which act directly on cAMP and cGMP
might be expected to be potent agents in modulating EIB. Very
little has been published concerning their effects in asthma,
let alone EIB. Austen and coworkers (41) showed direct stimulation of cAMP by PGE in pulmonary mast cells. Townley (42) showed
PGE to be a bronchodilator and $PGF_{2\alpha}$ a potent bronchoconstrictor.
Anderson found no effect of dextrapropoxyphone (43), a prostaglandin inhibitor, on EIB. Aspirin, a PGE inhibitor, may induce
asthma in some individuals and may also increase their EIB.

Other Drugs

Standardized marijuana containing known amounts of $\Delta 9$-tetra-
hydrocannabinol has been shown to hasten recovery from EIB (44)
with as rapid an effect as isoproterenol. Whether it would be
effective in its prevention if administered pre-exercise, however,
has not been studied. While not a suitable agent for therapeutic
use because of its psychotropic effects, related compounds such as
cannabinol and cannabidiol which lack CNS effects may be effective
agents. Sly (45) demonstrated weak inhibition of exercise by pretreatment with diethylcarbamazine palmoate, a drug which appears
to inhibit mediator release, though its precise mechanism of action
is not known.

Application to Patient Care

Patients with EIB as a physical handicap can be divided into
two groups. The first comprises those patients who have chronic
obstructive airway changes which are intensified by exercise.

The second consists of those individuals who, though they have
other allergic problems such as hay fever or middle ear dys-
function secondary to allergic rhinitis, have bronchospasm only
after exercise. Pharmacologic management of these two patient
populations will necessarily vary. Further, the choice of drug
in the United States may differ from that in the United Kingdom
or Canada since a number of potent agents have not been released
by the F.D.A. or are restricted to use in adults. Finally,
the reason for modifying EIB must be considered. The obvious
prescription of sympathomimetic amines in international competition
has been well publicized as a result of experiences in the 1972
Olympic Games and the 1975 Pan-American Games. Other considerations
which may influence the physician's choice of drug include the
route of administration, side effects and possible toxicity. For
instance, the use of freon propelled pressurized hand nebulizers, although an effective delivery system, has a higher abuse potential,
especially in adolescents (46). This was recognized only after a
700% increase in asthma mortality in adolescents (47) from their
abuse in the 1960's. For drugs administered orally, especially those
with short half lives, it is extremely important to administer
them sufficiently in advance of exercise that an optimal serum
concentration is present for pharmacologic effect. Generally,
most drugs are more rapidly absorbed in liquid formulations than
as tablets or capsules and this absorption is further modified by
such factors as dissolution rates of tablets and by the presence of
food in the stomach. A final consideration is that of the adverse
effects on sports performance such as interference with muscular
coordination, alertness, or timing. Drugs increasing ability to
exercise but decreasing performance would hardly be an asset to a
competitive athlete. Finally, there are individual preferences
from physician to physician. The following approach is one which
we have found to be useful.

Management of Patients with EIB and Asthma

The mainstay of management of asthma is theophylline, given
at appropriate intervals over 24 hours, sufficient to produce
a theophylline serum concentration of between 10 and 20 ug/ml
(48). Since there is considerable intersubject variation in
clearance and thus drug half life, one must establish a kinetic
pattern for each subject by taking multiple serum samples during
a dosing interval (49). Such a therapeutic program is effective
frequently in both controlling asthma and enabling the patient
to exercise normally.

If this is not effective, our second drug is cromolyn sodium,
administered by inhalation 5-20 minutes prior to exercise. This
is helpful in a majority of patients, and this combination is
acceptable in international athletic competition. For those who
fail to respond, the addition of an adrenergic such as metaproterenol or terbutaline administered orally has been shown to
be effective if given 1½ to 3 hours prior to exercise. No study
comparing optimal theophylline dosages with orally administered

sympathomimetic agents or their combination has been published.
We are currently involved in such a study but have not yet
reached a point where a definite conclusion can be drawn.
Aerosolized sympathomimetics administered before exercise are
extremely effective, but bear the hazard of abuse potential.
If required, they should be given by non-refillable prescriptions
only after a full discussion of adverse effects and consequences
of overdosage with the patient (and with the parents, if the
patients is a minor).

Management of Patients with only EIB

The use of theophylline or theophylline containing combinations
one to two hours prior to exercise is effective in many patients.
The effectiveness should be tested by a repeat exercise test
performed after administration of medication.

If this is not effective, add cromolyn sodium 5-20 minutes
prior to exercise to the theophylline medication. Again, test
effectiveness by a repeat exercise test after medication.

If this combination is not effective, place on full therapeutic
dosgae of theophylline (round the clock therapy) and treat in the
same manner as patients who have chronic asthma and EIB.

Summary

Exercise induced bronchospasm appears to be asthma in microcosm
with similar pulmonary physiological changes to acute asthma but
in a time frame of minutes as opposed to days. As a model of
asthma it is a useful non-pharmacologic, non-immunologic technique
to provide insights into its pathophysiology and to evaluate
drug effects. Drugs affecting asthma appear to have similar
effects on EIB. Drugs which have a beneficial affect on EIB include
beta adrenergic agonists, theophylline, cromolyn sodium, atropine,
some alpha adrenergic antagonists and possibly prostaglandin E.
Drugs adversely affecting EIB include beta antagonists, acetylcholine, alpha agonists and possibly prostaglandin F_2 .
Corticosteroids which are very effective in controlling chronic
asthma topically or systemically seem to be exceptions for they
have minimal effectiveness in EIB. Agents effective for clinical
use include the longer acting beta adrenergic agents and theophylline. Metaproterenol, terbutaline and salbutamol are active
orally if administered 1½ to 3 hours before exercise or by inhalation 10 minutes before exercise. Theophylline is effective
when administered in a dose which provides a serum concentration
of between 10 and 20 ug/ml at the time of exercise. Cromolyn
sodium is more variable and while it may be extremely effective
for some patients when inhaled 5 to 20 minutes before exercise,
is not helpful for others. The use of theophylline plus cromolyn,
or theophylline, a beta adrenergic agent and cromolyn, may be
effective in some patients in whom a single drug is not effective.
Other agents, such as inhaled atropine or thymoxamine, while
effective, are not available for clinical use.

It is the physician's obligation to identify the allergic

patient with EIB in order to minimize physical handicaps and
facilitate normal physical, social and recreational activity.
The appropriate use of drugs enables individuals with EIB to
lead a normal life including active participation in recreational
and competititve athletic events (50).

ACKNOWLEDGMENTS

The authors gratefully acknowledge the permission of Dr. E.R.
McFadden, Jr. and The New England Journal of Medicine for Figure
21.1B and Dr. J.L.L. Morse and the American Review of Respiratory
Disease for use of Figure 21.4. They are also very indebted to
Ms. Kathy Seese for her persistence in preparing the manuscript.

REFERENCES

1. Bierman CW, Pierson, WE and Shapiro GG: JAMA 234:295, 1975.
2. McFadden, ER Jr, Kiser R and deGroot, WJ: NEJM 288:221, 1973.
3. Cropp, GJA and Schmultzler, IJ: ,Pediatrics 56:860, 1975.
4. Eggleston, PA, Beasley P and Guerrant, JG: J Allergy Clin
   Imm 57:175, 1976.
5. Konig P and Godfrey S: J Allergy Clin Immunol 54:280, 1976.
6. Eggleston PA: Pediatrics 56:856, 1975.
7. Pierson WE and Bierman CW: Pediatrics 56:890, 1975.
8. Goldberg ND, Haddox MK, Nicol SE, et al: New Directions in
   Asthma, American College of Chest Physicians, 1975, p103.
9. Austen KF, Lewis RA, Wasserman SI and Goetzl EJ: Ibid, p187.
10. Jenne, JW: Ibid, p391.
11. McNeill R.S., Nairn JR, Miller JS and Ingram CG: Quart J Med
    35:55, 1965.
12. Heimlick EM, Strick L, Busser RJ: J Allergy 37:103, 1966.
13. Godfrey S, Silverman M, Anderson S: J Allergy Clin Immunol
    52:199, 1973.
14. Sly RM, Heimlick EM, Ginsberg J, et al: Ann Allergy 26, 253,
    1968.
15. Sly RM, Mayer J: Ann Allergy 26:253, 1968.
16. Morse, JLL, Jones NL, Anderson GD: Am Rev Resp Dis 113:89,
    1976.
17. Godfrey S and Konig P: Pediatrics 56:930, 1975.
18. Sly RM, Pediatrics 56: 910, 1975.
19. Anderson SD, Silverman M, Konig P, and Godfrey S: Brit J Dis
    Chest 69:1, 1975.
20. Kiechel F, Pollack J, Cooper D. and Winberger M: J Allergy
    Clin Immunol 57:250, 1976.
21. Simons FER, Bierman CW, Sprenkle AC, Simons KJ: Pediatrics
    56:916, 1975.
22. Zaid G and Beall GN: NEJM, 275:580, 1966.
23. Sly RM, Heimlick EM, Busser RJ, et al: J Allergy 40:93, 1967.
24. Irving MH, Britton BJ, Wood WG, et al: Nature 248:533, 1974.
25. Patel KR, Kerr JW, MacDonald EB, et al: J Allergy Clin Immunol
    57:285, 1976.
26. Jones RS, Wharton MJ, Buston MH: Arch Dis Childhood 38:972,
    1963.
27. Kiviloog, J: Pediatrics 56:940, 1975.

28. Kershnar H, Katz R, Tashkin D, et al: J Allergy Clin Immunol
    57:261, 1976.
29. Bierman CW and Soyka L: Pediatrics 55:586, 1975.
30. Simonsson BG, Skoogh BE, Ekstrom JB: Thorax 27:169, 1972.
31. Sly Rm: Ann Allergy 29:362, 1971.
32. Eggleston PA, Bierman CW, Pierson WE, et al: J Allergy Clin
    Immunol 50:57, 1972.
33. Silverman M, Konig P and Godfrey S: Thorax 28:574, 1973.
34. Pierson WE, Bierman CW, Shapiro GG: in preparation.
35. Anderson SD, McEvoy JDS and Bianco S: Am Rev Respir Dis 106:
    30, 1972.
36. Haynes RL, Ingram RH Jr, McFadden ER Jr: Am Rev Resp Dis, in
    press.
37. Konig P, Jaffe P and Godfrey S: J Allergy Clin Immunol 54:14,
    1974.
38. Frears J, Hodgson S and Friedman M: Arch Dis Child 50:387,
    1975.
39. Hodgson SV, McPherson A and Friedman M: Postgraduate Med J
    50 (Suppl 4) 69, 1974.
40. Pierson WE, Bierman CW, Kelley VC: Pediatrics 54:282, 1974.
41. Orange RP, Austen WG, and Austen KF: J Exp Med 134:136s,
    1971.
42. Adolphson RL and Townley RG: J Allergy Clin Immunol 45:119,
    1970.
43. Anderson SP, Dolton R, Lindsay DA, et al: Aust Nzlnd J Med
    4:312, 1974.
44. Tashkin DD, Shapiro BJ, Lee YE, et al: Am Rev Resp Dis 112:
    377, 1975.
45. Sly RM: J Allergy Clin Immunol 53:82, 1974.
46. Bierman CW, Pierson WE: Pediatrics 54:668, 1974.
47. Speizer FE, Doll R, Heaf P and Strang LB: Br Med J 1:339,
    1968.
48. Bierman CW, Commentary Pediatrics: in press.
49. Ellis EF, Koysooko R, Levy G: Pediatrics, in press.
50. Committee on Drugs: Am Acad Ped, Pediatrics 52:886, 1973.

DISCUSSION

Goldman: Did you say that there was an added effect from drug and placebo?

Bierman: There was a beneficial effect of placebo compared to no drug.

Godfrey: I am glad to hear that you have converted to believing cromolyn does something. The half life of protection by cromolyn is about three-fourths of an hour so that with two half lives in an hour and a half, there is not much protection from exercise induced asthma after that. In comparing the effect of different drugs the striking thing about atropine was the tremendous bronchodilitation it produced. Salbutamol and theophylline also dilated; cromolyn and placebo did not. There is a much higher baseline with atropine than with the other drugs. I believe that atropine does affect exercise induced asthma, but how much it does is still open to doubt (Fig. 1).

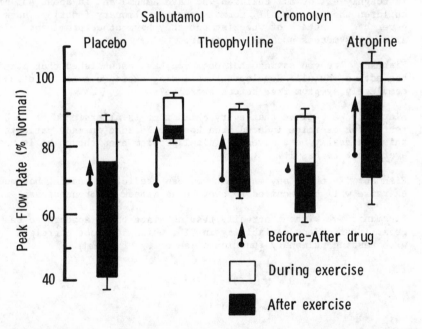

Fig. A. The effects of drugs on exercise induced asthma, the values being expressed as a percentage of the expected peak flow rate. The arrow indicates the bronchodilitation due to the administration of the drug, occurring at rest, before the exercise test. The bars indicate the mean ± SEM. (Reprinted from Anderson et al., British J. of Dis. of the Chest, 69:1, 1975.)

Cropp: I agree that in the assessment of the effectiveness of
therapeutic agents on exercise induced asthma we always have to
study the patient before drug treatment and again after the drug.
However, the assessment should be before exercise as well as repeatedly after exercise. When we looked at our data on the effectiveness of cromolyn and isoproterenol it appeared that isoproterenol was very much more effective in preventing exercise induced
bronchospasm than cromolyn. But, when we related the lesser degree
of bronchospasm elicited by exercise to post-treatment pre-exercise
measurements both drugs were equally effective. In other words,
the additional benefits from isoproterenol were the results of
pre-exercise bronchodilation rather than more effective prevention
of the exercise induced response.

Fishman: Will every asthmatic if pushed hard enough develop asthma?

Bierman: The answer may depend upon which test for pulmonary functions is employed. Looking at parameters such as FEV_1, FEF_{25}.
FEF_{75} and peak flow (PEFR) we see exercise induced asthma developing
in roughly 82% of all children who have asthma and in about 45% of
children who have totally normal resting pulmonary function, have
never had an attack of wheezing but they have other prominent
allergic symptoms such as hay fever.

Fishman: Are you saying that once you have established that a child
has asthma, he will develop asthma during exercise even if he is
completely symptom free before exercise?

Bierman: We believe that every child that is allergic ought to be
tested for exercise induced bronchospasm because in many patients
this can really be a severe clinical problem even though he is not
aware that he has it.

Fishman: Is there any way that you can predict by testing how much
exercise will be required to provoke an attack of bronchospasm?

Bierman: Not without actually testing since there appears to be
great intersubject variability in EIB, which does not correlate
with resting pulmonary function or severity of asthma.

Discussion

Godfrey: May I try to answer Dr. Fishman's question on the pre-dictability of an asthma attack? If an asthmatic child exercises for 6 minutes on a treadmill or by free range running and gets his heart rate up to about 160 he will wheeze. Whether he wheezes after exercise at a lesser level is a more difficult question. Our data suggests that the heavier the work the more the obstruction, provided the running is continuous. But with intermittent exercise the response is much less predictable.

McFadden: Dr. Fishman, do you mean to ask at what level of obstruc-tion will symptoms develop? Or are you asking what will happen in terms of lung function abnormalities?

Fishman: No, I am trying to understand the extent to which one can predict the occurrence of exercise-induced asthma. I am now convinced that the designation "post-exercise asthma" is a misnomer.

Cropp: In my opinion not every asthmatic falls on the same dose response curve in regard to the development of exercise induced asthma. In a patient who is exquisitely responsive to exercise, we can reproduce asthma very consistently provided that the patient starts off with the same lung function. When we test such patients on successive days with different levels of exercise we can demon-strate an increasing degree of exercise induced bronchospasm with increasing work loads up to a level at which we reach a maximum degree of exercise induced asthma. However, not every subject will fall on this curve. Some may have a threshold that is not the same on every day. The milder the phenomenon is in a given subject the less reproducible it is. Similarly, the temporal response to exercise is not the same in every subject. Children develop the greatest deterioration in function within two to three minutes, while adults usually develop their maximum reduction five to ten minutes after exercise. There are also some children who get progressively worse for one hour, and then spontaneously improve. Only about 5-10% of asthmatic children when stressed strenuously will get progressively worse for up to one hour after the comple-tion of exercise. As many as 30% of adults show progressive deterioration. It appears that those patients who get progressive-ly worse are those who have evidence of more small airway involve-ment than the ones who get worse very rapidly and then quickly recover.

Fishman: Do these views of "dose-response curves" imply that the lungs of an asthmatic can be regarded as though they were an isolated tracheao-bronchial preparation? By analogy, that you can write Starling-like curves for each patient? If this is so, then the asthmatic should be characterized by the position and slope of the "dose-response"curve without having to exercise to the point of an overt episode of bronchospasm?

McFadden: That is true. We do not need to get someone symptomatic to reach an end point.

Fishman: Will each patient write the same dose-response curve,
day after day, except when his course is interrupted by an
episode of asthma which moves him temporarily to another curve?

McFadden: I don't think the data is in. The question has to be
answered by a formal study which will be very tedious to do. One
has to consider existing obstruction and how much that influences
the dose response relationship. It would take a large number of
exercise trials in any given patient and a large number of patients
to come to those kinds of answers. We have studied twenty people
twice a day on two different days. We found that as their baseline varied their response varied. If they were very well or
normal by our standards, their response was apt to be just an
increase in residual volume. If only residual volume was abnormal,
the response was apt to be a significant change in all aspects of
lung function but no symptoms developed. If residual volume was
large and a maximum and expiratory flow rate reduced, the subject
was apt to get a moderately severe attack of asthma. If he had a
compromised FEV_1, he was apt to get a severe attack of asthma and
he was apt to deteriorate over a period of time before he got
better. We went to the arms and legs study because it is easier to
control. I don't agree that a fixed duration of exercise is
necessary. I submit that the response seen is related to the size
of the muscle mass exercised and to the stress applied to that
muscle mass for some quantity of time.

Godfrey: We also think there is no set and predictable amount of
exercise required. If you go on too long you probably run through
it. As far as the combination of intensity and duration of
exercise is concerned we compared running for short times very hard
and longer times less hard and the results were similar.

Wasserman: I think that we have to keep in mind that the blood is
essentially drained from the arms during arm exercise when the arms
are elevated. The subjects had an oxygen consumption of 1.7
liters/minute which is a very high oxygen consumption for arm
exercise in terms of the relative mass. The minute ventilation
relative to the oxygen consumption of your subjects was three times
that of what it was with leg exercise. They were apparently receiving a lot of pain from their acidotic and ischemic arms. Thus
after the arm exercise there would be a great post-exercise lactic
acidosis. The pH and bicarbonate would drop as the lactate went
up. I wonder if post-exercise bronchospasm is more related to
post-exercise lactic acidemia rather than the during-exercise
lactic acidemia. Have any of you measurements on post exercise
lactate and pH?

McFadden: [H+] data I showed were from the fifth minute of recovery.
It climbed as you indicated it would. The other thing we thought

about was were we making the arms so ischemic that we were liber-
ating something else.

Rankin: It seems to me that there is a part missing in this
story. Very extensive studies have been done during exercise and
equally extensive studies have been done several minutes after
exercise, but I have seen very little data on the dramatic transition from exercise to rest when the lactic acid is at its highest.
If the asthmatic were to diminish his exercise gradually and not
stop it abruptly so adjustments in lactic acid could occur and his
muscles would still use it, would that prevent asthma?

Godfrey: Some children get such severe exercise-induced asthma
that we have to stop while they are still running. I don't believe
that running down would have significant effect. As Dr. Fishman
pointed out the asthma is really beginning during exercise and is
probably being masked.

McFadden: I think, Dr. Rankin, that your point may be that if
they stop or run down before they develop any mechanical changes,
what then would happen?

Godfrey: That would be akin to warming up in an athletic event.
I postulate that you could slowly discharge your mast cells or whatever in the warm up period. May be that is what happens when kids
play football--they gradually trickle out their mediator while they
are protected by their sympathetic drive and therefore, they don't
get wheezy with intermittent exercise.

Forster: Can occupational activities induce asthma?

McFadden: As a matter of fact you can get asthma with forms of
activity like lifting bricks.

Reed: Your story about the cross country skier implied that well
trained subjects might have to undergo a lot more exercise to
provoke asthma than a sedentary person would. I wondered if there
is any systematic data on the value or lack of value of physical
fitness in preventing exercise-induced asthma?

Cropp: K.D. Fitch (Pediatrics, 56:904, 1975) studied this and
concluded that while physical training will not cure exercise
induced asthma it will raise the threshold above which it becomes
clinically significant.

Godfrey: Fitch (Fitch, K.D., Morton, A.R. & Blanksby, B.A. Arch.
Dis. Child., 51:190, 1976) trained some Australian children to
improve their physical fitness and aerobic capacity. He then
exercised them on the treadmill and found they still got exercise-
induced asthma. But the critical experiment would be to do a dose
response curve before and after training because if the exercise is
on the flat part of the dose response curve you can't really be

sure about the effect of training.

Jankowski: What happens to arterial blood gas during exercise?

McFadden: There are individuals whose oxygen tension goes up
during exercise, the mechanism of which is not known. There are
others whose oxygen tension goes down. The net effect, however, of
both groups is that after they stop exercising and develop the
airway obstruction they have a moderate fall in PO_2.

Sampson: Is the hypothetical release of mediators from mast cells
in the lung, complete and total? Is the time course for recovery
of the ability to undergo exercise-induced bronchospasm would be
consistent with the ability of mast cell to replete or replenish
their mediators whatever they are.

Adkinson: The question of whether the release of mediators is
complete in vivo is difficult. There are some studies showing that
compound 40/80 applied directly to one limited section of a membrane
of a rat mast cell can release mediators only from granules adjacent
to that particular part of the membrane. This suggests the possibility of partial release, at least in this artificial system. The
dose response curves of antigen-induced mediator release in vitro
are typical sigmoid-shaped curves; the time required for maximum
release is to some degree a function of the antigen concentration
employed. Optimal concentrations of antigen may release mediators
nearly completely within 15-20 minutes. Reconstitution of preformed mediators such as histamine is slow and probably takes many
hours. Assuming complete degranulation, it would surely take a
considerably longer period of time than 30 minutes to reconstitute
intracellular histamine. To the best of my knowledge, there is no
information about the time course for re-synthesis of the SRS-A
precursor.

Godfrey: The half time for recovery of response is about 3/4 of
an hour so we were looking for something with a re-synthesis half
time of about 3/4 hour.

McFadden: That is not evidence for mediator release or re-
synthesis. No one has established to my knowledge that mediators
even get released.

Sampson: I was asking the question in terms of the model.

Godfrey: Yes, it's a model but it is supported by the fact that
cromolyn is effective and the only known action of cromolyn is to
prevent mediator release.

Adkinson: One point relevant to this issue is that during the discharge process, biochemical mechanisms are desensitized in a way
that requires a recovery period; they are, therefore, unresponsive
to restimulation for a period of time. Recovery from this state

of responsiveness does not depend upon re-synthesis of mediators at all.

McFadden: In an antigen challenge, when the mast cell is fired does the antigen disassociate from the IgE and have to reassociate or does the Fc fragment disassociate from the membrane? Does the esterase have to regenerate?

Adkinson: The working hypothesis at our institution is that bridging of two surface-bound IgE antibodies by a single antigenic molecule is sufficient to trigger maximum release of histamine from circulating human basophils. Under appropriate conditions, the antigen-complexed IgE molecules together with the basophil Fc receptor will undergo cap formation and eventual endocytosis (Becker et al., J.E.M., 138:394-409, 1973). Requirements for esterase regeneration have not yet been studied to the best of my knowledge.

Sampson: I wonder if exercise-induced bronchospasm in patients with viral infections or some other disorders of the airways is similar or identical to that in asthmatic patients.

Bierman: Our asthmatic patients who had viral infections, had more severe exercise-induced bronchospasm for a period of four to six weeks.

Sampson: Do you know if non-asthmatic patients with viral infections have exercise induced bronchospasm?

Bierman: We haven't looked.

McFadden: Perhaps Dr. Reed would care to comment on some of his earlier studies that viral infection lowers the threshold for a number of stimuli, histamine and methacholine, for instance.

Reed: We haven't looked at exercise but did find that respiratory infections lower the threshold of both normal and asthmatic subjects to methacholine. Empey, et al., (Am. Rev. Resp. Dis., 113:131, 1976) found that respiratory infections lowered the threshold of normal persons to histamine.

Godfrey: Ian Gregg in serial studies of a small number of asthmatics finds that when they get a viral infection their exercise-induced asthma becomes much more marked for a while.

Eggleston: I have described a group of children with seasonal allergy who had a great deal more exercise-induced asthma in season than out of season (Eggleston, D.A., Ped., 56:856, 1975). I have since looked more extensively at a group of young adults and did not consistently find that phenomenon.

Bierman: Do you think there is a difference between children and adults?

Eggleston: There may be, but there is a great deal of variation between repeat tests in the same subjects and that may have accounted for the observation too.

Haynes: You observed that asthmatic individuals with respiratory tract infections have a greater degree of exercise-induced asthma than when not infected. We know that a major factor influencing an asthmatic's exercise response is the baseline state of his airways, particularly residual volume (Haynes, R.L., Ingram, R.H., and McFadden, E.R., Jr. Proceedings of the Eastern Society ATS, 2:10, 1975). Could not the increased exercise responsiveness of your subjects be on the basis of worsened baseline pulmonary function with respiratory infection rather than the infection per se?

Bierman: We have data on airway function by spirograms where the baselines have been the same. We don't have residual volume and conductive studies.

Reed: During infections, baselines may be different nevertheless. Studies currently in progress by our group suggest that both normal and asthmatic subjects have small airway obstruction 3-7 days after a rhinovirus infection at the time that their methacholine response is greater.

Cerny: It seems to me that the difference in the effects of swimming versus other types of exercise might give some clue as to a more mechanical type of mechanism. I was a little disappointed in Dr. McFadden's study showing that the increase in ventilation alone doesn't bring on the attack, since repeated FVC maneuvers can also cause obstruction.

McFadden: That is a different mechanism. It is a reflex that can be blocked with atropine. It is due to changing volume history and it may be related to a discrepancy between airway and parenchymal recovery phenomenon similar to normal relative hysteresis. That does not appear to be the mechanism operating in exercise-induced asthma.

Godfrey: Furthermore, there is a very simple observation that during exercise tests we keep repeating the FVC tests every two or three minutes. At first they get worse and then better. If the obstruction was being induced by the deep breathing maneuvers themselves you would expect it to get worse and keep on getting worse.

McFadden: I would like to come back to the swimming experiment. It seems to me that it is an extremely complex situation depending on which muscle groups are used in swimming and how the stroke is applied. Is that a recovery stroke, can I ask the work

physiologists? Is this intermittent work? Are the legs dead
weight? Has anyone performed swimming, for instance, in a water
treadmill to quantitate the subjects' speed, etc.? How was it
done? Fish and Morton did it by monitoring heart rates.

Godfrey: We did it in the swimming pool of the Imperial College
in London by monitoring heart rates and by having the children
swim around with Douglas bags on their backs in which we collected
oxygen so that we could measure their $\dot{V}O_2$.

McFadden: Does the fact that the body has a density that is almost
the same as the water explain things?

Godfrey: I don't know, but swimming is a very special case doing
a strange kind of exercise in a strange position in a strange
medium.

Grimby: Bronchoconstriction induced by the combination of exercise
and cold air is quite frequent. Have you looked at the effect of
cold air on exercise-induced bronchospasm?

Bierman: We did all of our screening tests free running out of
doors and we found definite seasonal effects with more marked
bronchoconstriction during cold weather than when it is warm.

McFadden: I would ask how far the air has to get down the tracheobronchial tree before it gets warmed. Does exercise overwhelm
the ability to humidify and heat the inspired air?

Cropp: I think the receptor for cold has to be very high up in
the respiratory passages, probably in the nose or possibly in the
posterior pharynx because Burton passed thermistors down the
trachea, and even when the inspired air was at $-70°$, air was warmed
to body temperature by the time it reaches the carina (Armstrong,
H.G., Burton, A.C., and Hall, G.E. J. Aviat. Med., 29:593, 1958).
Stimulation of nasal receptors can elicit bronchospasm. I think
there is no reason not to believe that very cold air in the nose
elicit this response.

Eldridge: This has been done. It was reported at an Atlantic
City meeting about ten years ago. Air at approximately $0°$, in
the pharynx caused measurable increase in airway resistance in
susceptible subjects. It could be blocked with atropine.

Cropp: Certain forms of athletic activities and recreational
activities are hardly ever associated with exercise-induced asthma.
For instance, in Colorado, downhill skiing rarely provokes
exercise-induced bronchospasm. Long distance running or cross
country skiing is very prone to elicit bronchospasm.

Grimby: How well have you standardized the time of the day when
the experiments were done?

Cropp: We always do them at a standard time early in the afternoon.

Godfrey: In our experiments with 80 children a small increase in
exercise-induced asthma before lunch and before tea has been noted.

Reed: DeVries and colleagues challenged asthmatic patients with
histamine every four hours for 24 hours and found much greater
sensitivity at night than during the day (Basel, Int. Arch.
Allergy & Appl. Immunol., 20:93, 1962).

Adkinson: I would like to comment on Dr. McFadden's acidosis
hypothesis in terms of facilitation of mediator release. The pH
optimum for mediator release in both peritoneal mast cells and
human basophils falls between 6.8 and 7.2. Furthermore, most of
the enzymes in the prostaglandin synthetase system have pH optimums
in the acidic range. This is also true for the phospholipases
that release the arachidonic acid precursor from the cell membrane.
So here are two theoretical ways in which the increase in [H+]
seen after exercise might potentiate mediator release. I have a
comment and a question for Dr. Bierman. You have reported that
some nonasthmatic patients, who are atopic individuals by virtue
of having allergic rhinitis or other IgE-mediated disorders, can
have pronounced exercise-induced asthma. These are patients who
are absolutely without asthmatic symptoms except when they
exercise. This to me suggests that there may be a risk factor
linked to the atopic constitution. Perhaps we ought not to associate exercise-induced bronchospasm exclusively with the asthmatic
state per se, but realize that there are other predisposing factors
as well.

Bierman: Many of these patients are unaware that they have post
exercise bronchospasm, but frequently they will cough with exercise.
Perhaps we are identifying a group who is not now asthmatic but is
at risk of becoming asthmatic in the future. An exercise test may
help predict the development of asthma.

Godfrey: We certainly have seen a group who were asthmatic, in
the past and who are not now clinically asthmatic, but wheeze on
the treadmill. I would be fairly happy now to say that a person
is an asthmatic if exercise provokes asthma. If you ask them
"do you have asthma," they may say "no." But if you say, "do you
wheeze" quite often they will tell you that they do when they get
a cold or something like that.

Cropp: Another epidemiological fact that may be pertinent to this
is that 40-50% of hay fever patients have exercise-induced
bronchospasm, and if 40-50% of hay fever patients eventually
develop asthma (Jones, R.S. Brit. Med. J., 2:972, 1966), it is
very possible that those patients with hay fever who show the
reactivity to exercise are those patients who later may develop
bronchospasm.

Reed: I don't know the sources of the statement that 30-40% of people with hay fever eventually develop asthma. The studies that I know of reported rates of 2 to 5% (Broder, et al. J. Allergy Clin. Immunol., 53:127, 1974. Hagy, G.W. and Settipane, G.A. J. Allergy Clin. Immunol., 48:200, 1971). A substantial number of people with hay fever do, however, have abnormal airway responses to histamine or methacholine aerosol (Parker, K.D., Bilbo, R., and Reed, C.E. Arch. Int. Med., 115:462, 1965). Could I pursue this analogy between the antigen-induced mediator and the hypothetical mediator release from exercise by asking a question? Sensitive individuals challenged with antigen by aerosol will often have a second wave of airway obstruction four to eight hours after recovery from the immediate reaction. Does one ever observe a second wave of obstruction after vigorous exercise in a patient prone to exercise-induced asthma?

Godfrey: We looked for it many times and we have never seen it.

McFadden: We have not seen it either.

Cropp: We have not seen it, but we have seen patients who have developed extreme exercise-induced asthma who were then treated with medications which elicited bronchodilation for longer than a couple of hours, and who three or four hours later would re-develop bronchospasm; I don't think that this proves that we are dealing with a secondary type of airway obstruction. In general, I would agree with Simon, but I think that exercise-induced asthma can last for hours. It is rare, but it can.

Godfrey: I don't believe that. It might in adults but I don't recall ever seeing a child where it has not begun to wear off within a half an hour and be significantly better by an hour.

McFadden: It can persist for three hours or more in an adult.

Godfrey: We have been talking mainly about allergic (atopic) subjects but Silverman and Turner-Warwick (Clin. Allergy, 2:137, 1972) compared allergic asthmatics and asthmatics in whom no antigens could be demonstrated. They found as much exercise-induced asthma in the intrinsic as the extrinsic groups. Interestingly, the blocking by cromolyn was a little less effective in the intrinsics than the extrinsics.

Part V
Pulmonary Gas Exchange

22

Pulmonary Gas Exchange: Introduction

Peter D. Wagner

The first four sessions of this Exercise Symposium have dealt in considerable detail with mechanical properties of the lung, the control of these properties, and the control of ventilation in general. Little has been said about the state of the pulmonary circulation during exercise or about the final end-product, pulmonary gas exchange. Few would deny that the pulmonary circulation and pulmonary gas exchange are as important areas for study as mechanics and control, yet only 20% of this meeting is devoted to some 50% of the physiology. This is not an oversight on the part of the organizers but rather a reflection of the current state of our knowledge of the pulmonary circulation and of pulmonary gas exchange during exercise. The reason for this unbalanced state of affairs seems fairly clear: insufficient methodology. Not only are the airways more accessible than the blood ways, but the techniques available for investigating the airways during exercise are considerably more direct than those available for examining the circulation. While we know what happens to the arterial P_{O_2} and P_{CO_2} during exercise, there is little known about the mechanisms of the changes in blood gases with exercise. This is because multiple factors influence the arterial P_{O_2} and P_{CO_2} and generally available techniques are incapable of differentiating these factors unequivocally in a given patient.

THE PULMONARY CIRCULATION DURING EXERCISE

1. <u>Relationships Between Vascular Pressures and Bloodflow</u>

We are all familiar with West's concept of the topographical inequality of perfusion in the lung and its gravitational mechanism (27). In this scheme, perfusion per unit of lung volume increases progressively from the apex down towards the base because pulmonary arterial pressure increases hydrostatically (zone II) or because transmural capillary pressure increases (zone III). Recruitment of unopened capillaries, distension of capillaries that are already open or both must accommodate this increase in perfusion, but the relative importance of these two mechanisms remains one of the most long-standing unresolved issues in the field (20).

315

Glazier and his coworkers (8) used rapid-freezing techniques to obtain evidence that while recruitment and distension were of similar importance in zone II, distension predominated in zone III, a finding that is intuitively comfortable for many. Warrell and his coworkers (25) entered into the debate by statistically analyzing the pattern of capillary filling also using the rapid-freezing preparation and concluded that there was considerable random variation in capillary filling within regions likely to be supplied by a single arteriole. These data were interpreted as evidence against the concepts advanced by Permutt and coworkers (20) that critical arteriolar opening pressures were of primary importance in determining capillary perfusion. Warrell's data suggested that the capillary bed did not respond passively and uniformly to changes in pulmonary arteriolar pressure and thus that local capillary factors were also important in the determination of regional perfusion. More recently West and coworkers (30) showed how a distribution of critical capillary opening pressures might explain Warrell's data.

The basic experimental approaches of Permutt's group on the one hand and West's on the other deserves some mention because they are reasonably removed from the physiological state of affairs in exercising human subjects. In both cases the experimental model was an open-chested anesthetized dog preparation. Permutt's dogs underwent double heart bypass and this enabled the group to measure relationships between pulmonary arterial and left atrial pressures, alveolar pressure and pulmonary bloodflow. In West's approach, essentially the same variables were measured, but much of the information was obtained through rapid-freezing techniques which allowed West and his group to examine the micro-structure of the subpleural region of the lung. Most of these data have been reported in terms of capillary dimensions and red cell concentrations in the alveolar capillaries.

A fresh approach to this problem was begun some 10 years ago by Drs. Wagner and Filley in Denver (24). They developed a preparation in which the subpleural alveoli and their capillaries were directly visualized through a transparent window in the chest wall. While the data from such preparations were necessarily less quantitative than those of either Permutt or West, they were obtained under considerably more physiological conditions and therefore complement the approaches of the previous groups. In this symposium Dr. Wagner brings his methods to bear on the question of capillary recruitment and changes in bloodflow with changes in pulmonary arterial pressure.

The issues discussed so far are set in a framework of a network of pulmonary capillary segments. In other words capillaries are conceived as a system of interconnected tubes. The alternative formulation of Fung and Sobin (7) of the capillary bed as a sheet of blood rather than as a network deserves mention. Sheet flow theory has produced some interesting predictions of the pressure flow characteristics of the pulmonary capillary bed, one of which is that the pressure in the pulmonary capillary is much closer to pulmonary arterial than to pulmonary venous. Although Fung and

Sobin have not specifically investigated the response of their
"sheet" to exercise, it is possible that such a study might provide
predictions that could be tested and thus help in evaluating
whether we should think of the capillary sys tem as a sheet or as a
network.

2. Pulmonary Capillary Blood Volume

Whether the capillary circulation in the lung responds during
exercise by distension, recruitment or both, there is widespread
agreement that in normal subjects at least the capillary blood
volume is increased. The evidence is more indirect than that obtained in the studies of pressure-flow properties described above,
but on the other hand it has been obtained under physiological
conditions in man. This evidence consists almost entirely of
estimates of the capillary blood volume made from measurements of
the diffusing capacity (transfer factor) (13,15,16). The approach
used is that pioneered by Roughton and Forster (22) in which the
reduction in diffusing capacity for carbon m onoxide with increasing arterial P_{O_2} is exploited. It is generally accepted that the
reaction rate (θ_{CO}) between carbon monoxide and hemoglobin falls
as P_{O_2} in blood is raised, and based upon the formulation (derived
by Roughton and Forster)

$$\frac{1}{DL_{CO}} = \frac{1}{DM_{CO}} + \frac{1}{VC \cdot \theta_{CO}}$$

it is possible to estimate the membrane diffusing capacity (DM_{CO}) and
the capillary blood volume (VC) from measurements of diffusing
capacity (DL_{CO}) under conditions in which θ_{CO} is varied in a known
manner. The theory and application of this approach have been well-
reviewed by Forster (5).

By separately controlling pulmonary arterial pressure and total
pulmonary bloodflow, Baker and Daly (2) were able to establish in
dogs that the increase in diffusing capacity that occurred on exercise was related only to the increase in pulmonary arterial pressure and not to the concurrent increase in total pulmonary bloodflow. This conclusion agrees with the West model of regional perfusion depending on pulmonary arterial pressure, if we assume that
regional perfusion and regional capillary volume are at least
qualitatively related. It is worth noting that methods based on
diffusing capacity measurements cannot differentiate between recruitment and distension as mechanisms responsible for the increase in pulmonary capillary blood volume during exercise, and in
any case are probably of limited usefulness in lungs containing
ventilation-perfusion inequality. Dr. Wagner is again in a position to provide us with some direct information concerning the
capillary volume response to changes in arterial pressure.

VENTILATION-PERFUSION INEQUALITY AND GAS EXCHANGE DURING
EXERCISE

1. Changes in the Topographical Distribution of Bloodflow

It is well known that pulmonary arterial pressure rises during
exercise even in normal subjects and that total pulmonary vascular
resistance falls. The fall in resistance is undoubtedly the result
of vascular recruitment and/or distension and there is widespread
agreement that this occurs to a relatively greater degree in the
upper regions of the lung associated with the increase in pulmonary arterial pressure. In other words, the topographical distribution of perfusion becomes more uniform and this has indeed
been found to be the case (4,29).

The result of the topographical distribution of perfusion becoming more uniform during exercise forms the basis of a very
common statement made concerning pulmonary gas exchange during
exercise, and that is that the distribution of ventilation-
perfusion ($\dot{V}_A/\dot{Q}$) ratios becomes more even during exercise (1,18).

This seems a good place to point out that the correct statement
is that the topographical distribution of ventilation-perfusion
ratios as detected with radioactive gases becomes more uniform
with exercise. Since radioactive gas methods have limited spatial
resolution, not all of the lung can be sampled and the areas that
are sampled are to a varying extent necessarily averaged. The
topographical distribution of $\dot{V}_A/\dot{Q}$ will accurately reflect the
functional distribution of $\dot{V}_A/\dot{Q}$ only if the areas that cannot be
resolved with the topographical approach are truly homogeneous
and in addition represent accurately any areas of lung that cannot be sampled.

Thus it is not at all a foregone conclusion that the functional
distribution of ventilation-perfusion ratios narrows upon exercise, even if the topographical distribution becomes more uniform.
In fact as will be discussed, the alveolar-arterial P_{O_2} difference
(AaD$_{O_2}$) generally widens on exercise which suggests, but does not
prove, that at the functional level the amount of ventilation-
perfusion inequality is increasing.

What happens to the distribution of ventilation-perfusion ratios
at the functional level remains one of the important unanswered
questions in exercise physiology, and half of today's session is
devoted to reports of data obtained using methods designed to
assess this particular issue.

2. Changes in the Arterial P_{O_2} and Alveolar-Arterial P_{O_2}
Difference

Aside from the issue of changes in the distribution of ventilation and perfusion, there is another important and really still unresolved question concerning gas exchange during exercise. This
is the mechanism of changes in arterial P_{O_2} and in the AaD$_{O_2}$.
Changes in ventilation-perfusion inequality are only one of several factors that may affect both the arterial P_{O_2} and the AaD$_{O_2}$
and more will be said about this in Dr. Gledhill's paper in this
session.

In studying normal subjects, most workers have found that the arterial P_{O_2} remains constant even with severe exercise but that the AaD_{O_2} progressively increases with increasing exercise loads. Even those who have observed an initial decrease in AaD_{O_2} in mild exercise find a substantial increase in that variable during severe exercise (26).

A different situation is seen in patients with cardiopulmonary disease undergoing exercise. While the alveolar-arterial difference widens as in normal subjects, the arterial P_{O_2} is usually seen to fall.

In order to explain these changes both in normal subjects and in patients with cardiopulmonary disease, one has to be aware of several important interacting factors that can affect the arterial P_{O_2} and AaD_{O_2}: 1) It has been found that the arterial P_{O_2} and AaD_{O_2} will change with changes in total ventilation, total pulmonary bloodflow and mixed venous P_{O_2} even if the distribution of ventilation-perfusion ratios remains unaltered (28). 2) Changes (either an improvement or worsening) in $\dot{V}_A/\dot{Q}$ relationships will alter the arterial P_{O_2} and AaD_{O_2} if the total ventilation and total bloodflow and venous P_{O_2} remain constant. 3) The effect of a given magnitude of shunt on the arterial P_{O_2} depends upon the venous P_{O_2} which in turn is related to the balance between oxygen uptake and cardiac output, a balance which changes during exercise. 4) The alveolar-arterial P_{O_2} difference will increase should there be failure of alveolar-endcapillary diffusion equilibration.

It is essentially impossible to sort out the quantitative or even qualitative importance of these various mechanisms from studies in which only the arterial P_{O_2} and AaD_{O_2} are measured. Some authors (18) choose to resolve the paradox of a widening AaD_{O_2} in the face of lessening topographical ventilation-perfusion inequality by ascribing the increase in AaD_{O_2} to failure of diffusion equilibration, but there is no good evidence to support this contention in normal subjects exercising at sea level.

More incisive tools for analyzing gas exchange are required to sort out the mechanisms that lead to alterations of arterial P_{O_2} and AaD_{O_2} during exercise and a first approach to this problem will be described in the ensuing session, applied to both normal subjects and patients with either chronic obstructive pulmonary disease or interstitial lung disease. The problem that is posed is how to partition the alveolar-arterial oxygen difference and so assign quantitative importance to the various factors referred to above. In this way a physiological explanation of changes in arterial P_{O_2} in going from rest to exercise may become available.

PARTIAL PRESSURE DIFFUSION EQUILIBRATION DURING EXERCISE

A topic of both physiological interest and clinical importance arises in the context of the preceding discussion and justifies a review of its own. This is the question of whether during exercise either in normal subjects or patients with cardiopulmonary disease alveolar-endcapillary partial pressure differences

are likely to develop on the basis of incomplete diffusion
equilibration.

A considerable amount of theoretical evidence has been accumu-
lated since the original work of Christian Bohr (3), and it allows us to develop a feel for the conditions necessary for development of alveolar-endcapillary diffusion differences in P_{O_2}.
More recently attention has been devoted to carbon dioxide, and
several theoretical studies indicate that CO_2 may be equally as
vulnerable to diffusion limitation as oxygen, a point to be taken
up later.

The question of whether failure of diffusion equilibration ever
limits gas exchange during exercise has been asked repeatedly at
the experimental level over the years but a definitive answer is
still not available. This is because virtually all techniques
designed to examine the diffusing properties of the lungs are affected to some extent by the co-existing presence of ventilation-
perfusion inequality.

Perhaps the first question to ask is whether exercise provides
conditions that are likely to result in failure of diffusion
equilibration. Most workers believe that if such differences develop during exercise they do so because the red cell transit time
is reduced due to the increased red cell velocity associated with
the increased cardiac output. However as discussed earlier,
capillary blood volume is known to increase along with cardiac
output (although not by as much in a relative sense). Mean red
cell transit time, equal to the ratio of capillary blood volume to
capillary bloodflow, will thus fall but a reasonable estimate is
only to about one half of the normal value of 0.75 sec (21). This
is because it is basically agreed that a four-fold rise in cardiac
output is associated with about a two-fold rise in capillary blood
volume. There is considerable theoretical evidence (11,12,23)that
partial pressure diffusion equilibration for oxygen is essentially
complete in approximately one quarter of a second so that the
available average transit time of about 0.4 seconds is sufficient
for diffusion equilibration for oxygen. For carbon dioxide, the
situation is not as clear cut. It used to be thought that because
CO_2 diffuses 20 times as rapidly as does oxygen through an aqueous
membrane, partial pressure equilibration of CO_2 would occur some
20 times sooner than it would for oxygen. While the factor of 20
is established, the conclusion that the rate of partial pressure
equilibration is 20 times greater for CO_2 than O_2 is clearly incorrect. Due to a number of factors (particularly the greater
capacity of the blood for CO_2, the more linear CO_2 dissociation
curve, and the finite rates of chemical reaction for CO_2 in the
blood) diffusion equilibration for CO_2 may in fact be slower than
for oxygen (11,23). In fact some aspects of CO_2 exchange in the
lung require several seconds for completion. For example the pH
of the plasma changes very slowly (6,11) due to the absence of
carbonic anhydrase from the plasma. This causes changes in the
P_{CO_2} of arterial blood once it has left the lungs and as a result
measurements of arterial P_{CO_2} made with blood gas electrodes several minutes after collection may not accurately reflect the P_{CO_2}

of the blood leaving the pulmonary capillaries. It should be
noted that while these differences are relatively large compared
to the total arterial-venous P_{CO_2} difference, they remain small in
an absolute sense and are currently virtually impossible to detect clinically.

It has been suggested that the "anomalous" P_{CO_2} gradient between
alveolar gas and arterial blood described by Jones and coworkers
(14), by Gurtner, et al. (10) and by others is at least in part
caused by this kind of mechanism (6) although Gurtner has another
theory (10) based upon a non-uniform distribution of hydrogen ions
within the pulmonary capillary. This interesting issue remains to
be resolved.

Overriding all of the considerations discussed above is the un-
questionable fact that not all red cells will be permitted the
same contact time for gas exchange in the pulmonary capillaries.
Cells that take longer than average to pass through the capillary
will do well, but those that take less will be liable to problems
in coming into diffusion equilibrium with alveolar gas. With his
photographic methods for direct observation of the pulmonary
capillaries, Dr. Wagner may be able to throw some light on this
problem.

While reduction in capillary transit time is the most widely believed mechanism likely to give rise to incomplete diffusion
equilibration in the lung, another pathophysiological possibility
is the leakage of fluid across the capillary endothelium which
may occur as the pulmonary arterial pressure rises during exercise.
If fluid were to accumulate in the interstitial space around the
capillaries and increase the distance for diffusion of gases between alveolar gas and the red cells one could imagine that diffusion equilibration might be compromised. In normal subjects this
is a somewhat unlikely hypothesis since even if there is leakage
of fluid, that fluid has direct access to the lymphatic drainage
system. Moreover a number of people believe on the basis of ultra-
structural observations of the alveolar wall that since the lymph-
atics appear to cluster on one side of the capillary, fluid leakage is unlikely to give rise to problems in diffusion under all
but the most severe circumstances. It is however conceivable that
in patients with cardiovascular insufficiency on exercise such
that the left atrial and/or pulmonary arterial pressures are
grossly elevated leakage of fluid might be a factor in impairing
gas exchange. This could be through the mechanism of increasing
the distance for diffusion of gases but may also be on the basis
of impairing the ventilation of terminal lung units through the
narrowing of airways, particularly in the dependent regions of
the lung where the vascular pressures are likely to be highest.

Facilitated Diffusion

Finally in the context of diffusion limitation is the controversial subject of facilitated diffusion. Dr. Gurtner, who is the
main proponent of this theory, will address us on this topic in
this session.

Briefly, he and his colleagues have hypothesised (9) that a pulmonary carrier exists for the gases oxygen and carbon monoxide in lung tissue. Following Longmuir's original suggestion (17) that cytochrome P-450 may be this carrier, Dr. Gurtner and his colleagues have sought evidence to support the concept of facilitated diffusion in the lung. Measurements of the variation of carbon monoxide diffusing capacity with inspired carbon monoxide tension (19) and experiments in which drugs known to inhibit cytochrome P-450 were given have been performed. Perhaps two fundamental questions need to be answered. Is facilitated diffusion unequivocally present as a mechanism involved in pulmonary gas exchange, and secondly if so what is its clinical relevance to both normal subjects and patients with cardiopulmonary disease? We will undoubtedly hear more about this interesting development in the years to come.

(This work supported by NIH grants HL 17731 and HL 00111).

REFERENCES

1.   Astrand, P. D. and K. Rodahl. Textbook of Work Physiology, McGraw Hill, New York, 1970, pp. 225-226.
2.   Baker, D. H. and W. J. Daly. J. Appl. Physiol. 28: 461-464, 1970.
3.   Bohr, C., Skand. Arch. Physiol. 22: 221-280, 1909.
4.   Dollery, C. T., N. A. Dyson, and J. D. Sinclair. J. Appl. Physiol. 15: 411-417, 1960
5.   Forster, R. E.   Phys. Rev. 37: 391-452, 1957.
6.   Forster, R. E. and E. D. Crandall, J. Appl. Physiol. 38: 710-718, 1975.
7.   Fung, Y. C. and S. S. Sobin.   J. Appl. Physiol. 26: 472-488, 1969.
8.   Glazier, J. B., J.M.B. Hughes, J. E. Maloney and J. B. West. J. Appl. Physiol. 32: 346-356, 1972.
9.   Gurtner, G. H. and B. Burns.   Nature 240: 473-475, 1972.
10.   Gurtner, G. H., S. H. Song and L. E. Farhi. Resp. Physiol. 7: 173-187, 1969.
11.   Hill, E. P., G. G. Power and L. D. Longo. Am. J. Physiol. 224: 904-917, 1973.
12.   Hlastala, M. P. Resp. Physiol. 15: 214-232, 1972.
13.   Johnson, R. L., Jr., W. S. Spicer, J. M. Bishop and R. E. Forster. J. Appl. Physiol. 15: 893-902, 1960.
14.   Jones, N. L., E.J.M. Campbell, G.J.R. McHardy, B. E. Higgs and M. Clode. Clin. Sci. 32: 311-327, 1967.
15.   Lawson, W. H., Jr., J. Appl. Physiol. 29: 896-900, 1970.
16.   Lewis, B. M., T. H. Lin, F. E. Noe and R. Komisaruk. J. Clin. Investig. 37: 1061-1070, 1958.
17.   Longmuir, I. Symposia of 6th European Conference on Microcirculation, Basel. 1971. pp. 3-7.
18.   Margaria, R. and P. Cerretelli. Chap. 2 in Exercise Physiology (Edited by H. B. Falls), Academic Press, New York,1968, pp. 70-71.

19. Peavy, H., M. Jaberi, B. Burns and G. Gurtner, Fed. Proc. 33: 421, 1974 (Abs).
20. Permutt, S., P. Caldini, A. Maseri, W. H. Palmer, T. Sasamori and K. Zierler. Chap. 26 in The Pulmonary Circulation and Insterstitial Space (Edited by A. F. Fishman and H. H. Hecht), Univ. of Chicago Press, 1969. pp. 375-387.
21. Roughton, F.J.W. Am. J. Physiol. 45: 621-633, 1945.
22. Roughton, F.J.W., and R. E. Forster. J. Appl. Physiol. 11: 290-302, 1957.
23. Wagner, P. D. and J. B. West. J. Appl. Physiol. 33: 62-71, 1972.
24. Wagner, W. W. and G. F. Filley. Vascular Dis. 2: 229-241, 1965.
25. Warrell, D. A., J. W. Evans, R. O. Clarke, G. P. Kingaby and J. B. West. J. Appl. Physiol. 32: 346-356, 1972.
26. Wasserman, K. and B. J. Whipp. Am. Rev. Resp. Dis. 112: 219-249, 1975.
27. West, J. B. J. Appl. Physiol. 17: 893-898, 1962.
28. West, J. B. Resp. Physiol. 7: 88-110, 1969.
29. West, J. B. and C. T. Dollery. J. Appl. Physiol. 15: 405-410, 1960.
30. West, J. B., A. M. Schneider and M. M. Mitchell. J. Appl. Physiol. 39: 976-984, 1975.

23

Ventilation to Perfusion Distribution During Exercise in Health[1]

Norman Gledhill, A. B. Froese, & Jerome A. Dempsey

The primary function of the lungs is to exchange oxygen and carbon dioxide by enabling pulmonary blood and alveolar gas to equilibrate across a blood/gas interface. Optimal function would occur with the precise matching of aerated alveolar gas and mixed venous blood throughout the lungs. However, there are a number of factors which could oppose the attainment of such a condition, especially when the stress of muscular work is added. For example, the lung interface is an extremely complex and heterogenous anatomical structure which also has a functional inhomogeneity created by gravity-related variations in alveolar size, regional ventilation and pleural and perfusion pressures. Muscular work imposes additional stresses on the lung; energy requirements increase up to twenty-fold, arterial to mixed venous O_2 and CO_2 contents widen, and pulmonary blood flow rises. That is, mixed venous blood requires more oxygenation and de-acidification during exercise, yet the lung has less time to accomplish the task. Despite these potential problems, in healthy man arterial blood PO_2 and PCO_2 are maintained near resting levels with remarkable stability even during very heavy exercise.

A number of beneficial adaptations are known to occur in the lung during muscular work which are critical to preserving arterial blood gas homeostasis. The linear rise in alveolar ventilation with increasing metabolism is well documented and is, of course, critical to maintaining adequate levels of alveolar PO_2 and PCO_2. Changes in the pulmonary capillary blood volume are also important. Total pulmonary blood flow may vary from 5 litres per minute at rest to 25 litres per minute in heavy exercise (44). Resistance in the pulmonary circulation is remarkably low at rest, and during exercise it can actually drop with both an opening of new vessels (recruitment) and an increase in the calibre of those

1. Key Abbreviations: $P\bar{c}O_2$ - mixed end-capillary oxygen tension.
   A-a$\bar{D}O_2$ - alveolar to arterial oxygen difference.
   A-$\bar{c}DO_2$ - alveolar to mixed end-capillary oxygen difference.

Supported by MRC Grant MA-5363, NIH Grants HL17540 and HL00149, and York University, Faculty of Arts.

already open (distension) (23,24,39,45,46). The result is an
increase in the pulmonary capillary blood volume to the extent that
this volume is always in excess of the increased stroke volume seen
during exercise (28). Pulmonary arterial pressure increases only
slightly during light exercise and there is no further increase with
more strenuous exercise (19,20,27,64). As a result of these accom-
modations, the transit time of a red blood cell in the pulmonary
capillary bed only drops to approximately .5 seconds in moderate
to heavy exercise, which is more than enough time for alveolar-
capillary diffusion equilibration to occur (28,48).

While the distribution of V_A/Q ratios certainly play a key
role in determining gas exchange during exercise, currently available data has not permitted delineation of this role. A number of
techniques have been developed to evaluate the distribution of V_A or
Q in the lung but it is not possible to evaluate pulmonary gas
exchange from the information they provide (8,11,12,14,32,34,41,
43,66). Until recently, the most definitive information has been
obtained from radioactive scanning techniques (6,7,61). These
studies have indicated that in normal subjects in the upright
position, blood flow is distributed in the lungs such that the apex
is underperfused relative to the base (1,13,61). This is thought
to be due to the effect of gravity on interrelationships between
alveolar, arterial, and venous pressures (1,62). Alveolar ventilation per unit lung volume is also greater at the base than at
the apex (7,61). The accepted explanation for this is based on
the existence of a pleural pressure gradient which leads to
regional variations in end-expiratory alveolar volumes. This
causes regional differences in compliance, which results in preferential ventilation of the dependent zones (25,31,62). However,
the rate of increase in Q from the apex to the base is greater
than the rate of increase in V_A, resulting in a high V_A/Q ratio at
the apex and a low V_A/Q ratio at the base (13,61,62).

During exercise, blood flow and ventilation are reported to
increase relatively more to the apex than to dependent regions.
Thus, there is less of a regional inhomogeneity in the distribution
of V_A and Q, and topographically, the distribution of V_A/Q ratios
appears to be more uniform (6,13,61). The trend to topographical
homogeneity in V_A and Q progresses with increasing intensity of
exercise until they are virtually evenly distributed throughout
the lung at heavy workloads (6).

It has been established that at rest, the distribution of Q
is directly related to the pulmonary arterial (Pa) pressure (7,15,
60) but it is felt that the changes in Pa pressure reported during
exercise are not of sufficient magnitude to completely account for
the topographical redistribution of Q (13). However, as Bryan et
al. point out, the total pressure in a flowing system is the sum
of the static pressure, as recorded with a cardiac catheter, plus
the stagnation pressure due to kinetic energy. During exercise
the latter component, which is velocity dependent, may well account
for the topographical redistribution of perfusion (13).

Although early reports indicated that the frequency of breathing does not alter the distribution of ventilation in the lungs

(4), several authors (5,7,35) have since observed an increased
uniformity in $\dot{V}_A$ when inspiratory flow is increased. Bake et al.
(5, and this Symposium, Chapter 16) proposed that this is the
reason for the increased topographical uniformity seen in exercise.
The pattern of redistribution has been explained in terms of
regional differences in mechanical time constants which become
significant at high flow rates.

It is difficult, however, to reconcile this increased uniformity in the matching of ventilation to perfusion with the widening
of the A-a DO_2 which accompanies exercise (2). Due to the disproportionate increase in $\dot{V}_A$ relative to $\dot{Q}$, the P_AO_2 rises, while the
P_aO_2 stays constant or perhaps increases slightly. Consequently,
with increasing workloads there is a progressive increase in the
A-a DO_2 up to 25 to 30 mmHg in heavy exercise (2,30,57). Assuming
no impairment of diffusion during exercise, which, in light of the
calculations of Staub et al. (48) appears to be a tenable assumption
for normal subjects, possible explanations for this apparent inconsistency are: 1) despite a more even topographical matching of
ventilation and perfusion, intraregional inhomogeneity of $\dot{V}_A/\dot{Q}$
ratios may increase substantially in exercise without being detected by the radioactive tracer technique; 2) the increased A-a DO_2
may be caused by an increase in anatomical shunt fraction during
exercise and/or a marked desaturation of the shunted blood fraction.
However, with previously available techniques it has not been
possible to examine these alternatives.

Recently, a new method has been developed by Wagner et al. (56)
for measuring the distribution of ventilation-perfusion ratios,
based on the steady state elimination of six inert gases with varying solubilities. By infusing the dissolved inert gases intravenously, sampling arterial blood and expired gas, and measuring
cardiac output and minute ventilation, it is possible to derive the
position, shape and dispersion of log normal distributions of
ventilation and blood flow. In addition, the true intrapulmonary
shunt (perfused but unventilated alveoli) and amount of ventilation
to unperfused gas exchange units are determined. Unlike the radioactive tracer technique, which yields information regarding the
amount of ventilation and perfusion per unit lung volume, the inert
gas technique determines the amount of blood and gas coming together at specific $\dot{V}_A/\dot{Q}$ ratios, so that gas exchange can be
calculated and the functional significance of the distribution
assessed. This information can then be used to evaluate the above
options.

The Distribution of $\dot{V}_A/\dot{Q}$ Ratios During Exercise: Methods

We employed the multiple inert gas washout technique with minor
modifications to determine the distribution of $\dot{V}_A/\dot{Q}$ ratios of five
healthy male subjects in the sitting position at rest and during
steady state graded exercise on an electrically braked bicycle
ergometer corresponding to oxygen uptakes of approximately 1.0, 1.5
and 2.0 litres/minute. The subjects ranged in age from 23 to 31.
All had normal pulmonary function, blood gases and acid-base status.

Catheters were inserted for the sampling of arterial blood, for dye dilution cardiac outputs and for infusion of the inert gas solution. In each condition, following at least 15 minutes of infusion, simultaneous samples of arterial blood and mixed expired gas were collected in duplicate for the determination of inert gas retention and excretion, and traditional measurements of gas exchange were made concurrently.

The collection, preparation and analysis of the inert gas samples were similar to that reported by Wagner et al. (54). The standard deviation in the measurement of chromatograph peak heights expressed as a percent of the mean peak height was $\pm 0.75\%$. When the error involved in the extraction process was included, the average error in the analysis of the inert gases in blood was $\pm 2.5\%$ (range = 1.3 to 3.5%). Unlike the original procedure of Wagner et al. (54) acetone was not measured in the present study. Thus, the distributions were recovered using only 5 gases; SF_6, ethane, cyclopropane, halothane and diethyl ether. With this modification the highest $\dot{V}_A/\dot{Q}$ ratio which could be differentiated from true dead space was 15. Solubilities of each gas in blood were determined for each subject, and they were very similar to previously reported values (55).

Considerable effort was made to ensure that a steady state of gas exchange existed during all sampling times. The average difference between repeat measurements of $\dot{V}_A$ expressed as a percent of the mean was $\pm 2.8\%$, and for the dye dilution cardiac outputs, this figure was $\pm 7.1\%$. Polarographic blood-gas electrodes were calibrated with gas of known composition prior to each measurement, and a blood-gas correction factor was determined for PO_2 (1.02 $\pm$ .005) by comparing tonometered blood samples with these mixtures. The standard deviation of duplicate measurements was as follows: PO_2 ± 1.7 mmHg; PCO_2 ± 1.1 mmHg; pH $\pm$ .005.

All calculations were performed on a computer, using the program of Wagner and Evans to recover the distributions. A smoothing constraint (52) was incorporated in the numerical analysis such that the function became a linear one with a formal solution. Using this approach, the recovery of the distributions is stable in the face of the present level of experimental error. Olszowka (38) has shown recently that the recovered distribution is not a unique solution to the inert gas data, but one member of a family of distributions, all of which satisfy the basic data. Wagner and Evans (53) recognize this problem, but they showed that with narrow distributions similar to those in the present study, little uncertainty exists in describing the parameters of the distribution and there are virtually no differences among gas exchange values calculated from the possible distributions.

The cardiopulmonary data of the subjects at rest and during the three levels of exercise were consistent with similar values in the literature and are summarized in Table 23.1.

Table 23.1. Cardiorespiratory Data of Five Young Healthy Males at
Rest and During Three Levels of Exercise (Mean ± SD)

		Exercise $\dot{V}O_2$ L/min		
	Rest	1.0 - 1.2	1.4 - 1.6	2.0 - 2.2
$\dot{V}_{E\ BTPS}$ L/min	8.1 ±1.9	32.8 ±3.7	40.6 ±7.4	59.3 ±3.7
$\dot{Q}$ L/min	5.5 ±1.3	12.6 ±1.1	13.5 ±3.0	17.8 ±1.2
PaO_2 mmHg	88.7 ±1.5	91.4 ±2.2	89.4 ±3.8	89.8 ±3.2
A-a DO_2 mmHg	10.4 ±0.9	17.1 ±4.5	19.1 ±0.4	21.6 ±1.1
$PaCO_2$ mmHg	38.4 ±1.6	36.1 ±1.1	35.7 ±4.0	36.0 ±0.7
pH_a	7.41 ± .01	7.41 ± .02	7.40 ± .02	7.39 ± .06
V_D/V_T	.34 ± .09	.20 ± .06	.16 ± .05	.16 ± .06

Changes in $\dot{V}_A/\dot{Q}$ During Exercise

A summary of the changes in $\dot{V}_A/\dot{Q}$ observed at rest and during
the three levels of exercise appears in Table 23.2. During exer-
cise there was an increase in the $\dot{V}_A/\dot{Q}$ at the mean of the $\dot{V}_A$ and
$\dot{Q}$ distributions ($\overline{V}_A$, $\overline{Q}$) and this increase progressed with increasing severity of exercise. Exercise also resulted in a slight,
but progressive increase in the log standard deviation of the
$\dot{V}_A$ and $\dot{Q}$ distributions (SDV, SDQ), indicating increasing inhomogeneity in the distribution of $\dot{V}_A/\dot{Q}$ ratios.

Table 23.2. The Distribution of Ventilation and Perfusion at Rest
and During Three Levels of Exercise

			Exercise $\dot{V}O_2$ L/min					
	Rest		1.0 - 1.2		1.4 - 1.6		2.0 - 2.2	
η	$\bar{X}$	SD	$\bar{X}$	SD	$\bar{X}$	SD	$\bar{X}$	SD
	5		4		3		3	
$\bar{Q}*$	.92	.10	1.98	.21	2.46	.53	3.20	1.0
SDQ	.36	.03	.45	.03	.45	.06	.50	.01
$\bar{V}**$	1.05	.11	2.46	.24	3.09	.76	4.15	1.2
SDV	.36	.03	.48	.04	.49	.08	.54	.03

*$\bar{Q}$ =the $\dot{V}_A/\dot{Q}$ at the mean of the $\dot{Q}$ distribution
** $\bar{V}$ = the $\dot{V}_A/\dot{Q}$ at the mean. of the $\dot{V}_A$ distribution
For example, .92 is the $\dot{V}_A/\dot{Q}$ ratio at the mean of $\dot{V}_A$ distribution.

The distributions of the subject R.H., age 31, seated at
rest were very similar to the group mean and appear in Figure 23.1.
Ventilation and blood flow in litres/minute, when plotted
against $\dot{V}_A/\dot{Q}$ on a logarithmic scale are distributed log normally.
Each point represents the amount of blood or gas going to gas
exchange units at the $\dot{V}_A/\dot{Q}$, and summation of all points will give
the total alveolar ventilation or pulmonary blood flow. The lines
joining the points are included only for clarity. The $\dot{V}_A/\dot{Q}$ ratios
at the mean of the $\dot{V}_A$ and $\dot{Q}$ distributions were .84 and .94
respectively. The log standard deviation of both distributions
was .34. All the blood flow and ventilation is confined to the
$\dot{V}_A/\dot{Q}$ range .5 to 2.1. Also, there was no intrapulmonary shunt,
and the V_D/V_T ratio was .34. (Note: As will be explained later
in this paper, anatomical shunt is not detected by this method.)
Figure 23.2 illustrates the effect of moderate exercise in the
sitting position on the distributions of $\dot{V}_A$ and $\dot{Q}$. The sitting
distributions of subject R.H. at rest and during exercise at a $\dot{V}O_2$
of 1.1 L/min are plotted against $\dot{V}_A/\dot{Q}$. With exercise, total
ventilation and cardiac output increased substantially. However,
since ventilation increased out of proportion to blood flow, the
$\dot{V}_A/\dot{Q}$ at the mean of the $\dot{Q}$ distribution increased from .84 to 1.95
and the $\dot{V}_A/\dot{Q}$ at the mean of the $\dot{V}_A$ distribution increased from
.94 to 2.52. In addition, the log S.D. of the $\dot{Q}$ distribution
increased from .34 to .47 and the log S.D. of the $\dot{V}_A$ distribution
increased from .34 to .53. Thus, the range of $\dot{V}_A/\dot{Q}$ ratios at which
gas was being exchanged increased from a span of 0.5 to 2.1 at rest

to 0.9 to 7.8 during exercise. There was no intrapulmonary shunt
in either condition and the V_D/V_T ratio decreased from .34 at rest
to .12 during exercise.

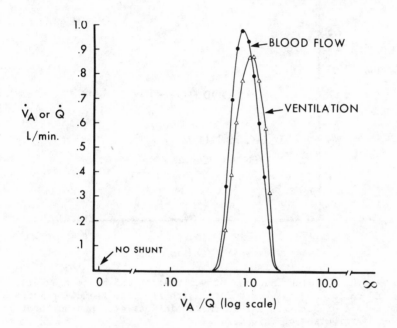

Figure 23.1. The distribution of ventilation and blood flow in a
young healthy male sitting at rest. Each point represents the
amount of blood or gas going to gas exchange units at that $\dot{V}_A/\dot{Q}$
and summation of all points gives the total ventilation or blood
flow.

Functional Effects of the Observed Changes

We now know that during exercise there was an increase in
the $\dot{V}_A/\dot{Q}$ at the mean of the $\dot{V}_A$ and $\dot{Q}$ distributions together with
an increase in their log standard deviation. From routine calcu-
lations of gas exchange it is now possible to analyze the effect
of these adaptations in $\dot{V}_A/\dot{Q}$ distribution on blood-gas homeostasis
and the observed widening of the A-a DO_2.

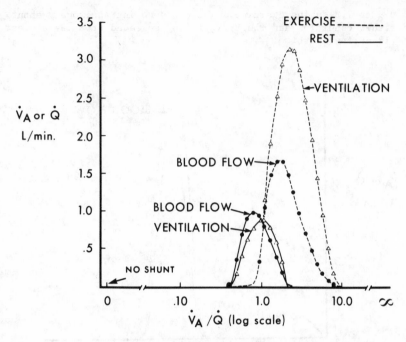

Figure 23.2. The distributions of ventilation and blood flow at rest and during moderate exercise. With exercise the distributions shifted to a higher V_A/Q and there was in increased non-uniformity in the distribution of $\dot{V}_A/\dot{Q}$ ratios.

The lung may be viewed as a number of gas exchanging units arranged in parallel. If the composition of inspired gas and mixed venous blood are known it is possible to calculate the composition of alveolar gas and end-capillary blood from any gas exchange unit with a known $\dot{V}_A/\dot{Q}$ ratio using the following relationship:

$$\frac{\dot{V}_A}{\dot{Q}} = K \, \frac{Cc_{O_2} - C\overline{v}_{O_2}}{P_{I}_{O_2} - P_{A}_{O_2}}$$

In the recovered lung with 50 compartments and $\dot{V}_A/\dot{Q}$ ratios, the inspired gas composition is known, and the mixed venous content of O_2 can be determined from the measured $\dot{V}_{O_2}$. (A similar calculation is made for CO_2.) Therefore, compartmental gas exchange can be calculated for the recovered distributions and these values appear in Table 23.3.

TABLE 23.3 Compartmental Gas Exchange Values at Rest[1] and During Exercise[2] in Subject R.H.

$\dot{V}_A/\dot{Q}$	Rest				Exercise			
	$P_cO_2\,P_AO_2$ mm Hg	$P_cCO_2\,P_ACO_2$ mm Hg	C_cO_2 vol %	C_cCO_2 vol %	$P_cO_2\,P_AO_2$ mm Hg	$P_cCO_2\,P_ACO_2$ mm Hg	C_cO_2 vol %	C_cCO_2 vol %
.49	73.3	43.0	19.3	51.9				
.57	80.2	42.4	19.6	51.5				
.67	87.1	41.6	19.7	51.0				
.79	93.7	40.7	19.9	50.6				
.93	99.8	39.7	20.0	50.0	72.4	46.7	21.0	47.5
1.10	105.3	38.6	20.0	49.4	79.9	45.3	21.4	46.7
1.29	110.1	37.3	20.1	48.7	87.4	43.7	21.6	46.0
1.52	114.4	36.0	20.1	47.9	94.4	41.9	21.8	45.1
1.79	118.2	34.5	20.2	47.1	100.8	40.0	22.0	44.2
2.10	121.5	33.0	20.2	46.2	106.5	37.9	22.1	43.2
2.49					111.5	35.8	22.1	42.2
2.93					115.9	33.7	22.2	41.1
3.45					119.7	31.5	22.3	39.9
4.06					123.0	29.3	22.3	38.7
4.88					126.0	27.1	22.3	37.5
5.63					128.6	25.0	22.4	36.2
6.63					130.9	22.9	22.4	34.9
7.80					132.8	20.9	22.4	33.6

[1] $\dot{V}O_2$ = 298 ml/min., $\dot{V}CO_2$ = 245 ml/min., $\dot{Q}$ = 5.8 l/min., $\dot{V}_E$ = 8.24 l/min., overall $\dot{V}_A/\dot{Q}$ = .93, PaO_2 = 90.2 mmHg, $PaCO_2$ = 39.0 mmHg, $P\bar{v}O_2$ = 39.2 mmHg, $P\bar{v}CO_2$ = 44.7 mmHg, PIO_2 = 146 mmHg, Hb = 14.5 mg %.

[2] $\dot{V}O_2$ = 1.1 l/min., $\dot{V}CO_2$ = 1.06 l/min., $P\bar{v}O_2$ = 31.7 mmHg, $P\bar{v}CO_2$ = 51.9 mmHg, PaO_2 = 89.4 mmHg, $PaCO_2$ = 36.5 mmHg, $\dot{Q}$ = 11.7 l/min., $\dot{V}_E$ = 29.03 l/min., overall $\dot{V}_A/\dot{Q}$ = 2.19, Hb = 16.0 mg %.

In examining the gas exchange values within a given lung, it is apparent that with higher compartmental $\dot{V}_A/\dot{Q}$ ratios, the end-capillary oxygen tension increases in a complex non-linear manner. For the resting distribution, with a normal mixed venous O_2 content of 14.8 volume %, most of the effect of a higher $\dot{V}_A/\dot{Q}$ ratio occurred between a ratio of .49 ($C\bar{c}O_2$ = 19.0 volume %) and 1.1 (CcO_2 = 20.0 volume %). Beyond a $\dot{V}_A/\dot{Q}$ ratio of 1.1, higher $\dot{V}_A/\dot{Q}$ ratios resulted in only minimal additional increases in the end-capillary O_2 content. Thus, in essence, in the resting lung, a $\dot{V}_A/\dot{Q}$ ratio of greater than 1.0 resulted in wasted ventilation with respect to additional oxygenation. This is due to the fact that gas exchange was occurring on the flat portion of the oxygen dissociation curve where hemoglobin is almost fully saturated.

By comparing the gas exchange values in the resting and exercising lungs, it is possible to examine the effect of the changes in $\dot{V}_A/\dot{Q}$ during exercise. It is apparent that the increase in overall $\dot{V}_A/\dot{Q}$ from rest to work resulted in the loss of the lowest $\dot{V}_A/\dot{Q}$ compartments so that no gas was exchanged at a $\dot{V}_A/\dot{Q}$ ratio of below 0.9 as compared with .5 at rest. However, due to the increased desaturation of mixed venous blood during exercise, it was necessary to have a considerably higher $\dot{V}_A/\dot{Q}$ ratio in order to achieve end-capillary O_2 tensions equal to those at rest. For example, during exercise, with a $P\bar{v}O_2$ of 31.7 mmHg, it was necessary to have a $\dot{V}_A/\dot{Q}$ of 2.1 to achieve the same end-capillary PO_2 (105 mmHg) as was observed at a $\dot{V}_A/\dot{Q}$ of 1.1 at rest when the $P\bar{v}O_2$ was 39.2 mmHg. Nevertheless, due to the increased $\dot{V}_A/\dot{Q}$, the end-capillary O_2 tensions are for the most part higher during exercise. A slight hemoconcentration, which is commonly reported in exercise, was also observed in the current study (Hb = 14.5 gm % at rest and 16.0 gm % during exercise) and it is reflected in an increased O_2 carrying capacity in exercise.

Once more examining an individual lung, it can be seen that since the CO_2 dissociation curve is essentially linear, the over-ventilation in high $\dot{V}_A/\dot{Q}$ compartments removes CO_2 from blood in the same proportion as the corresponding underventilation in low $\dot{V}_A/\dot{Q}$ compartments fails to remove it. This is especially evident during exercise, where the offloading of CO_2 steadily increases with higher $\dot{V}_A/\dot{Q}$ ratios.

Comparing the resting and exercise distribution again, it is apparent that when the $\dot{V}_A/\dot{Q}$ at the mean of the blood flow distribution shifted from .87 up to 1.98 from rest to exercise the end-capillary CO_2 tensions corresponding to these mean $\dot{V}_A/\dot{Q}$ ratios decreased from 47 mmHg to 39 mmHg respectively. This is consistent with a number of earlier reports which point out the effectiveness of a high $\dot{V}_A/\dot{Q}$ for CO_2 elimination (17,36,39).

If each compartment had the same $\dot{V}_A/\dot{Q}$ ratio and therefore, the same PO_2 and PCO_2 at equilibration, there would be no difference between the resultant mixed alveolar and mixed end-capillary O_2 tensions. On the other hand, since the $\dot{V}_A/\dot{Q}$ ratio was not the same in all compartments, the PO_2 and PCO_2 varied between compartments as seen in Table 23.3. Therefore, even though equilibrium is assumed to have been achieved in each compartment, an alveolar

to end-capillary O_2 difference developed. This is due to the fact
that compartments with high $\dot{V}_A/\dot{Q}$ ratios, by virtue of this high
ratio of alveolar ventilation to blood flow, affect gas tensions
more than blood, whereas compartments with low $\dot{V}_A/\dot{Q}$ ratios affect
blood tensions more than gas. That is, arterial blood is weighted
by the lower O_2 tensions, and alveolar gas is weighted by the
higher O_2 tensions. Thus, inhomogeneity in $\dot{V}_A/\dot{Q}$ ratios causes the
mixed alveolar gas tensions to deviate from the mixed end-capillary
tension, i.e., an A-c̄ DO_2 develops.

In the resting distribution, a degree of inhomogeneity (log
standard deviation of the distribution) exists in a normal lung such
that there is an A-c̄ DO_2 of approximately 5 mm Hg. During exercise,
an increase in the dispersion of the distribution was observed such
that gas exchange occurred over a wider range of $\dot{V}_A/\dot{Q}$ ratios, and
the result was a greater difference between the alveolar and mixed
end-capillary O_2 tensions, i.e., an increased A-c̄ DO_2 during
exercise, which accounts for at least a portion of the A-a DO_2
during exercise.

Since the amount of blood flow and ventilation going to each
$\dot{V}_A/\dot{Q}$ compartment is known, they are used to weight the blood and
gas effluents, which can then be summed to give overall gas exchange values for the lung. In subject R.H. at rest, the resultant
mixed end-capillary PO_2 was 93.4 mmHg, and the $P\bar{c}CO_2$ was 39.8 mmHg.
During exercise the $P\bar{c}O_2$ increased to 97.6 mmHg, and the $P\bar{c}CO_2$ dropped
to 38.2 mmHg. Thus, the overall result in exercise is that the
lowest $\dot{V}_A/\dot{Q}$ compartments with the least oxygenated effluent are
dropped, there is a minimal increase in the PO_2 of blood flow from
the highest $\dot{V}_A/\dot{Q}$ compartments, and a net improvement in mixed end-
capillary PO_2.

In order to assess the independent effects of the adjustments
in $\dot{V}_A/\dot{Q}$ occurring during exercise the recovered distributions were
manipulated mathematically to separate out the effects of observed
changes in the $\dot{V}_A/\dot{Q}$ and dispersion of the distribution and the results are summarized in Table 23.4.

Table 23.4.   The Effect of Removing the Changes in $\dot{V}_A/\dot{Q}$ Observed
During Exercise

	Recovered	If $\dot{V}_A/\dot{Q}$ had not increased	If the dispersion had not increased
$P\bar{c}O_2$ mmHg	97.6	47.4	103.5
$P\bar{c}CO_2$ mmHg	38.2	90.4	36.0
A-c̄ DO_2 mmHg	8.6	8.0	5.0

If the cardiac output and dispersion of the distribution had
changed as observed, but the overall $\dot{V}_A/\dot{Q}$ had not increased from
the sitting value, (i.e., the $\dot{V}_A$ had increased in proportion to $\dot{Q}$),
the mixed end-capillary PO_2 would have been considerably lower at

47.4 rather than 97.6 mmHg, the $P\bar{c}CO_2$ would have been considerably higher at 90.4 mmHg rather than 38.2 mmHg, and the $A-\bar{c}$ DO_2 would still have increased to the exercise level. Also, there would have been a marked effect on gas transfer, with $\dot{V}CO_2$ dropping from 1064 ml/min to 554 ml/min, and $\dot{V}O_2$ dropping from 1130 ml/min to 938 ml/min.

If the alterations in cardiac output and overall $\dot{V}_A/\dot{Q}$ had changed as observed during exercise, but the dispersion of the $\dot{V}_A/\dot{Q}$ distribution had remained at the sitting level, the mixed end-capillary PO_2 would have been 103.5 mmHg rather than 97.6 mmHg, the $A-\bar{c}$ DO_2 would have been narrower (5.0 mmHg rather than 8.6 mmHg), and the $P\bar{c}CO_2$ would have been 36.0 mmHg rather than 38.2 mmHg. Also there would have been a small improvement in both the $\dot{V}O_2$ and $\dot{V}CO_2$.

Thus, this analysis demonstrates that the major portion of the improvement in gas exchange observed from the sitting distribution to the exercise distribution was due to an increase in overall $\dot{V}_A/\dot{Q}$. On the other hand, during exercise, there was also a slight increase in the dispersion of the distribution, and this alteration partially negated the above improvements in gas exchange and created a small net increase in the alveolar to arterial oxygen difference.

Partitioning of the Alveolar to Arterial Oxygen Difference

As exercise intensity increased, A-a DO_2 widened progressively in all subjects to a mean value of $\sim$22 mmHg at the highest work-load. This progressive increase in A-a DO_2 during exercise agrees with most published findings (2,30,57) although some studies have reported a narrowing of A-a DO_2 in light exercise followed by a subsequent widening as workload progresses (26,63).

The factors which might contribute to the observed A-a DO_2 at rest and during exercise are: a limitation in diffusion, the anatomical shunting of blood, and non-uniformity in the matching of $\dot{V}_A$ and Q throughout the lung. Previous investigators have calculated that for normal subjects, both at rest and during exercise, diffusion is not limited (2,47,51). The mean transit time of a red cell traversing the lung at exercise levels similar to the highest intensity observed in the current study has been estimated at approximately .5 seconds (28,48). This is well in excess of the .35 seconds reported to be the minimum time required for complete equilibration (47). Even if the theoretical distribution of transit times postulated by Johnson et al. existed (SD = $\pm$0.1 sec.), 95% of the distribution of transit times would still be equal to or greater than .35 seconds (29). It can therefore be assumed that in the current study, diffusion limitation was not one of the factors which contributed to the A-a DO_2. Thus the remaining factors which may have contributed to the A-a DO_2 are anatomically shunted blood and/or non-uniformity in the matching of blood and gas throughout the lung.

The inert gas technique does not detect the true anatomical shunt from bronchial and thebesian admixture. Blood from these sources, although low in O_2 and high in CO_2, has already been equilibrated with alveolar air in the previous passage through the lung. Under steady state conditions, there is no further exchange of inert gases in the bronchial or coronary circulation, and therefore, from an inert gas point of view, the blood is still arterialized and gives the appearance of non-shunted blood. Therefore, calculations of gas exchange from this technique give mixed end-capillary values prior to the admixture of anatomical shunt. It should be pointed out, however, that since the highly insoluble gas SF_6 is virtually eliminated from venous blood in the presence of even small amounts of alveolar gas, its presence in arterial blood is a very sensitive index of intrapulmonary shunt. No intrapulmonary shunt was detected in the normal subjects either at rest or during exercise.

Since the difference between the measured PaO_2 and $P\bar{c}O_2$ predicted from the distribution is due to anatomically shunted blood, it is possible to use this information to calculate the anatomical shunt fraction from the formula $(\dot{Q}_s/\dot{Q}_T) = Q_s/Q_T = (C\bar{c}O_2 - CaO_2)/(C\bar{c}O_2 - C\bar{v}O_2)$.

Such calculations show that both at rest and during exercise anatomical shunt of less than 1% of the cardiac output can account for the entire difference between the predicted $P\bar{c}O_2$ and the measured PaO_2. These estimates are quite compatible with those reported by several authors, who have calculated flow through the thebesian veins to be between 0.25 and 0.4% of the total cardiac output (4,33,37,40) and bronchial venous flow to be less than 1% of the cardiac output (3,21,20).

The measured arterial and calculated end-capillary oxygen tensions for the recovered distributions appear in Table 23.5, together with the alveolar to mixed end-capillary and alveolar to arterial oxygen differences.

Table 23.5. Calculated Mixed End-Capillary and Measured Arterial Oxygen Tensions for the Distributions Recovered at Rest and During Exercise

	n	$P\bar{c}O_2$ mmHg	P_aO_2 mmHg	A-ē DO_2 mmHg	A-a DO_2 mmHg
Rest	5	93.0	88.7	6.7	10.4
Exercise	4	98.9	91.4	9.3	17.1

It can be assumed that both at rest and during exercise there is no impairment of diffusion (1,9,10). The difference between the mixed end-capillary O_2 tension and the measured arterial O_2 tension seen in Table 23.5 is due to anatomically shunted blood. Therefore, of the total A-a DO_2 at rest (~10 mmHg), approximately 4 mmHg is due to anatomically shunted blood, and of the A-a DO_2 during exercise (~17 mmHg), approximately 8 mmHg is due to this shunt. The remaining portion of the A-a O_2 difference in both

cases must be due to non-uniformity in the distribution of $\dot{V}_A/\dot{Q}$
ratios, and its effect is seen in the A-$\bar{c}$ DO_2. During exercise,
an increase in both the dispersion of the distributions and the
A-$\bar{c}$ DO_2 was observed, and these changes progressed with increasing
intensity of exercise. Thus, of the measured A-a O_2 difference at
rest, approximately 4 mmHg was due to anatomically shunted blood,
and the remaining 6 mmHg was due to non-uniformity of the $\dot{V}_A/\dot{Q}$
ratios throughout the lung. Of the measured A-a O_2 difference
during exercise, approximately 8 mmHg was due to anatomically
shunted blood, with the remaining 9 mmHg being due to non-uniformity
of $\dot{V}_A/\dot{Q}$ ratios.

The Paradox of Topographical Uniformity of $\dot{V}_A/\dot{Q}$ Ratios and An Increased A-a DO_2

Considering the type and intensity of exercise employed in
this study, it is reasonable to assume that the increased topographical homogeneity of $\dot{V}_A$ and $\dot{Q}$ observed by earlier investigations
also occurred here. For example, according to the calculations of
Bryan et al., with the two to three-fold increase in cardiac output observed in the current study, the stagnation pressure would
increase as much as four to nine times (13). Thus, the increment
in the total perfusion pressure, although not sensed by a cardiac
catheter, would be expected to result in a topographical redistribution of perfusion. Likewise, Bake et al., (5) reported a
uniform redistribution of ventilation at inspiratory flow rates
greater than 1.5 litres/sec., and all exercise flow rates in the
present study were in the range of 1.2 to 2.8 litres/sec. as compared with approximately .3 litres/sec. at rest.

We are therefore left with the contradictory conclusions that
during exercise the distributions of $\dot{V}_A$ and $\dot{Q}$ became more uniform
topographically, while at the same time there was a decreased uniformity in the distribution of $\dot{V}_A/\dot{Q}$ ratios throughout the lung.
These seemingly incompatible observations can be reconciled by
postulating an intraregional inhomogeneity in $\dot{V}_A/\dot{Q}$ ratios.

The assessment of ventilation-perfusion ratios using radioactive tracers is basically an insensitive technique, in that the
measurements are made over a relatively large volume of lung in a
two-dimensional plane, and the average ratio of gas to blood is
assigned to all gas exchange units within that volume. However,
there is mounting evidence which indicates that at rest there is
considerable inhomogeneity in the $\dot{V}_A/\dot{Q}$ ratios of intraregional gas
exchange units.

Engel et al. (16) reported recently that ventilation varies
considerably within parallel lung units subtended from peripheral
airways and results in an intraregional inhomogeneity of gas
tensions. Wood et al. (65) observed a reduction in the A-a DO_2
when SF_6 was substituted for nitrogen in 21% oxygen. They concluded that since increased gas density promotes convective diffusion, convective mixing and asynchronous ventilation, SF_6
breathing diminished alveolar O_2 concentration differences between
peripheral lung units. Consequently there was a reduction in

intraregional $\dot{V}_A/Q$ variance which accounted for the observed reduction in the A-a DO_2 (30).

Additional evidence supporting the existence of intraregional variance in $\dot{V}_A/\dot{Q}$ ratios are the findings that within small lung regions, considerable non-uniformity exists in ventilation (49), elastic properties and pressure-volume relationships (50), and alveolar size (42). Therefore, it is likely that although radio-active tracer studies detect a base-to-apex redistribution of $\dot{V}_A$ and $\dot{Q}$ during exercise, they are missing the existing intraregional $\dot{V}_A/\dot{Q}$ inequalities.

Although an increased dispersion was observed in both the distributions of $\dot{V}_A$ and $\dot{Q}$ versus $\dot{V}_A/\dot{Q}$ it is not necessary to postulate a changing distribution of $\dot{Q}$ as well as $\dot{V}_A$. A limitation of the multiple inert gas technique lies in the manner in which the distributions are expressed. That is, since the dependent variable appears on both the ordinate and abscissa any observed changes in the $\dot{V}_A$ and $\dot{Q}$ distributions could have resulted from changes in either $\dot{V}_A$ or $\dot{Q}$ alone. Thus, the intraregional mal-distribution of $\dot{V}_A$ proposed above could account for the observed increase in inhomogeneity of both the $\dot{V}_A$ and $\dot{Q}$ distributions. It is important to note that the presence of intraregional $\dot{V}_A/\dot{Q}$ in-equality during exercise would account for the observed increase in the A-a DO_2.

<u>Summary</u>

Studies employing radioactive tracers have suggested that during exercise in the upright position, the $\dot{V}_A/Q$ ratio becomes more uniform from the top to the bottom of the lung. However, it is difficult to reconcile an increased uniformity in the matching of blood and gas with the increased A-a O_2 difference which accompanies exercise. For normal subjects it is doubtful that the increase is due to a diffusion impairment. The two remaining explanations are: a greater contribution from anatomically shunted blood; or, contrary to the radioactive tracer studies, less uni-formity in the distribution of $\dot{V}_A/\dot{Q}$ ratios.

The multiple inert gas washout technique of Wagner et al. (56) was used to determine the distribution of $\dot{V}_A$ and $\dot{Q}$ in five young healthy males at rest and during graded exercise on a bicycle ergometer. With increasing severity of exercise there was a pro-gressive increase in the $\dot{V}_A/\dot{Q}$ ratio at the mean of the $\dot{V}_A$ and $\dot{Q}$ distributions and there was a slight but progressive increase in the non-uniformity of $\dot{V}_A/\dot{Q}$ ratios. From the point of view of gas exchange, the important change was a shift to higher $\dot{V}_A/\dot{Q}$ ratios.

Traditional indices of gas exchange (a) measured during exer-cise and (b) predicted from the recovered $\dot{V}_A/\dot{Q}$ distributions, were used to calculate the magnitude of the anatomical shunt and to partition the alveolar to arterial PO_2 difference. Both at rest and during exercise, an anatomical shunt of less than 1% of the cardiac output could account for the entire difference between the calculated $P\dot{c}O_2$ and the measured PaO_2. With an A-a DO_2 of 10 mmHg at rest, approximately 4 mmHg can be attributed to the effect of anatomical shunt, with the remainder being due to the non-uniformity of ventilation-perfusion ratios. During exercise, although the anatomical shunt fraction is virtually unchanged, its decreased O_2 saturation results in a greater desaturation from the end-capillary to the arterial PO_2, such that shunt can account for approximately 8 mmHg of an A-a DO_2 of 17 mmHg. The remaining 9 mmHg is due to the increased non-uniformity of the distributions of $\dot{V}_A$ and $\dot{Q}$ during exercise--an increase which progresses as exercise becomes more severe. It is proposed that the increased non-uniformity of $\dot{V}_A/\dot{Q}$ ratios during exercise is due to an increased intraregional inhomogeneity of $\dot{V}_A$ distribution.

REFERENCES

1. Anthonison, N.R. and J. Milic-Emili. J. Appl. Physiol. 21: 760-766, 1966.
2. Asmussen, E., and M. Nielson. Acta. Physiol. Scand. 50:153-166, 1960.
3. Aviado, D.M., M. de Burgh Daly, C.Y. Lee, and C.F. Schmidt. J. Physiol. 155:602-622, 1961.
4. Bachofen, H., H.J. Hobi and M. Scherrer. J. Appl. Physiol. 34:137-142, 1973.
5. Bake, B., L. Wood, B. Murphy, P.T. Macklem and J. Milic-Emili. J. Appl. Physiol. 37:8-17, 1974.
6. Bake, B., J. Bjure and J. Widimsky. Scand. J. Clin. Lab. Invest. 22:99-106, 1968.
7. Ball, W.C., P.B. Stewart, L.G.S. Neusham and D.V. Bates. J. Clin. Invest. 41:519-531, 1962.
8. Berggen S.M. Acta Physiol. Scand. Suppl. 11:1-92, 1942.
9. Bevegard, S., A. Holmgren and B. Jonsson. Acta. Physiol. Scand. 49:279-298, 1960.
10. Chiodi, H. In: The Regulation of Human Respiration, ed. D.J. Cunningham and B.B. Lloyd. Oxford, Blackwell 1963, pp. 363-378.
11. Bjorkman, S. Acta. Med. Scand. Suppl. 56:1934.
12. Bradley, E.C. and J.W. Barr. Am. Heart J. 78:643-648, 1969.
13. Bryan, A.C., L.G. Bentivoglio, F. Beerel, H. MacLeish, A. Zidulka and D.V. Bates. J. Appl. Physiol. 19:395-402, 1964.
14. Comroe, J.H. and W.S. Fowler. Am. J. Med. 10:408-418, 1951.
15. Dawson, A., K. Kaneki and M. McGregor. J. Clin. Invest. 44:999-1008, 1965.
16. Engel, L.A., L.D.H. Wood, G. Utz and P. Macklem. J. Appl. Physiol. 35:18-24, 1973.
17. Farhi, L.E. Resp. Physiol. 3:1-11, 1967.
18. Finley, T.N. J. Clin. Invest. 40:1727-1734, 1961.
19. Fishman, A.P., H.W. Fritts and A. Cournand. Circulation. 22:220-225, August 1960.
20. Freedman, M.E., G.L. Snider, P. Brosloff, S. Kimelblot and L.N. Katz. J. Appl. Physiol. 8:37, 1955.

21. Fritts, H.W., A. Hardewig, D.E. Rochester, J. Durand and A. Cournand. Circulation. 23:390-398, 1961.
22. Fritts, H.W., P. Harris, C.A. Chidsey, R.H. Clauss and A. Cournand. J. Clin. Invest. 39:1841-1850, 1960.
23. Fung, Y.C. and S.S. Sobin. J. Appl. Physiol. 26:472-488, 1969.
24. Glazier, J.B., J.M.B. Hughs, J.E. Maloney, et al. J. Appl. Physiol. 26:65-76, 1969.
25. Glazier, J.B., J.M.B. Hughes, J.E. Maloney, M.C.F. Pain and J.B. West. Lancet. 2:203-204, 1966.
26. Hesser, C.M. and G. Matell. Acta. Physiol. Scand. 63:247-256, 1965.
27. Holmgren, A., B. Jonsson and T. Sjostrand. Acta. Physiol. Scand. 49:343-363, 1960.
28. Johnson, R.L., W.S. Spicer, J.M. Bishop and R.E. Forster. J. Appl. Physiol. 15:893-902, 1960.
29. Johnson, R.L., H.F. Taylor and A.C. DeGraff. J. Clin. Invest. 44:789-800, 1965.
30. Jones, N.L., G.J.R. McHardy, A. Naimark and E.J.M. Campbell. Clin. Sci. 31:19-29, 1966.
31. Kaneko, K., J. Milic-Emili, M.B. Dolovich, A. Dawson and D.V. Bates. J. Appl. Physiol. 21:767-777, 1966.
32. Lenfant, C. J. Appl. Physiol. 18:1090-1094, 1963.
33. Lenfant, C. J. Appl. Physiol. 19(2):189-194, 1964.
34. Martin, C.J., F. Cline and H. Marshall. J. Clin. Invest. 32:617-621, 1953.
35. Martin, R.R., N.R. Anthonisen and M. Zutter. Clin. Sci. 43:319-329, 1972.
36. Markello, R. Anaesthesiology Review. Sept. 11-29, 1974.
37. Mellemgaard, K., N.A. Lassen and J. Georg. J. Appl. Physiol. 17:778-782, 1962.
38. Olszowka, A.O. Resp. Physiol. 25: 191-198, 1975.
39. Permutt, S., P. Caldine, A. Maseri, et al. Chicago: U. of Chicago Press, 1969, pp. 375-387.
40. Ravin, M.B., R.M. Epstein and J.R. Malm. J. Appl. Physiol. 20(6):1148-1152, 1965.
41. Riley, R.L. and A. Cournand. Theory. J. Appl. Physiol. 4: 77-101, 1951.
42. Robertson, C.H., D.L. Hall and J.C. Hogg. J. Appl. Physiol. 34:344-350, 1973.
43. Rochester, D.F., R.A. Brown, Jr., W.A. Wichern, Jr., and H.W. Fritts, Jr. J. Appl. Physiol. 22:423-430, 1967.
44. Rowell, L.B. Circulation. Med. & Sci. in Sports. 1:15-22, 1969.
45. Sobin, S.S., Y.C. Fung, H.M. Tremer, et al. Circ. Res. 30: 440-450, 1972.
46. Sobin, S.S., H.M. Tremer and Y.C. Fung. Circ. Res. 26:397-414, 1970.
47. Staub, N.C. J. Appl. Physiol. 18:673-680, 1963.
48. Staub, N.C., J.M. Bishop and R.E. Forster. J. Appl. Physiol. 17:21-27, 1962.

49. Suda, Y., C.J. Martin and A.C. Young. J. Appl. Physiol. 24: 480-485, 1970.
50. Sugihara, T., C.J. Martin and J. Hildebrandt. J. Appl. Physiol. 30:874-878, 1971.
51. Turino, G.M., E.H. Bergofsky, R.M. Goldring and A.P. Fishman. J. Appl. Physiol. 18:447-456, 1963.
52. Wagner, P.D. Letter to the Editor. J. Appl. Physiol. 38: 950-951, 1975.
53. Wagner, P.D. and J. Evans. Fed. Proc. 35(3):478, 1976.
54. Wagner, P.D., R.B. Laravuso, R.R. Uhl and J.B. West. J. Clin. Invest. 54:54-68, 1974.
55. Wagner, P.D., P.F. Nauman and R.B. Laravuso. J. Appl. Physiol. 36:600-605, 1974.
56. Wagner, P.D., H.A. Saltzman and J.B. West. J. Appl. Physiol. 36(5):588-599, 1974.
57. Wasserman, K., A.L. Van Kessel and G.G. Burton. J. Appl. Physiol. 22:71-85, 1967.
58. West, J.B. Philadelphia, F.A. Davis, 1965, chapter 4, pp. 55-87.
59. West, J.B. Resp. Physiol. 7:88-110, 1969.
60. West, J.B., C.T. Dollery and B.E. Heard. Circ. Res. 17:191-206, 1965.
61. West, J.B. and C.T. Dollery. J. Appl. Physiol. 15:405-410, 1960.
62. West, J.B., C.T. Dollery and A. Naimark. J. Appl. Physiol. 19:713-724, 1964.
63. Whipp, B.J. and K. Wasserman. J. Appl. Physiol. 27:361-365, 1969.
64. Widimsky, J., E. Berglund and R. Malmberg. J. Appl. Physiol. 18(5):983-986, 1963.
65. Wood, L.D.H., A.C. Bryan, S.K. Bau, T.R. Wing and H. Levison. J. Appl. Physiol. Accepted for publication.
66. Yokoyama, T. and L.E. Farhi. Resp. Physiol. 3:166-176, 1967.

DISCUSSION

Wasserman: An increased VA:Q dispersion during exercise—as you showed—would result in an increase in dead space:tidal volume ratio. However, you showed a decrease in VD:VT with increasing work. How can you explain this discrepancy?

P. Wagner: The increased dispersion is small and although it would result in an increase in alveolar dead space this increase would be small and would be masked by the large increase in tidal volume tending to lower the measured physiologic VD to VT.

Gledhill: With increased inhomogeneity, the Bohr CO_2 dead space would increase, but not the true dead space as determined by the inert gases, and since the VT increases so much during exercise the result is a decrease in the VD/VT ratio.

Wasserman: Whipp and Wasserman (J. Appl. Physiol., 27:361-365, 1969), showed a decrease in alveolar to arterial oxygen tension gradient (A-a DO_2) during mild exercise. Your data showed a rise in A-a DO_2 at all work levels studies. Can this discrepancy be explained by plotting individual, rather than mean data, and could this be due to a wide disparity in fitness in the subjects.

Gledhill: The data I showed was from Dempsey et al. (Resp. Physiol. 13:62-89, 1971; J. Appl. Physiol., 21:1807-1819, 1969) which agrees with our current findings. That is, all individual subjects showed a consistent widening of the A-a DO_2 during mild exercise regardless of the fitness level. Your earlier data is shown on this slide (Wasserman et al., J. Appl. Physiol., 27:361-365, 1969) and indicates that there was also no narrowing of the A-a DO_2 gradient with mild work.

Wasserman: The data shown on that slide was not corrected for temperature. When we did correct for temperature, the A-a DO_2 gradient narrowed. Did you correct for temperature?

Gledhill: Yes, all values were corrected to 37°C.

Wasserman: Perhaps there is a difference in technique. In what position were the subjects exercised.

Gledhill: Both rest and exercise measurements were made in the sitting position.

24

Ventilation-Perfusion Inequality & Gas Exchange During Exercise in Lung Disease

Peter D. Wagner

In comparing gas exchange during exercise and rest, it is apparent that a large number of factors, which by themselves each affect the arterial P_{O_2} and P_{CO_2}, may change simultaneously. Usually, oxygen uptake ($\dot{V}_{O_2}$) increases as does cardiac output ($\dot{Q}_T$) and minute ventilation ($\dot{V}_E$), mixed venous P_{O_2} falls while mixed venous P_{CO_2} rises, and the distribution of ventilation and perfusion may be altered. It is also believed that the average contact time of the red cell for gas exchange falls and consequently a gas exchange unit in which partial pressure equilibration between alveolar gas end-capillary blood is marginal even at rest is likely to develop alveolar-end capillary differences during exercise attributable to incomplete diffusion equilibration.

It is clearly a difficult problem to sort out the quantitative interactions occurring in individual patients so as to arrive at a complete explanation for the arterial P_{O_2} and P_{CO_2} during exercise. At the center of this problem lies the difficulty in identifying the nature and amount of ventilation-perfusion ($\dot{V}_A/\dot{Q}$) inequality on the one hand, and the amount of hypoxemia due to failure of diffusion equilibration on the other. This is particularly so when both abnormalities co-exist. Exchange of "diffusion-limited" gases such as carbon monoxide is seriously affected by $\dot{V}_A/\dot{Q}$ inequality; conversely any increase in the alveolar-arterial P_{O_2} difference (AaD_{O_2}) during exercise cannot be assumed to be due to failure of diffusion equilibration on one hand or to worsening $\dot{V}_A/\dot{Q}$ relationships on the other.

A partial solution to these problems is offered by the method of multiple inert gas elimination (4,6). Under steady-state conditions it is possible to derive considerable quantitative information about the functional distribution of ventilation and blood flow and with this information it is possible to predict quantitatively the exchange of O_2 and CO_2 on the explicit assumption that diffusion equilibration is complete. Since the other interacting factors are allowed for in this prediction scheme, application of the inert gas method can test the hypothesis that incomplete diffusion equilibration is a significant factor in the genesis of hypoxemia in a given patient. The physiological basis of this scheme is the known order of magnitude difference in the rates of diffusion equilibration of inert gases on the one hand and oxygen on the other. Inert gases reach alveolar-capillary partial pressure

345

equilibration within the first few 100ths of a second (1) while oxygen requires approximately one-quarter of a second for the same degree of partial pressure equilibration (2,3,7).

The objectives of the studies reported here were to determine if, during the mild exercise that patients with severe chronic obstructive pulmonary disease (COPD) and chronic interstitial lung disease (CILD) can tolerate, changes in the $\dot{V}_A/\dot{Q}$ distribution from the resting state could be detected, and in addition what mechanisms were responsible for hypoxemia during exercise.

METHODS

Eighteen patients were studied. All had advanced pulmonary disease with grossly abnormal indices of mechanical lung function. Ten (Table 24.1) had COPD of various causes and 9 had CILD. All patients were free of recent acute changes such as respiratory infections. None of the patients with COPD had significant acute reversibility of airways obstruction when given Isoproterenol.

Patients were prepared by catheterization of the pulmonary artery (Swan-Ganz No. 7F, inserted percutaneously via an antecubital vein), insertion of a radial or brachial arterial cannula, and insertion of a peripheral venous line. The peripheral venous line was used for administration of the dissolved inert gas mixture. Pulmonary artery pressure and EKG were monitored continuously throughout the study. Minute ventilation and respiratory frequency were measured minute by minute during collection periods, and cardiac output was measured at these times using indocyanine green and a Giford densitometer.

The mixture of dissolved inert gases was prepared as described previously (4) and infused at 2.5 mls/min for a total period of about 2 hours. After waiting initially 30 minutes for equilibration, resting arterial and pulmonary arterial blood and mixed expired gas samples were taken simultaneously for measurement of P_{O_2} and P_{CO_2}, inert gas concentrations (5), and acid-base status. Duplicate measurements were made of all variables within 5 minutes.

The above sampling procedure was repeated during a steady level of exercise. The level of exercise was that developed by the patient as a compromise between discomfort and the ability to maintain a steady state for 10 minutes. Duplicate samples were taken during the last 5 minutes of exercise at which time oxygen uptake was usually between 2 and 4 times resting values (Table 2).

Finally resting measurements were repeated exactly as above, after allowing the patient 30 minutes to recover from exercise.

RESULTS

a. Chronic Obstructive Pulmonary Disease

Patients 1, 2 and 3 (Table 24.2) had the features of type A COPD while patients 4 through 9 had the features of type B COPD. Patient 10 was classified as mixed type A and B. The resting $\dot{V}_A/\dot{Q}$

Table 24.1. Patients with Chronic Obstructive Pulmonary Disease

Patient Number	1	2	3	4	5	6	7	8	9	10
Age, years	62	64	46	64	55	49	53	44	60	53
Weight, Kg	96.8	64.5	52	68.6	93.2	77.7	85.5	100.0	105.0	59.0
Height, Cm	185	170	163	168	188	180	178	180	175	193
Surface area, M^2	2.20	1.75	1.58	1.75	2.20	1.97	2.03	2.19	2.20	1.84
TLC, Liters	8.8	8.4	8.1	5.2	5.1	9.3	6.5	6.1	6.7	9.3
FRC, Liters	6.6	7.2	5.9	4.3	3.7	8.2	3.8	4.1	3.0	8.0
RV, Liters	5.4	6.2	4.5	3.5	2.6	7.4	3.4	3.4	2.0	6.9
VC, Liters	3.4	2.2	3.6	1.7	2.5	1.9	3.1	2.7	4.7	2.4
FVC, Liters	2.3	1.0	2.8	1.5	2.4	1.9	3.0	2.6	4.5	2.2
% FEV_1	37	39	43	39	48	29	59	58	58	19
MMEFR, L/sec	0.2	0.1	0.4	-	0.3	0.2	2.2	0.7	0.9	0.1
R_{aw}, cm H_2O/L/sec	4.0	3.2	2.4	3.3	5.3	10.8	3.1	-	1.3	-
C_L, L/cm H_2O	.140	.170	-	-	-	.348	-	-	.248	.410
PTP at TLC, cmH_2O	9.9	7.5	-	-	-	5.7	-	-	27.9	3.3
DLCO,% Predicted	100	44	38	-	78	17	119	105	52	37

PATIENTS WITH CHRONIC INTERSTITIAL LUNG DISEASE

Patient Number	1	2	3	4	5	6	7	8	9
Age, years	44	27	31	48	72	58	49	72	40
Weight, Kg	72.0	80.0	84.0	82.0	77.0	76.4	97.3	68.2	79.5
Height, Cm	175	180	171	188	170	165	185	173	174
Surface Area, M^2	1.87	1.98	1.97	2.06	1.89	1.81	2.21	1.81	1.94
TLC, Liters	3.3	4.5	4.3	3.1	4.8	3.7	5.4	2.2	3.2
FRC, Liters	2.0	2.7	1.6	1.7	2.5	2.5	2.1	1.2	1.9
RV, Liters	1.0	0.5	1.2	0.9	1.4	1.8	1.8	0.9	1.1
VC, Liters	2.3	4.0	3.1	2.2	3.4	1.9	3.6	1.3	2.1
FVC, Liters	2.3	4.0	3.0	2.3	3.3	1.9	3.7	1.2	2.0
% FEV_1	88	80	79	92	86	83	70	89	86
MMEFR, L/sec	5.3	10.0	6.4	10.7	12.5	7.5	5.8	2.8	1.8
R_{aw}, cm H_2O/L/sec	-	-	-	-	-	0.6	0.3	-	1.8
PTP at TLC, cm H_2O	-	-	-	-	-	47	46	51	-
DLCO% Predicted	23	33	35	27	60	49	55	56	70

distributions contained areas of normal $\dot{V}_A/\dot{Q}$ in all cases. In addition areas of low (L), high (H) or both (HL) $\dot{V}_A/\dot{Q}$ were noted in each case as indicated in Table 24.2. Only 1 patient (number 5) had a physiologically significant shunt. The degree of hypoxemia was variable, but the calculated values agreed well with those measured with the oxygen electrodes (Table 24.2, Figure 24.1).

During exercise, there were no significant changes in the $\dot{V}_A/\dot{Q}$ distributions in any of the patients, but it should be remembered that the level of exercise was slight. In particular the basic $\dot{V}_A/\dot{Q}$ pattern (L, H, or HL) remained unchanged in going from rest to exercise, and the arterial P_{O_2} and P_{CO_2} calculated from the

Table 24.2.   Patients with Chronic Obstructive Pulmonary Disease

Patient Number	1	2	3	4	5	6	7	8	9	
Clinical Type	A	A	A	B	B	B	B	B	B	
$\dot{V}_A/\dot{Q}$ Pattern	L	H	H	HL	HL	HL	L	HL	L	
% Shunt	0.0	0.3	0.8	0.0	12.4	0.0	0.0	0.0	0.0	
REST:										
Measured PaO_2 mmHg	71	67	66	69	44	56	55	41	64	
Predicted PaO_2 mmHg	66	76	58	64	44	49	50	43	57	
Measured $P\bar{v}O_2$ mmHg	41	31	32	37	30	32	30	31	31	
$\dot{V}_{CO_2}$ ml/min	160	130	160	210	290	200	260	220	170	2
$\dot{V}_{O_2}$ ml/min	200	170	200	260	380	260	320	300	220	2
$\dot{V}_E$ L/min	12.1	6.5	11.8	16.1	11.9	8.7	10.6	10.0	10.8	
$\dot{Q}_T$ L/min	6.8	3.4	4.1	4.2	8.3	7.4	7.3	7.9	4.7	
EXERCISE:										
Measured PaO_2 mmHg	62	62	61	58	37	49	34	37	56	
Predicted PaO_2 mmHg	56	66	61	53	40	46	35	38	55	
Measured $P\bar{v}O_2$ mmHg	34	29	28	30	24	29	17	22	20	
$\dot{V}_{CO_2}$ ml/min	270	170	390	490	390	390	750	740	870	3
$\dot{V}_{O_2}$ ml/min	330	220	480	600	520	500	990	1000	1030	4
$\dot{V}_E$ L/min	17.8	7.5	24.8	28.0	15.6	16.2	20.3	29.1	32.9	1
$\dot{Q}_T$ L/min	9.0	3.3	6.4	6.5	8.8	10.5	10.9	14.0	8.3	
REST:										
Measured PaO_2 mmHg	66	67	65	71	41	50	49	40	63	
Predicted PaO_2 mmHg	60	78	57	76	41	58	50	46	56	
Measured $P\bar{v}O_2$ mmHg	39	31	30	39	30	34	32	32	30	
$\dot{V}_{CO_2}$ ml/min	170	130	170	200	280	220	310	230	210	1
$\dot{V}_{O_2}$ ml/min	210	160	210	250	360	300	360	320	280	1
$\dot{V}_E$ L/min	11.9	6.5	12.1	16.0	12.5	9.4	12.7	10.2	10.8	
$\dot{Q}_T$ L/min	6.8	3.4	4.3	4.0	8.3	7.8	6.0	7.6	3.8	

Table 24.2 (continued)

	PATIENTS WITH CHRONIC INTERSTITIAL LUNG DISEASE								
Patient Number	1	2	3	4	5	6	7	8	9
$\dot{V}_A/\dot{Q}$ Pattern	HL	L	HL	L	L	L	HL	L	L
% Shunt	10.4	10.6	5.2	4.9	0	2.3	0	9.6	0
REST:									
Measured PaO_2 mmHg	50	56	53	69	63	65	54	106*	78
Predicted PaO_2 mmHg	51	59	60	67	66	77	55	104	81
Measured $P\bar{v}O_2$ mmHg	29	37	37	42	35	36	32	31	39
$\dot{V}_{CO_2}$ ml/min	210	170	190	200	210	230	200	160	160
$\dot{V}_{O_2}$ ml/min	300	250	240	260	250	260	260	200	190
$\dot{V}_E$ L/min	13.6	10.7	12.2	11.3	9.2	18.3	10.6	18.5	8.8
$\dot{Q}_T$ L/min	5.0	6.5	4.7	5.6	4.3	3.8	4.0	4.0	4.0
EXERCISE:									
Measured PaO_2 mmHg	35	45	40	64	54	54	43	56**	68
Predicted PaO_2 mmHg	45	54	55	76	51	72	48	64	64
Measured $P\bar{v}O_2$ mmHg	17	27	24	34	24	32	25	25	27
$\dot{V}_{CO_2}$ ml/min	580	640	630	630	650	380	590	180	730
$\dot{V}_{O_2}$ ml/min	670	900	740	650	750	480	670	230	870
$\dot{V}_E$ L/min	38.8	31.8	35.6	44.2	30.2	32.3	23.7	18.0	29.1
$\dot{Q}_T$ L/min	5.7	14.7	7.3	8.1	8.4	6.4	7.1	4.3	10.7
REST:									
Measured PaO_2 mmHg	57	51	56	78	60	71	57	88*	88
Predicted PaO_2 mmHg	64	55	60	79	55	75	59	83	87
Measured $P\bar{v}O_2$ mmHg	30	37	31	42	31	35	34	29	38
$\dot{V}_{CO_2}$ ml/min	220	200	220	190	230	200	150	150	170
$\dot{V}_{O_2}$ ml/min	290	250	300	240	300	240	190	170	200
$\dot{V}_E$ L/min	14.6	11.9	13.5	14.0	9.2	18.0	9.7	16.1	9.7
$\dot{Q}_T$ L/min	4.1	7.0	4.7	4.4	4.8	4.2	3.3	3.6	4.2

* Resting values obtained at $F_{IO_2} = 0.5$
** Actually, resting at $F_{IO_2} = 0.21$

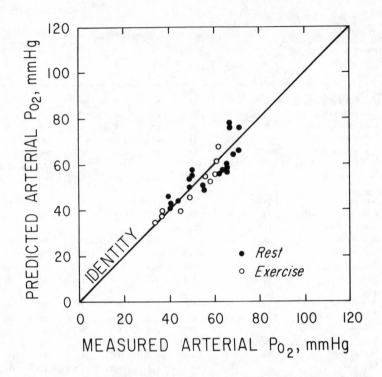

Figure 24.1. Relationship between measured arterial P_{O_2} and that predicted from the $\dot{V}_A/\dot{Q}$ inequality and shunt determined by the inert gas technique. The results are for 10 patients with chronic obstructive pulmonary disease both at rest and during exercise. Note that both at rest and during exercise there is no systematic difference between the measured and predicted values. This is evidence that $\dot{V}_A/\dot{Q}$ inequality and shunt account for all of the hypoxemia in these patients and that failure of diffusion equilibration is not a factor.

recovered distributions agreed well with the measured values (Table 24.2, Figure 24.1).

On returning to resting conditions, the distribution patterns remained unchanged and the arterial blood gases essentially returned to their previous values, again with good agreement between the predicted and measured arterial P_{O_2} and P_{CO_2}.

b. Chronic Interstitial Lung Disease

In spite of generally similar levels of hypoxemia, the patients with CILD had generally different $\dot{V}_A/\dot{Q}$ distributions from the patients with COPD above. While virtually all of the ventilation

and much of the blood flow was present in a relatively narrow range
of normal ventilation-perfusion ratios, substantial amounts of perfusion were present as both shunt and areas of extremely low ventilation-perfusion ratios (0.01 and less). This is to be contrasted
with the results in COPD where even those patients having areas of
low $\dot{V}_A/\dot{Q}$ did not have regions that were so poorly ventilated in relation to bloodflow. In addition the shunt was generally higher
(Table 24.2) in CILD. While the arterial P_{O_2} in these patients
varied between about 50 and 80 mmHg, the degree of hypoxemia at
rest was well predicted from the $\dot{V}_A/\dot{Q}$ distributions together with
shunt (Table 24.2, figure 24.2).

During exercise, there was little or no change in the $\dot{V}_A/\dot{Q}$ distribution. When a change was seen, it was found to take the form
of a broadening of the distribution in the normal range of $\dot{V}_A/\dot{Q}$.
There was a slight shift of the mean of the distribution towards
a higher $\dot{V}_A/\dot{Q}$, consistent with the relatively greater increase in
total ventilation than cardiac output. However the size of the
shunt and the amount of perfusion in very poorly ventilated areas
remained unchanged from the resting values.

The important finding during exercise was that the measured distributions generally did not account for all of the hypoxemia, unlike the situation seen in patients with COPD undergoing exercise.
In virtually every patient, the measured arterial P_{O_2} was repeatably
lower than the value calculated from the $\dot{V}_A/\dot{Q}$ distribution. This
is illustrated in Figure 24.3.

On return to resting conditions, the degree of hypoxemia was
similar to that seen prior to exercise and the predictability of the
arterial P_{O_2} was equally as good. The distribution patterns when
altered during exercise returned to the resting configurations in
each case.

DISCUSSION

Blood Gases at Rest and During Exercise

All patients had hypoxemia at rest breathing room air. In every
patient of both groups arterial P_{O_2} fell during exercise and returned to control values after exercise. The mean fall in arterial
P_{O_2} on exercise was 8.2 mmHg (range 4 to 21) in the patients with
COPD and 10.6 mmHg (range 5 to 15) in the patients with CILD. The
major function of the ensuing discussion is to elucidate the roles
of the various interacting factors contributing to the initial
resting hypoxemia and the fall in arterial P_{O_2} with exercise.

Mechanism of Hypoxemia at Rest

Figures 24.1 and 24.2, expressing the data contained in Table
24.2, demonstrate that in both groups of patients all of the hypoxemia was fully explained by the measured $\dot{V}_A/\dot{Q}$ inequality and shunt.
Recalling that this scheme involves the explicit assumption of diffusion equilibration, these results provide good evidence that there
is no measurable failure of diffusion equilibration for oxygen.

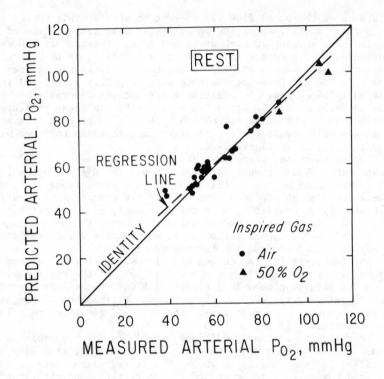

Figure 24.2. Relationship between measured P_{O_2} and that predicted from the $\dot{V}_A/\dot{Q}$ inequality and shunt estimated by the
inert gas technique in 9 patients with chronic interstitial
lung disease at rest. There is no statistical difference between measured and predicted values, suggesting that all of
the hypoxemia at rest in these patients is explained by the
observed inequality and shunt.

Overall hypoventilation was also not a factor (except possibly in
patient 2 with COPD) with values of minute ventilation ($\dot{V}_E$) either
normal or considerably above normal. Thus the reasons for hypoxemia at rest in both groups were ventilation-perfusion inequality
(of which several different patterns were observed) and shunt (particularly in CILD). The lower than normal values for mixed venous
P_{O_2} generally observed in both groups of patients at rest is in ac-
cord with the behavior of the lung in the presence of $\dot{V}_A/\dot{Q}$ inequalit
as discussed by West (8).

Changes in the $\dot{V}_A/\dot{Q}$ Distribution with Exercise

When the effects of errors of the method were considered, there
were with one exception no significant changes in the extent or

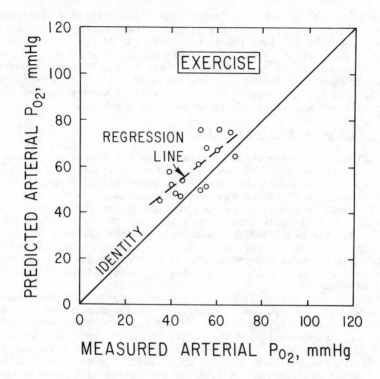

Figure 24.3. Relationship between measured arterial P_{O_2} and that predicted using the inert gas data measured during exercise in patients with chronic interstitial lung disease. A systematic difference (P<0.01) is seen with the predicted arterial P_{O_2} being higher than the measured value. This is evidence that failure of diffusion equilibration contributed to hypoxemia during exercise in these patients.

pattern of $\dot{V}_A/\dot{Q}$ inequality in both groups of patients. The exception occurred in the patients with CILD and took the form of a slight broadening and shift towards higher $\dot{V}_A/\dot{Q}$ ratios of the units with normal $\dot{V}_A/\dot{Q}$ at rest, consistent with the relatively greater increase in minute ventilation than cardiac output during exercise (Table 24.2). Superimposed upon the already moderately severe $\dot{V}_A/\dot{Q}$ inequality present at rest, these changes are of little importance to overall gas exchange.

Changes in Venous P_{O_2} During Exercise

Direct sampling of mixed venous blood from the pulmonary artery revealed that mixed venous P_{O_2} ($P_{v_{O_2}}$) fell in every patient during exercise. The mean fall was by 7.2 mmHg (range 2 to 13) in COPD

patients, and by 9.6 mmHg (range 4 to 13) in patients with CILD.
The fall in venous P_{O_2} with exercise is well known and mostly reflects a relative increase in the ratio (R) of $\dot{V}_{O_2}$ to cardiac output. The data of Table 24.2 can be plotted to illustrate the relation
ship between R' (= $R_{exercise}/R_{rest}$) and $P_{v_{O_2}}$. This was found to be
linear such that for R' = 2, the measured fall in $P_{v_{O_2}}$ was 12 to 13
mmHg. If extrapolated to R' = 1, no fall in venous P_{O_2} was antici-
pated from this relationship as would be expected.

Mechanism of Hypoxemia During Exercise

(1) Chronic obstructive pulmonary disease: Figure 24.1 shows that
just as at rest, all of the hypoxemia was accounted for by $\dot{V}_A/\dot{Q}$
inequality and shunt when present. Hypoventilation and diffusion
impairment on the other hand did not contribute to hypoxemia.
The fall in arterial P_{O_2} from resting values (by a mean of 8.2
mmHg) could be fully explained by the fall in venous P_{O_2} which in
turn was the result of the relatively greater increase in $\dot{V}_{O_2}$ than
cardiac output. In particular $\dot{V}_A/\dot{Q}$ relationships did not measur-
ably worsen under the conditions of this study and cannot thus be
invoked as a mechanism for reducing the arterial P_{O_2} at this level
of mild exercise.
(2) Chronic interstitial lung disease: Figure 24.3 shows that there
was a small but systematic discrepancy between measured and predicted arterial P_{O_2} (P<0.01). During exercise the combined effects
of ventilation-perfusion inequality and shunt accounted for a mean
of 83% of the total alveolar-arterial P_{O_2} difference and the remainder, 17%, has been ascribed to failure of alveolar-endcapillary
diffusion equilibrium. A feel for the effect of the independent but
interactive fall in venous P_{O_2} can be had by comparing the actual
fall in arterial P_{O_2} on exercise to that predicted from the measured $\dot{V}_A/\dot{Q}$ inequality and shunt (reflecting primarily the fall in
$P_{v_{O_2}}$ since the changes in the $\dot{V}_A/\dot{Q}$ distribution were negligible).
The mean measured fall in arterial P_{O_2} was 10.6 mmHg (Table 24.2)
(excluding patient 8 who was not exercised) while the mean predicted fall in arterial P_{O_2} for the same patients was 6.4 mmHg. Thus
to a first approximation half of the fall in arterial P_{O_2} with
exercise in these patients with advanced CILD is the result of a
reduction in venous P_{O_2}, while the remainder appears to be the result of failure of diffusion equilibration. $\dot{V}_A/\dot{Q}$ relationships did
not worsen significantly and did not therefore contribute directly
to the fall in arterial P_{O_2}.
It will be recalled that the $\dot{V}_A/\dot{Q}$ distribution patterns in patients
with interstitial lung disease consisted mostly of two groups of lung
units: those with essentially normal $\dot{V}_A/\dot{Q}$ ratios and those with very
low or zero $\dot{V}_A/\dot{Q}$ values (<0.01). Since in the latter group end-
capillary P_{O_2} is within a fraction of a mmHg of venous P_{O_2} even
when diffusion equilibration is complete, it is difficult to see
how failure of diffusion equilibration in these units could be responsible for the discrepancy between predicted and measured arteria
P_{O_2} values. In fact this very point suggests that little can be
said about the diffusing properties of these poorly ventilated units

Consequently the discrepancy between predicted and measured arterial P_{O_2} is in all probability related to the group of well-ventilated and perfused units, although it is impossible to be more specific than this about the distribution of diffusing properties in relation to $\dot{V}_A/\dot{Q}$ amongst these units.

A final consideration relates to the magnitude of the "diffusion component" to hypoxemia – only some 17% of the total alveolar arterial difference during exercise. While this is only a small fraction of the total alveolar-arterial difference, its existence implies considerable reduction in the average diffusing properties of the areas concerned. Theoretical studies indicate that for regions of approximately normal $\dot{V}_A/\dot{Q}$, the diffusing properties must on the average be reduced to about 1/5 of normal (2,7) to explain the observed alveolar-endcapillary differences. It is stressed that this is an average estimate and it is possible (if not even probable) that these diffusing properties are themselves unevenly distributed so that relating them to global variables such as the $D_{L_{CO}}$ is not profitable at the present time.

SUMMARY

In 10 patients with chronic obstructive pulmonary disease, and 9 with chronic interstitial lung disease the mechanisms of hypoxemia at rest and during exercise were studied with a multiple inert gas elimination method. Repeatable and distinct patterns of V_A/Q inequality and shunt were found both at rest and during exercise in the two groups, and the amount of inequality and shunt completely explained the resting arterial P_{O_2} in both groups. During mild steady-state exercise (increase in mean $\dot{V}_{O_2}$ by a factor of 2.6) no clinically significant changes occurred in the $\dot{V}_A/\dot{Q}$ distribution in either group, but the arterial P_{O_2} fell by 8.2 and 10.6 mmHg in the patients with COPD and CILD, respectively. In the COPD group this fall was completely accounted for by the observed fall in mixed venous P_{O_2} which resulted from the relatively greater increase in $\dot{V}_{O_2}$ than cardiac output. None of the hypoxemia could be attributed to failure of diffusion equilibration. In the CILD group on the other hand about one-half of the fall in P_{O_2} with exercise was explained by the fall in venous P_{O_2}, the remainder being attributed to failure of diffusion equilibration in well-ventilated and well-perfused gas exchange units. Even though the diffusional component of the alveolar-arterial difference was only a small fraction of the total (17%) it is stressed that even this small amount implies substantial impairment of diffusing properties in the regions concerned.

ACKNOWLEDGMENTS

It is a pleasure to acknowledge a number of coworkers without whom the collection of data in these patients would have been impossible. My thanks goes to Dr. Jack Clausen, Dr. David Dantzker, Dr. Larry DePolo, Dr. Ronald Dueck, Dr. Vincent Tornabene, Dr. Karl Wasserman, and Dr. J. B. West (Supported by NIH Grants HL 17731 and HL 00111).

REFERENCES

1.   Forster, R. E.   Chap. 33 in Handbook of Physiology, Respira-
      tion, Vol. 1. Amer. Phys. Soc., Washington, D. C. 1964.
2.   Hill, E. P., G. G. Power and L. D. Longo. Am. J. Physiol.
      224: 904-917, 1973.
3.   Hlastala, M. P. Resp. Physiol. 15: 214-232, 1972.
4.   Wagner, P. D., R. B. Laravuso, R. R. Uhl, and J. B. West.
      J. Clin. Invest. 54: 54-68, 1974.
5.   Wagner, P. D., P. F. Naumann, and R. B. Laravuso. J. Appl.
      Physiol. 36: 600-605, 1974.
6.   Wagner, P. D., H. A. Saltzman and J. B. West. J. Appl.
      Physiol. 36: 588-599, 1974.
7.   Wagner, P. D., and J. B. West. J. Appl. Physiol. 33: 62-71,
      1972.
8.   West, J. B. Resp. Physiol. 7: 88-110, 1969.

DISCUSSION

Goldman: Were any measurements of diffusing capacity for CO made
in the interstitial lung disease patients?

P. Wagner: Yes, all patients had a gross decrease in DL_{CO} to a
mean of 60% of predicted. However, in the presence of severe VA:Q
inequality, these changes are difficult to interpret.

Gee: Was DL_{CO} per litre alveolar volume changed?

P. Wagner: I haven't shown these data in that form, but appropriate
data will be available in the proceedings.

Wasserman: We found a reduced DL per VA in these same patients
with alveolar proteinosis, presumably due to theconsiderable amount
of insoluble proteinoceous material in alveoli.

Dempsey: You showed a discrepancy between measured and predicted
arterial PO_2 of $\sim$ 10 mmHg and explained this on the basis of an
estimated diffusion defect which was $\sim$ 17% of the A-a DO_2, which
you stated was a trivial defect. Isn't this in fact a very large
defect?

P. Wagner: The discrepancy between the measured and predicted
arterial oxygen tension was small. In terms of diffusing properties
of the lung it is large, I agree.

25

Is There Carrier-Mediated Oxygen Transport in the Lung?

Gail H. Gurtner, Carlos J. Mendoza,
Hannah H. Peavy, & Barry Burns

It may seem odd to pose the question in the title of this paper more than 50 years after J. S. Haldane's hypothesis on O_2 secretion by the lung had apparently been disproved by the experiments of August Krogh. However, we have made some experimental observations which may indicate that Haldane was in part correct.

Over the past few years we have been involved in a series of experiments which lead us to believe that there is a facilitated transport system for oxygen and carbon monoxide in the lung and placenta. Facilitated transport systems provide a carrier mediated alternative path for diffusion which can operate over and above the path of simple diffusion. We, unlike Haldane, believe that the mechanism which assists in the transfer of O_2 and CO operates on the existing electrochemical gradient of permeant, and requires no other input of free energy--except that required for the maintenance of cell membrane structure. We have never observed transport against an electrochemical potential gradient, as would be possible with "active transport". This series of investigations began with the observation that O_2 crossed the sheep placenta far more rapidly than inert gases. The rate limiting processes for O_2 and inert gas exchange appear to be qualitatively different; that for O_2 being the rate of delivery of O_2 and that for inert gases and other substances being the small permeability of placenta (1).

The carrier may be cytochrome P-450 as suggested by Longmuir for O_2 transport in the liver (2). The evidence in favor of cytochrome P-450 as the carrier are the effects on gas exchange of compounds which bind to the cytochrome. These compounds, some of them drugs, markedly decrease transplacental O_2 transfer while not affecting inert gas transfer (3). Cytochrome P-450 present in the liver, lungs, placenta, kidney and adrenals. This cytochrome binds reversibly both O_2 and CO; the reaction rate with CO has been measured and is considerably faster than the reaction rate of CO with hemoglobin (4,5). The O_2 association rate with P-450 for mammalian liver P-450 has been reported to be 20 times faster than the CO association rate (6). It is intuitively obvious that the reaction rate may preclude a molecule from the role as a membrane carrier if the rate is not fast enough, e.g., if the rate were infinitely slow the gas would be bound and not released. Compounds which bind to cytochrome P-450 act to slow the association and

357

dissociation with CO, presumably by shielding the CO binding site (4,7). This may be the mechanism by which placental O_2 transport is reduced by such compounds. CO transfer in the placenta also is partially facilitated; we have demonstrated saturation kinetics of placental CO transfer and competition between O_2 and CO for the carrier (8,9).

All of our placental research has been performed on the sheep placenta, which because of the large distances between maternal and fetal vessels and small surface area, poses a formidable barrier with low diffusing capacity for eachange of materials by simple diffusion. We estimate that up to 80% of placental O_2 transfer may be mediated by the carrier (3). Other investigators have demonstrated carrier mediated transport of CO in the guinea pig placenta which because of the lack of fetal tissue layers offers a lesser barrier to simple diffusion. In this placenta the estimate of percentage of carrier mediated CO transport is approximately 30% (10).

Cytochrome P-450 is also present in the lung and appears to act as a carrier for CO. We have found that some drugs which interact with cytochrome P-450 decrease the diffusing capacity for CO (DLCO). We have also observed saturation kinetics for CO transfer. Saturation of a pulmonary carbon monoxide carrier would be manifested by decrease in the DLCO as the inspired carbon monoxide concentration is varied. We have demonstrated this phenomenon using single breath and rebreathing methods for DLCO (11). Since these methods measure only the disappearance of CO from the lung during a transient state, there is a possibility that the altered rate of disappearance may represent binding of CO to tissue cytochromes which do not act as CO carriers but represent a sink for CO which could be saturated as the CO concentration is increased. Because of this, we measured steady-state DLCO at four different inspired CO levels in dogs. The steady-state DLCO is a true measure of gas to blood transfer and is not affected by binding of CO to carrier or non-carrier molecules in the lung tissue. The dogs were anesthetized with phenobarbital, a drug which does not alter DLCO or placental O_2 transfer. They were paralyzed and ventilated at constant rate. For each DLCO measurement we measured inspired, expired, end tidal CO concentration as well as the back pressure of CO in the blood. Since the animals varied in size, the DLCO at the different CO concentrations were normalized by dividing by the DLCO measured using an inspired CO concentration of 1000 ppm. The results are shown in Figure 25.1.

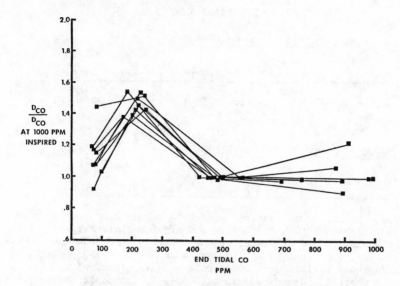

Fig. 25.1. The ratio of steady-state DLCO measured at various
inspired CO concentrations divided by the DLCO measured at 1000
ppm inspired CO is plotted against end tidal CO concentration.
The mean normalized DLCO measurements made at the lowest CO concentration as well as the group measured at 500 ppm inspired CO
were significantly different from the measurements made at 1000
ppm (P < .001). The measurements made at an inspired CO concentration of 2000 ppm were not significantly different from those
made at 1000 ppm.

The decrease in DLCO as end tidal CO concentration is increased from 200 to 500 ppm is nearly identical in the steady-
state and single breath measurements reported in reference 11.
This indicates that the single breath and rebreathing measurements
also reflect true facilitated transport of CO.

Saturation kinetics for CO transfer as well as the decreases
in DLCO caused by drugs which bind to cytochrome P-450 can be
correlated with the presence of the cytochrome in the lung. This
is clearly demonstrated by comparing the measurements made in the
newborn lamb, which has less than 1/10th the adult concentration
of pulmonary cytochrome P-450, with the same measurements made
in the adult sheep. These results are shown in Tables 25.1 and
25.2.

DRUG EFFECTS ON DLCO IN SHEEP

DLCO (Normoxia)

	Control	SKF 525A
Adult Sheep	30.7 (N = 6)	20.4 (N = 6)
	.0025 > P	
Newborn Lambs	1.46 (n = 9)	1.36 (n = 6)
	N.S.	

Table 25.1.   DLCO was measured by a rebreathing technique at an initial FACO of 400 ppm before and after administration of SKF 525A buffered to pH 7.4. The adult dose of the drug was 1000 mg, the lamb dose was 100 mg. On the basis of mg/kg body weight or mg/M^2 body surface area, the lambs actually received a larger dose. Note that DLCO decreased significantly in the adult sheep, but did not change in the lambs who lack cytochrome P-450.

SATURATION KINETICS FOR PULMONARY CO TRANSFER

	t 1/2 (sec)		DLCO(ml/min / mm Hg)	
	FACO 65 ppm	FACO 650 ppm	FACO 65 ppm	FACO 650 ppm
Adult Sheep (N = 9)	4.6	5.1	32.2	24.9
	P < .025		P < .001	
Newborn Lambs (n = 3)	20	19.66	1.16	1.18
	N.S.		N.S.	

Table 25.2.   DLCO measured by the rebreathing technique in adult sheep and newborn lambs. Note that DLCO at an initial FACO of 65 ppm was significantly larger than at 650 ppm. This was partly due to an increased rate of CO disappearance at the lower CO concentration, but was also related to an increased volume of distribution of CO in the lung due to the rapid uptake of CO by the carrier (see reference 11 for details). No such effects were seen in the newborn lambs who lack cytochrome P-450. This is evidence that cytochrome P-450 is responsible for the changes in DLCO observed in the adult sheep and that facilitated CO transport can be correlated with the presence of cytochrome P-450.

The role of a carrier in pulmonary oxygen transfer is more
difficult to assess. Because of the large surface area for gas
exchange, the short distance between gas and blood, and the large
P_{O_2} gradient between alveolar gas and mixed venous blood, sufficient
O_2 exchange can occur by simple diffusion to satisfy metabolic
needs. There is no clear evidence that, under normal physiological
conditions, diffusion could become a rate limiting process in
pulmonary oxygen exchange. To test the hypothesis that O_2 transfer
might be partially carrier mediated, we had to devise experimental
conditions which were distinctly abnormal. To do this we used an
isolated dog lung preparation in which we could control mixed
venous and inspired P_{O_2} as well as pulmonary blood flow rate.

The pulmonary artery and vein of left lower lobe of lung of
an anesthetized dog was cannulated in vivo not allowing any air
in the blood vessels. The dog was then bled and the blood was
used to perfuse the lobe. The preparation is shown in Figure 25.2.

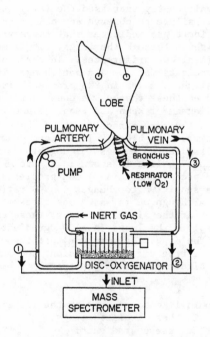

Fig. 25.2ı   Experimental setup for isolated lobe perfusions.
The lobe is suspended by adhesive discs, perfused with autologous
blood which is equilibrated with inert gas in the disc oxygenator,
and ventilated via the bronchus with various gas mixtures.
Partial pressures of gases in the blood and air phases are
measured with a semi-permeable membrane attached to the inlet of
a mass spectrometer (Bendix MA1). In these experiments, both O_2
and CO_2 were passing from alveolus to blood.

The lobe was suspended from rubber discs glued to the pleura with blood vessels dependent. Using this preparation, pulmonary blood flow of over 1000 cc/min without abnormal pulmonary artery pressure was achieved. The lung was respired with a mixture containing O_2, CO_2 and N_2 and some times Argon. P_{O_2} in the inspired gas was kept below 70 to minimize the effects of small changes in $\dot{V}/\dot{Q}$ ratios and shunts and also to optimally demonstrate any carrier system with a heme group which binds oxygen avidly. The blood coming from the lobe was deoxygenated in a disc type oxygenator through which inert gas was circulated. Partial pressures of O_2, CO_2 and inert gases were measured in pulmonary artery, vein and airway using membrane tipped probes connected to a mass spectrometer as described in other publications (1,3).

We measured (A-a) gradients before and after acute infusion of compounds known to bind to cytochrome P-450. In Table 25.3 we show the results.

The drugs significantly increased the (A-a) gradient for O_2 in all cases. The failure to observe any change in the (A-a) gradients for the inert gas indicates that there was no change in the anatomical shunt through the lungs. It is more difficult to interpret the (A-a) CO_2 differences. In three of six experiments the (A-a) gradients for CO_2 did not change; in the other three there were slight changes in CO_2 gradients from (1-3) mm Hg. In order to interpret these changes we constructed a $\dot{V}/\dot{Q}$ line using the O_2-CO_2 diagram of Rahn and Fenn. Since in our experiments CO_2 was crossing in the same direction as O_2, both blood and gas R lines were negative. The blood R lines were drawn from the combined O_2-CO_2 dissociation curves for dog blood from the Rahn-Fenn monograph. The $\dot{V}/\dot{Q}$ line is shown in Figure 25.3. It can be seen that it would predict that (A-a) CO_2 gradients for CO_2 would be nearly as sensitive to changes in $\dot{V}/\dot{Q}$ ratios as (A-a) O_2 gradients. Thus, although we may have observed small changes in $\dot{V}/\dot{Q}$ ratios in three of the six experiments, these changes are not large enough to explain the large (A-a) O_2 gradients after administration of the drug. We conclude that these gradients may well represent a true diffusion gradient and may indicate that under normal circumstances O_2 transport may be partially carrier mediated.

Finally, I would like to comment on the large (A-a) CO_2 gradients observed in these isolated lungs. Two possible explanations exist for these gradients:

(1)   They represent a manifestation of the step up in P_{CO_2} which we and others have observed between blood and alveolar gas during rebreathing. In the case where no net gas exchange occurs or during gas exchange occurs from alveolus (or tissue to blood), the mechanism causing the step up in P_{CO_2} (the charged membrane hypothesis) would predict that gradients would exist under these conditions (12-13).

Table 25.3

Results from the Isolated Lung Perfusion

Oxygenator equilibration gas	$\dot{Q}$ (ml/min)	$\dot{V}$ (ml/min)	End tidal gas tension					(A–a) gas tensions mmHg										Drug used and dose
			P_{O_2}	P_{CO_2}	PA	PN_2	PHe	Before drug					After drug					
								O_2	CO_2	A	N_2	He	O_2	CO_2	A	N_2	He	
A	440	2250	58	62	330	300		5	14	-10	15		15	16	-10	15		Metyrapone 500 mg
A	440	2250	58	62	330	300		4	20	-10	10		29	20	-10	10		Morphine 30 mg
He	530	2250	70	110	150	420	0	1	35	5	20	-30	22.5	35	5	20	-30	Metyrapone 1750 mg
A	530	1500	82	100	75			14	25	0			36	26	0			Analine 2000 mg
A	310	1500	58	62	330			5	10	-40			16	10	-30			Metyrapone 1000 mg
He	310	1500	150	60	75			20	10	5		-50	70	13	5		-50	SKF-525A 1500 mg

After the administration of the drugs, the (A–a) O_2 gradients increased markedly while those for the other gases did not change significantly. Drugs were infused directly into the perfusion circuit over 1–2 min. and were adjusted to the pH of the perfusate.

363

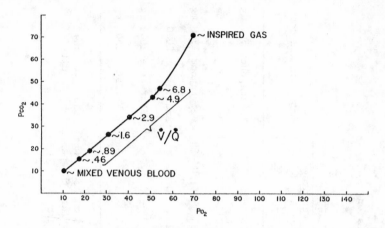

Fig. 25.3.   The $\dot{V}/\dot{Q}$ diagram for the isolated perfused lung lobes.
In the lower left hand corner the PO_2 and PCO_2 of the mixed
venous blood are represented, while at the upper right hand
corner these same values for the inspired gas are given. The
points in-between represent different ratios of $\dot{V}/\dot{Q}$ and corresponding gas tensions. Note that any change in the PO_2 due to a
variation in $\dot{V}/\dot{Q}$ would cause an almost equal change in PCO_2.

(2)   They represent $\dot{V}/\dot{Q}$ abnormalities present before the drug was
       infused.

     In an attempt to test these alternatives we equilibrated the
blood in the oxygenator with a CO_2 mixture and rebreathed the lobe
of lung. In these experiments under conditions of no net gas
exchange across the alveolar capillary membrane, (A-a) CO_2
differences also occurred similar in magnitude to those reported
in living dogs by us and several other groups of investigators.
It seems likely, therefore, that the charged membrane mechanism
was active and could explain part of the (A-a) CO_2 gradients
observed.

SUMMARY

     A specific O_2, CO transport system appears to be present in
the lung and placenta mediated by cytochrome P-450. The carrier
may be physiologically important in the placenta where from up to
80% of the fetal O_2 supply may be transported by the carrier. In
the lung, the physiological significance of the carrier is less
clear under normal circumstances. It may become important in
disease states.

REFERENCES

1. Gurtner, G.H. and B. Burns. J. Appl. Physiol. 35:728-734, 1975.

2. Longmuir, I.S. and S. Sun. Microvascular Res. 2:287-293, 1970.

3. Gurtner, G.H. and B. Burns. Nature 240:473-475, 1972.

4. Peterson, J.A. and B.W. Griffin. Arch. Biochem. and Biophys. 151:427-433, 1972.

5. Peterson, J.A., Y. Ishimura and B.W. Griffin. Arch. Biochem. and Biophys. 149:197-208, 1972.

6. Rosen, P. and A. Stier. Biochem. Biophys. Res. Comm. 51(3): 603-611, 1973.

7. Lipscomb, J.D. and I.C. Gunsalus. Drug Metab. Disp. 1(1): 1-5, 1973.

8. Gurtner, G.H. and B. Burns. Fed. Proc. 35:830, 1976.

9. Gurtner, G.H. and B. Burns. Physiologist 18:235, 1975.

10. Bissonnette, J.M. and W.K. Wickham. Physiologist 35:852, 1976.

11. Gurtner, G.H., H. Peavy, W. Summer and B. Burns. Proceedings of a symposium on Interstitial Processes in the Lung. Paris, May 30-31, 1974. Prog. in Resp. Research 8:166-176, 1975.

12. Gurtner, G.H., S.H. Song and L.E. Farhi. Resp. Physiol. 7:173-187, 1969.

13. Gurtner, G.H., D.G. Davies and B. Burns. In: Carbon Dioxide and Metabolic Regulations, Ed. G. Nahas and K. Schafer, Springer-Verlag, 1974.

DISCUSSION

Goldman: Considering reaction kinetics, are there any other possible explanations for your findings?

Gurtner: The single breath DL_{CO} measurements may have an alternate
explanation. During the breath-hold technique we are only measuring
a transient disappearance of carbon monoxide from the alveolar
volume and assume that it enters the blood. The apparent saturation
kinetics could be explained by binding of CO by Cytochrome P450 or
some other cytochrome in the lung parenchyma. With the steady-state
DL_{CO} measurements, there is true alveolar gas to blood transfer;
therefore, we feel that we have demonstrated true saturation kinetics for pulmonary CO_2 transport.

Gee: How migratory is Cytochrome P450?

Gurtner: The cytochrome is structurally part of the endoplasmic
reticulum and cannot be easily extracted without denaturation. Because of this, the concept is that the cytochrome must act as a
"fixed site" carrier. There is a possibility that the cytochrome
may have some motion about its point of attachment which might give
it some of the properties of a mobile carrier. Longmuir has observed that halothane inhibits tissue respiration in liver slices by
interference with an oxygen transport mechanism (Brit. J. Anesth.,
43:1036, 1971). This might be due to a direct effect of halothane
on the carrier or due to a physico-chemical effect of halothane
such as a change in the structuring of cell water, which might
affect motion of the carrier.

Gee: Have you tried the effects of colchicine because, like colchicine, many general anesthetics prevent the reassembly of micro-
tubules which regulate cell motion?

Gurtner: That is an interesting idea.

P. Wagner: Is there a physiological role for this mechanism?

Gurtner: I think that the carrier may be important to placental
oxygen exchange. We do not have enough information to speculate
on its physiological importance in the lung. I hope that your
inert gas method will answer the question.

J.H.G. Rankin: Much of the evidence for such facilitation is
largely based on results which indicate that various drugs which
block cytochrome P450 also inhibit the transplacental flux of
oxygen without affecting the flux of inert gases. This result
could also indicate that the drugs caused a non-specific decrease
in placental permeability thereby decreasing the flux of those substances (such as oxygen) which usually reached a steady-state
closer to the venous end of the capillaries.

Gurtner: The transplacental flux of oxygen decreases by as much as 80% after administration of drugs which bind to Cytochrome P450 while simultaneously measured argon transfer did not change. The failure of argon transfer to change seems to rule out distribution effects and shunt as the cause of the decreased O$_2$ transfer, leaving only diffusion impairment as the mechanism. As you have pointed out previously, non-specific, noxious effects of the drugs affecting permeability might lead to the same results if argon transfer were perfusion limited. Because of this possibility, we performed the experiments which indicated that inert gas transfer appears to be diffusion limited. If this is so, a generalized change in permeability would effect argon transfer as well as O$_2$ transfer. Thus, we are left with the conclusion that the drug specifically interfered with O$_2$ transport, probably by blocking facilitated diffusion.

J. Rankin: The reaction kinetics of CO with hemoglobin will vary with the oxygen and CO tension. Would the rate of association of CO with hemoglobin affect your results?

Gurtner: Yes, this would affect the DL$_{CO}$ measurements. In the experiments in which we demonstrated saturation kinetics for pulmonary CO transfer the alveolar and arterial PO$_2$ remained constant so that changes in DL$_{CO}$ with a changing inspired CO concentration could not be explained on that basis. At the CO concentrations used in these experiments (range of .015% to .2%) the value of Θ should be independent of CO concentrations (F.J.W. Roughton and R.F. Forster, J. Appl. Physiol., 11:268-276, 1957). Because of this, it is unlikely that the observed saturation kinetics are related to the reaction of CO with hemoglobin.

The question of whether the drugs such as SKF-525A which reduce DL$_{CO}$ might affect CO association with hemoglobin is an important one. We have not measured the CO reaction kinetics with hemoglobin in the presence of the drugs; however, none of them affects the O$_2$ dissociation curve. This is not proof that the drugs do not interact with hemoglobin but it seems unlikely.

26

Regulation of Pulmonary Capillary Blood Flow

Wiltz W. Wagner, Jr., & Leonard P. Latham

The lung is the essential link in the transport of oxygen from the air to the blood. The alveolar capillaries provide the critical air-gas interface in this process. From rest to maximal exercise, pulmonary blood flow increases five-fold and oxygen uptake increases by a full order of magnitude. This requires that the surface area for oxygen uptake expands by altering the ways in which the capillaries are perfused. The air-blood barrier must be thin for efficient oxygen transfer. But the thinness of the barrier sets the stage for water leakage from the capillaries. Indeed, the continual flow of lung lymph has been interpreted to mean that there is continual water filtration by the pulmonary microcirculation. Thus the capillaries must accommodate the massive increases in blood flow without permitting a rise in capillary blood pressure with its associated increase in transcapillary water flux which would impede oxygenation. The lung successfully manages this rather delicate balance under a wide variety of normal circumstances, but precisely how is not clear. Part of the problem in understanding these aspects of capillary function is that most of the methods used to study these vessels are indirect and difficult to interpret.

The purpose of this paper is to report some preliminary, direct, microscopic observations made of the pulmonary capillaries of the anesthetized dog during a variety of hemodynamic conditions and to attempt to relate these observations to the ways in which the pulmonary capillaries utilize their reserve when they respond to exercise.

Materials and Methods

The techniques we use to visualize the pulmonary microcirculation are complex and have been published in detail elsewhere (1,2). For these reasons we will deal only briefly with the methods here. Pentobarbital anesthetized adult dogs are used. Intermittent positive pressure respiration produces normal arterial oxygen tensions (PaO_2) > 100 torr under control conditions. Pulmonary artery pressures (Ppa) are measured by a high fidelity pressure transducer implanted in the main pulmonary artery. Cardiac outputs are measured by dye dilution techniques.

A transparent window implanted in the chest wall permits observations to be made of the pulmonary microcirculation on the uppermost surface of the lung. This surface is approximately 15 cm above the heart placing it in Zone II where Ppa is sufficiently high to pump blood through the capillaries after which the red cells spill into the veins where the pressure is low (3).

Observations are made with a surface illumination microscope. To record capillary a beam-splitting device incorporated into the microscope permits the observer to see the superimposed image of the lung on a sheet of drawing paper beside the microscope. A tracing is made on the drawing paper of the outlines of 4-10 adjoining alveoli and of only those capillaries within the outlines in which there is flow of red blood cells. To quantitate capillary perfusion the summed length (calibrated in μm) of the capillaries on each drawing is determined with a map-measuring tool. The area (μm^2) of the outlined alveoli (defined as field area) is planimetered. Capillary Perfusion Index (CPI) is expressed as the length of perfused capillaries per area of an average alveolar wall (approximately 10,000 μm^2 in our preparation):

$$CPI\ (\mu m) = \frac{\Sigma\ capillary\ lengths\ (\mu m)}{field\ area\ (\mu m^2)/10,000\ (\mu m^2)}$$

Red blood cell velocity varies significantly during the maneuvers. For technical reasons, we have not quantitated velocity changes. The changes are very obvious, however, so we can make statements with confidence concerning increases or decreases in red cell velocity from control levels.

Two challenges have been given to the pulmonary circulation to observe the response in the capillaries.
<u>Isocapnic hypoxia</u>.

A number of inspired gas mixtures of differing oxygen tensions are administered in random order to the animal during each study. The observer, who does not know which is being given to the animal, makes a separate drawing of the red blood cell perfused capillaries within the chosen alvoeli for each gas.

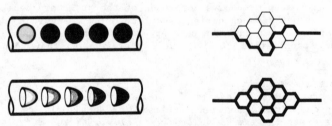

LONGITUDINAL RECRUITMENT   LATERAL RECRUITMENT

Figure 26.1. At rest (upper left) red cells move slowly and become oxygenated in first third of capillary pathlength. With increased cardiac output (lower left), cell velocity increases and entire capillary length is recruited for oxygenation, i.e. longitudinal recruitment. When Ppa is low (upper right), red cells perfuse only a few capillary channels (heavy lines). When Ppa increases (lower right) recruitment of parallel channels occurs, i.e. lateral recruitment.

Increased cardiac output.
     Isoproterenol is infused in doses from 1 to 60 µg/min to
elevate cardiac output.   By varying isoproterenol infusion it is
possible to elevate cardiac output from control levels up to values
4 times control.   The observer again makes drawings.
Results:
     Two patterns of response to hemodynamic alterations have been
observed as ways in which the capillaries utilize their reserve.
     Lateral recruitment.   This response is characterized by an
increase in the number of perfused segments (see Figure 26.1).
Velocity of the red cells through the capillaries may or may not
increase depending on the maneuver.   Mean capillary transmural
pressure or "flooding pressure" is probably high under these circumstances.   Clearly, lateral recruitment increases the area for
gas exchange, but this advantage may be offset to varying extent by
the increase in flooding pressure which tends to increase transcapillary water flux and thereby reduce the diffusing capacity of
the membrane.   We quantitate lateral recruitment using the Capillary Perfusion Index (CPI).
     Lateral recruitment seems to occur only during maneuvers that
elevate Ppa.   An example is shown in Figure 26.2 where arterial
oxygen tension was progressively lowered via isocapnic hypoxia.
The relationship between either CPI or Ppa and progressive hypoxia
is curvilinear; the curve swings upward between arterial oxygen
tensions of 60 and 70 torr, the point on the HbO_2 dissociation curve
where systemic arterial oxygen desaturation begins to occur.   The
CPI is about six times as great at a PaO_2 of 40 as during control (P<
0.001).   In every experiment, the magnitude of the increase in CPI
was significantly correlated in a linear relationship to the magnitude of the rise in Ppa.   Other maneuvers that elevated Ppa, e.g.
infusion of prostaglandin $F_{2\alpha}$, produced a similar increase in the
CPI.
     Longitudinal recruitment.   The red cells move faster through
the capillaries during exercise.   Roughton (4) calculated that the
increased erythrocyte velocity with exercise could diminish the red
cell capillary transit time by a factor of three.   The term
longitudinal recruitment means that the red cells recruit more
capillary path length for oxygenation.   In other words, at rest, the
red cells become oxygenated in about the first third of the capillary.   During exercise, the red cells use the whole capillary path
length for oxygenation.   Longitudinal recruitment permits more red
cells to pass through a given capillary per unit time and become
oxygenated.   Because significant arterial oxygen desaturation does
not occur even at maximum exercise, the reserve capillary path
length must be sufficient for the red cells to move faster yet still
become oxygenated.   This observation has been substantiated by Lee
(5) who has shown that O_2 uptake in the pulmonary capillaries is
linearly related to capillary blood flow even when systolic peak
flows are very high.
     Longitudinal recruitment as seen through the window is charac-
terized by an increase in the velocity of the red cells through the
capillaries (see Figure 26.1).   Maneuvers that raise cardiac output

cause a significant increase in erythrocyte velocity as observed
with our window preparation. Lateral recruitment does occur, but,
in the upper parts of the lung where we are making our observations,
there are substantial numbers of capillary segments left unperfused. The unperfused segments still amount to more than 50% of the
available capillaries when cardiac output reaches high values.
According to our current thinking, flooding pressure is low under
these circumstances because of the relatively low levels of lateral
recruitment, but "driving pressure," i.e., the pressure at the head
of the capillary net, must be high in order to drive the red cells
through the net so rapidly.

Maneuvers that cause a rise in cardiac output are primarily
associated with a rise in red blood cell velocity rather than
lateral recruitment. For example, during isoproterenol infusion
(Figure 26.3), there is little increase in the number of perfused
capillaries when output is raised to double or even triple control
values. However, red cell velocities increase in a very obvious
manner. Although for technical reasons we can not yet quantitate
velocities, the increases are sufficiently large and consistent,
that we are confident the change exists even though we cannot
quantitate it.

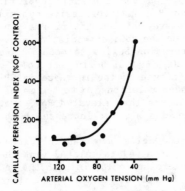
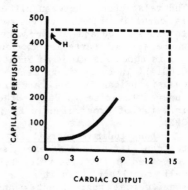

Figure 26.2. Lateral recruitment, quantified by capillary
perfusion index, increases in
curvilinear fashion during progressive hypoxia.

Figure 26.3. Even with large
increases in cardiac output
(liters/min), there is little
lateral recruitment. "H" indicates typical CPI at a PaO_2 of
40 torr.

Discussion

Our findings that increased Ppa is associated with lateral
recruitment and that increased cardiac output is associated with
longitudinal recruitment has been a consistent finding in a very
large number of animals (n > 200). Obviously it is a tenuous step
to relate drug induced changes in capillary perfusion patterns in
anesthetized dogs to the perfusion patterns present during exercise
in awake normal animals. We have made a correlation between Ppa

waveforms and pressures that may be of use in relating our findings
to exercise. In Figure 26.4, recordings of Ppa from an implanted
high-fidelity Konigsberg transducer are shown. We note that the Ppa
associated with lateral recruitment is characterized by: 1) high
diastolic pressure, 2) high mean pressure, and 3) a moderate
systolic pressure. In contrast, the Ppa associated with longitudinal recruitment is characterized by: 1) low diastolic pressure,
2) low mean pressure, and 3) high systolic pressure. We were
surprised to be unable to find in the literature Ppa waveforms in
awake exercising animals to compare to our pressure records. We,
therefore, measured Ppa with a high-fidelity manometer tipped catheter (Millar) in an unanesthetized, awake dog during rest and
exercise. The Ppa waveform during exercise (Figure 26.5) compared
to resting values is characterized by: 1) low diastolic pressure,
2) low mean pressure, and 3) high systolic pressure, a pressure
waveform very similar to the waveform we associate with longitudinal recruitment. The association between a specific Ppa waveform
and longitudinal recruitment in the anesthetized dog and the presence of the same specific Ppa waveform in the awake, exercising dog
suggests that longitudinal recruitment may be occurring during
awake exercise.

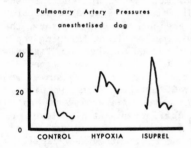

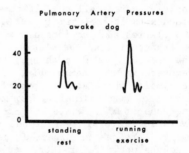

Figure 26.4. High fidelity recordings of Ppa in an anesthetized dog during hypoxia (associated with lateral recruitment) and during isoproterenol
infusion (associated with longitudinal recruitment).

Figure 26.5. High fidelity recordings of Ppa in an awake dog
running on a treadmill. Exercise waveform resembles isoproterenol waveform (associated
with longitudinal recruitment).

It is interesting to note that if the curve in Figure 26.3
comparing cardiac output to CPI is extrapolated linearly, it inter-
sects the crossing point of the dashed lines; the CPI of 450
(indicated by "H" in the figure) is the mean CPI response to a PaO_2
of 40 torr, a condition that produces near maximal recruitment in
Zone II. Projecting the same intersecting point to the absiccsa, a
cardiac output of about 15 liters/min is found, a value in the range
of the maximal cardiac output that an awake dog generates during
maximal treadmill exercise. This implies that maximal exercise may

be associated with near total lateral recruitment of the capillary
bed in all lung zones.

A number of unanswered questions remain about exercise and the
capillaries, especially how D_L changes during exercise. For example, Kotter et al., (6) measuring $D_{L,CO}$ in anesthetized dogs found
the dinitrophenol increased $\dot{V}O_2$ sevenfold and cardiac output by a
factor of 2.5, yet, $D_{L,CO}$ increased only 15%. In contrast Piper et
al. (7) found that DNP under similar conditions markedly increased
$D_{L,O2}$. From this and other work (8) it is not clear whether
exercise increases the area of the capillary bed (true $D_{L,O2}$) or
reduces nonuniformities in D_L/Q or $\dot{V}_A/Q$. The discrepancy between
$D_{L,CO}$ and $D_{L,O2}$ was shown again by Cross et al. (9) uring moderate
exercise (100 watts) in normal men where cardiac output increased
87%. In this study, $D_{L,CO}$ was unchanged with exercise (45 to 49 ml
min^{-1} $torr^{-1}$) while in contrast $D_{L,O2}$ increased 72%. In their
recent review, Forster and Crandall (10) conclude, "It is not clear
why $D_{L,CO}$ increases so little with exercise."

We can propose a solution to the issue of why $D_{L,O2}$ increases
rapidly with low to moderate exercise while $D_{L,CO}$ shows relatively
little change. Our data suggest that low to moderate rises in flow
utilize capillary reserve primarily in the form of decreased red
cell transit time (longitudinal recruitment). O_2 uptake increases
rapidly as red cell transit time is diminished, because desaturated
blood with its relatively low O_2 back pressure is washed through the
capillaries and provides a relatively large gradient favoring rapid
O_2 transport into the plasma. In contrast CO uptake is relatively
unaffected by such a change, because CO in the plasma is rapidly
removed by the hemoglobin, thus preventing back pressure from
developing which would oppose further CO uptake. Thus, we predict
that the longitudinal recruitment of moderate exercise favors an
increase in $D_{L,O2}$ while leaving $D_{L,CO}$ unaffected. At high levels of
exercise, lateral recruitment comes into play (see Figure 26.3);
$D_{L,CO}$ increases as expected, because recruitment of new capillary
segments would favor increased CO uptake.

Summary

Using challenges that either elevate cardiac output or pulmonary artery pressure, we have observed by direct in vivo microscopy
two distinct responses in the pulmonary capillary bed. Moderate
increases in cardiac output are primarily associated with increases
in red blood cell velocity (longitudinal recruitment). Increased
pulmonary artery pressures are primarily associated with recruitment of previous unperfused capillaries (lateral recruitment). We
have been unable to find any evidence of active regulation of blood
flow in the pulmonary microcirculation. Rather, we see evidence of
a simple, passive system that responds appropriately to the hemodynamic and O_2 uptake demands of exercise. By a combination of
longitudinal and lateral recruitment, capillary pressure is kept low
to prevent pulmonary edema while a large, vigorously perfused
surface area is provided for complete red cell oxygenation even
during maximal exercise.

REFERENCES

1. Wagner, W.W.: J. Appl. Puysiol. 26:375-377, 1969.
2. Wagner, W.W., and L.P. Latham: J. Appl. Physiol. 39:900-905, 1975.
3. West, J.B.: Ventilation/Blood Flow and Gas Exchange. Blackwell, Oxford, 1965.
4. Roughton, F.J.W.: Am. J. Physiol. 143:621, 1945.
5. Lee, G. de J., and A.B. DuBois: J. Clin. Invest. 34:138, 1955.
6. Kotter, D., A. Huch, H. Stotz, and J. Piiper: Single breath CO diffusing capacity in anesthetized dogs with increased oxygen consumption. Resp. Physiol. 6:202-208, 1969.
7. Piiper, J., A. Huch, D. Kotter, and R. Herbst: Pulmonary diffusing capacity at basal and increased O_2 uptake levels in anesthetized dogs. Resp. Physiol. 6:219-232, 1969.
8. Piiper, J.: Apparent increase of O_2 diffusing capacity with increased O_2 uptake in homogeneous lungs: theory. Resp. Physiol. 6:209-218, 1969.
9. Cross, C.E., H. Gong, C.J. Kurper-Shoek, J.R. Gillespie, and R.W. Hyde: Alterations of blood flow to the lungs diffusion surface during exercise. J. Clin. Invest. 52:414-421, 1973.
10. Foster, R.E., and E.D. Crandall: Pulmonary gas exchange. In Annual Review of Physiology, Vol. 38. E. Knobil, R.R. Sonnenschein, and I.S. Edelman, eds. Palo Alto, Annual Reviews, Inc., 1976.

DISCUSSION

P. Wagner: What is the local PO_2 in units you are looking at through your window preparation?

W. Wagner: We do not know the local PO_2 in the alveoli under the window. Certainly more O_2 would be extracted from the alveoli when there is massive recruitment.

Cropp: What was the temperature in the area of photography? Could the temperature of the light source have had an effect on the gas tension?

W. Wagner: We use optical filters. Experiments on mesentary using a thermister to measure temperature change showed that with the filtered light source there was less than a 0.1°C rise in temperature in a 100 μ arteriole. Furthermore, the light is only on for a brief period of time. However, the lung lives in a light-tight box and therefore any light at all may affect the preparation.

Bake: I did not see evidence of pulsatile flow in the film. Is this present?

W. Wagner: Although pulsatility is dampened by the time the blood reaches the pulmonary capillaries, flow is still pulsatile.   These were Nembutal anesthetized dogs with a heart rate of 180 beats/ min., thus pulsatility would be less than an awake animal with a rate of 70.

Fishman: You have not had to invoke neural or humoral factors to explain your findings.   How then do you explain the re-distribution seen in hypoxia.   Do the pulmonary capillaries constrict?

W. Wagner: Surface vessels seen in our preparation are less than 100 µ in diameter and not expected to have much smooth muscle. Probably for this reason we have never seen constriction of arterioles, capillaries or venules.   However, there must be changes in resistance and compliance upstream to cause the re-distribution of blood flow that is seen during hypoxia.

Fishman: Could this be out of your line of vision?

W. Wagner: Yes, I'm sure it is.

Discussion

Wasserman: Do you have any correlations of capillary flow simultaneously with the electrocardiogram in order to identify whether lateral recruitment accounts for more flow during systole?

W. Wagner: We don't see much in the way of vessels opening and closing between heart beats. It's primarily a change in velocity in already open segments. Apparently, once red cell flow gets established through certain pathway in a network, it is fairly stable. I don't believe there is much lateral recruitment with systole.

Wasserman: The transit times might be very discriminating because with lateral recruitment, the transit time would be expected to remain relatively constant whereas with longitudinal recruitment the transit times would change depending on the flow change. Effros, in our lab, compared transit times with increasing or decreasing flow in the isolated lung. The transit times remained constant. Thus, to accomodate changes in flow, it appears as though this is accomplished by a lateral recruitment, de-recruitment type of phenomenon.

W. Wagner: Effros made huge changes in flow and I would expect that the bed would either expand or contract markedly (via lateral recruitment) with his level of flow change.

Wasserman: As measured with the nitrous oxide uptake method, the normal situation in man is for pulmonary capillary blood flow to be virtually zero at the end of diastole, and then shoot-up to about 15 ℓ/min during peak flow in systole. With isoproterenol and exercise the increase is still greater (Wasserman, K., J. Britten and V. VanKennel: J. Appl. Physiol., 21:890-900, 1966).

W. Wagner: My guess would be that if you had massive changes in flow then you would see changes in the number of open vessels. Otherwise, with a relatively small flow change, such as on a beat to beat basis when stroke volume is low, the stable patterns would maintain a few channels open and alter rbc velocity which account for the humps and bumps you see when you measure it with a plethysmograph.

Cropp: One thing that surely controls or affects lateral vs. longitudinal recruitment, are the white cells in the pulmonary circulation where many of these cells are located at least at rest. Do you have any information whether longitudinal recruitment, as you see it with Isoproterenol for instance, is not associated with dislodging the marginated white cells while lateral recruitment is associated with the mobilization of these white cells; i.e., are the plugs taken out of these collateral channels.

377

W. Wagner: I don't have a specific answer. I can tell you that
if we inject epinephrine, which is a lateral recruiter, we can
see lodged white cells in the capillaries get bumped out. I would
expect that something like Isuprel which seems content to push
blood faster through already opened channels most likely would not
go searching around to find capillaries plugged with white cells
and try to open them up. Whereas, with a lateral recruiter, where
the pressure in the capillaries seems to go up, I'd expect the
added pressure would push the white cells out of the capillaries.

Cropp: One way to study this would be to measure the number of
white cells in the active circulation. Epinephrine increases
the white count enormously, and even mild exercise will triple
the white count. I wonder whether that would also be associated
with lateral recruitment?

W. Wagner: I think that's a fantastic idea, it's another way to
look at the same problem.

Kampine: I thought that was a beautiful demonstration and I
wondered if you'd done any systematic comparisons of your
measured perfusion index and changes in pattern of ventilation or
any studies of deliberate attempts to change mechanics.

W. Wagner: We have compared IPPB with spontaneous breathing and
what happens is, with spontaneous inspiration with a slight time
lag of about a third of a second, there is a surge of flow through
the capillaries following the peak of inspiration. When we put
the animal on a pump, there is a 180° change in the phasic
relationship between ventilation and perfusion, so that the flow
slows down with inspiration and then surges during expiration.

Kampine: Any change in the pattern of flow? Can you give us some
numbers on the perfused area with changes in ventilation?

W. Wagner: It is very difficult to quantitate perfusion since
the major change is in the rbc velocity, a parameter we can't
measure at this point. If we raise alveolar pressure the first
vessels that are affected are the ones that run out across the
open walls of the alveoli and corner vessels are protected.
There is still flow right around the edges of the alveoli. As
alveoli pressure is raised to higher and higher values, the
coroner vessels get turned off and then the arterioles and
venules get turned off. The vessels that cross an alveolar wall
seem to turn off at about the same alveolar pressure. The corner
vessels take more pressure to be turned off.

P. Wagner: It is possible that with longitudinal recruitment, say
when you give Isoproterenol, that although the red cells go
through faster, it is conceivable that they may go over a longer
path length at the same time, i.e., that they may see more alveoli?

W. Wagner: That's an intriguing question. I think that once there
is a flow channel established it runs over a constant distance
from an artery to a vein. Because isoproterenol causes mostly
increased velocity rather than lateral recruitment, the rbc
seems to go faster through an established path length.

Fishman: According to the pictures of Wearn who also examined
the circulation at the surface of the lung, as well as your
striking pictures, under some conditions the paths traversed by
blood cells may be shorter than others. This prospect raises the
question, "how many alveoli does a red cell see at rest as compared
to exercise"? As you recruit more channels laterally, does the
red cell go a longer distance? Would the longer path promote
equilibration in gas tensions between alveoli and blood? How
many alveoli does a pulmonary capillary see during exercise?
Wouldn't it be a terrible design if the red cell were fully
loaded with oxygen in one capillary and then had to waste its
time traversing another capillary? and another one? What if
it traversed a well-oxygenated alveolus first and then had to
traverse a hypoxic alveolus before reaching pulmonary veins?

P. Wagner: I would like to ask a question which relates to Dr.
Kampine's questions pertaining to positive airway pressure
(or alveolar pressure). In one preparation where we look at
steady-state gas exchange, in an intact normal lung in a paralyzed
ventilated normal dog, we apply a high positive airway pressure and
see that there are gas exchange units that develop very high
ventilation perfusion ratios. And yet, some areas in these dogs
also have normal VA:Q ratios. Thus, the units seem to separate
into two groups. Is there any reason why some units of lung
might have their blood flow essentially abolished while others
not, in at what at first sight is an isotropic lung?

W. Wagner: I don't know that capillaries in Zone II might be more
easily closed than in Zone III where capillary pressure is higher.
Another possibility might be the corner vessels could still exchange gas and be relatively immune to alveolar pressure. To
Dr. Fishman's interesting point of a set distance between arterioles
and venules, and that there is more than one alveolus between them
has been studied by Staub. He estimates an 800 micron distance
between arterioles and venules which he says is reasonably constant,
and therefore, depending upon the species and the alveolar size,
there would be anywhere from 4 to 10 alveoli that the rbc has
to cross. The statement was made on the first day of this conference that the lung is probably designed to handle exercise so that
when you have to run you don't go into pulmonary edema and you
stay pink. My notion would be that it's not a waste of time for
the red cell at rest to pick up its load of O_2 in one or two alveoli
and then spend time going across other alveoli because the extra
length provides the sort of elaborate reserve that the lung seems
to have. It is this reserve length that is recruited for

oxygenation during the increased rbc velocity of exercise.

P. Wagner: You did not see distension of the capillaries only
longitudinal and lateral recruitment. Could you comment on this?

W. Wagner: When there is lateral recruitment, there is obviously
enough distension of the capillary lumen to let a red cell through
but we have not observed enough distension to let two or three
red cells through.

P. Wagner: I really didn't mean distension in the sense of new
capillaries being distended and now having flow where they didn't.
Were previously open capillaries that had flow getting any wider?

W. Wagner: With a screw clamp on the aorta we can raise left
atrial pressure to 50 or 60 torr. Everything opens and what is
open may get big enough to let red cells just overlap but if
there is distension it is not massive. It looks like the sheet
flow system of Fung and Sobin. But in terms of gross distension
I just do not see it. However, this is a difficult question for
me to comment on because, if the vessel distends, it is most
likely distending down into the alveolus, which is the dimension
I cannot see very well. I do not think it distends much at all
in the plane of the alveolar wall, nor do, curiously, the arterioles
and venules. They seem to be like Permutt's idea of cellaphane
tubes, in that they are easy to collapse with alveolar pressure
but they very rapidly reach a plateau on their pressure volume
curve and it does not seem to matter how much pressure is
applied, they just do not seem to get any bigger.

Cropp: Many years ago, Dr. Burton made observations on the size
and distensibility of capillaries in the frog web. He observed
that capillaries were either open or closed, regardless of the
driving pressure that was applied. Even at 300 mmHg the capillary
would not distent (Burton, A.C., Personal Communication). I think
such observations along with your statement, because I believe
these small vessels are so non-compliant that they are either
collapsed and flat or they are open maximally.

W. Wagner: By open did he mean red cells going through them?

Cropp: Yes, but red cells are said to deform. I think pulmonary
capillaries are on the average slightly larger in diameter than
systemic capillaries, and thus the transit time of a red cell
through a systemic capillary may be longer. The only point that
I am trying to make is that there is evidence that systemic
capillaries do not distend with pressures of up to 100 or even
300 mmHg.

W. Wagner: If we inject fluorescent dye we see the dye going
through capillaries that red cells are not going through.

Apparently there is some plasma perfusion but we wouldn't consider
these vessels as being perfused capillaries because of the lack
of rbc. This may fit the lubrication theory where, if there is
not a layer of plasma, the red cells seize up in the vessel and
create an enormous resistance to flow. So, perhaps, there is some
dilation which is just enough to let the plasma get around
the red cell and lubricate it so it can flow again. But the
difference between open and closed may be very small indeed and
the lack of cell overlapping indicates little distension even at
high pressures.

Farber: Can you give any structural or any anatomical evidence
that might account for VA:Q's as high as 7 to 10 during exercise;
when at rest the VA/Q did not exceed 2?

Gledhill: There are differences in alveolar size at rest wherein
some alveoli are more fully distended than others. Dr. Bake
hypothesized from his data yesterday that those alveoli which
have greater distention at rest would have a lower resistance in
the accompanying airways which during exercise, due to the
increased inspiratory flow would receive preferential ventilation.
Presumably this is one reason for the increased inhomogeneity
between the lower VA:Q ratios and the higher VA:Q ratios. All of
the gas exchange compartments seem to shift to higher VQ ratios
but there may be a preferential re-distribution of ventilation
to the distended units, thus, creating some very high VA:Q ratios.

Cerny: Dr. Fishman's studies of a number of years ago apparently
showed both neural and humoral components to pulmonary vascular
control (Szidon, S.P. and A.P. Fishman, in The Pulmonary Circulation and Interstitial Space. A.P. Fishman and H.H. Hect, ed.,
Chicago Press, 1969, p. 239). What is the relationship of the
increased blood flow that you showed, to the exercise state
where you might have a neural and humoral component to the
regulatory mechanisms? Perhaps one way of looking at this would
be passively engorge the pulmonary bed and then simulate exercise
to see if you do get changes even with this passive engorgement.

W. Wagner: My use of Isoproteronol with beta 1 and beta 2
activities to simulate exercise makes me nervous. Dr. Fishman
indicates that the vessels get stiffer with increased sympathetic
activity, which obviously occurs with exercise. These conditions
must be different from a beta agonist relaxing the vessels. I
think it's an excellent point you raise and one we need to look
into rather soon.

Bake: One may divide the pulmonary vessels into alveolar and
extra-alveolar. Have you observed these two types of vessels
through your window? They ought to react differently, for example,
with respect to lung inflation or to closure of these vessels
at low lung volumes.

W. Wagner: In the movies I showed the alveoli appear to have
fairly thick walls, which is really an optical illusion. The
extra-alveolar vessels that run along in the space around the
alveoli are obviously less affected by over inflation of the lung
with positive pressure. The vessels crossing alveolar walls
turn off instantly with only 5-10 cm of water pressure, whereas
the extra-alveolar vessels require 20-50 cm of water pressure
to disturb their flow very much.

Tipton: This symposium is entitled, "Exercise and the Lung",
and yet it has been implied that all exercises are the same; however, there are vast differences between the physiological responses
from light to medium to exhaustive exercise. Dr. Gledhill,
your subjects were exercising at a $\dot{V}O_2$ of 2 litres, which was
approximately 50-60% of their Max $\dot{V}O_2$, and you concluded that
inhomogeneity and de-saturation were the potential mechanisms.
Is that conclusion valid at 90 or 95% Max? Dr. W. Wagner, you
alluded to a cardiac output of 15 litres in the dog in which the
heart rate must have bee in excess of 260 beats/m with an oxygen
consumption of approximately 100 ml per kg. Did you observe a
linear horizontal recruitment pattern in the transition from
light exercise to a cardiac output of 15 litres/min.?

W. Wagner: We couldn't reach 15 litres/min that is a number
from the literature. The best we could do with Isoproterenol
was about 9 litres/min.

Tipton: What about with exercise per se?

W. Wagner: We can't exercise the dogs.

Tipton: So this is an extrapolation.

W. Wagner: Yes.

Tipton: P. Wagner, you alluded to an oxygen consumption of 1 ℓ/min.
in your patients. What level of exercise was that in respect to
the total capacity of the patient? Did the patient reach a heart
rate of 150 to 180 beats/min? If we can quantify the workload we
can better relate your remarks to the kinds of changes we see
in 'hormal subjects" with exercise. The exercise level has to be
quantified in more rigorous terms than has been used throughout
this symposium.

P. Wagner: The exercise in the patients was as much as they
could tolerate. The heart rate attained was variable but well
over 100 and often around 140. The patients were continuously
monitored, especially since they had the Swanganz catheter in
place. K. Wasserman also studied some of the patients with
interstitial lung disease and perhaps could comment.

Wasserman: Four of these subjects that we studied had their oxygen uptake quantitated and exercised to their maximum tolerable work rate. Quantitation in terms of heart rate may be misleading in patients with respiratory disease as their heart rate at their maximum tolerable work rate may be only 100 bpm or less.

Gledhill: The workloads represented a range of approximately 50% of the $\dot{V}O_2$ Max in a trained subject to approximately 65% in an untrained subject. The anatomical shunt component and increased inhomogeneity component of the A-a DO_2 increased progressively from rest to the highest work load. Extrapolating to work loads of up to 90% of Max $\dot{V}O_2$, I would estimate that approximately 50% of the increase in A-a DO_2 at this level would be attributable to the shunt component and 50% to the distribution component.

Dempsey: I think that the principles that are stated, at least in the healthy individuals,--Norman with his functional data and Wiltz with his anatomical data--apply to very heavy exercise. For example, the A-a DO_2 continues to widen up to very heavy work with arterial PO_2 still staying constant. We see the same thing, i.e., PaO_2 staying at resting values, if we exercise people to exhaustion even at 11,000 ft. elevation. I believe that the two mechanisms that Norman's talking about, the small anatomical shunt and the increase in the dispersion of the distribution are still contributing to the further widening of A-a DO_2. He showed this up to 1 litre of VO_2, up to 2 and I think there's good reason to believe it continues on up. Wiltz talked about protection of capillary pressure under high flow conditions. Until recently it was thought, from indirect indicator dilution techniques, that extra-vascular lung water increased during exercise. Recent direct studies of wet/dry lung weight ratios in the dog has shown at maximum exercise in the dog lung that there is no evidence at all that there is an accumulation of extra-vascular lung water. I think that this is also an indication that capillary pressures and left-sided pressures are staying pretty normal. Otherwise, you're going to get leakage. So, I think that even under the high loads of exercise these concepts apply.

Fishman: There is an undercurrent of confusion in the literature concerning water accumulation in the lung. Some investigators have identified pulmonary edema experimentally by demonstrating an excessively-rapid turnover of water. This need not be pulmonary edema. During exercise many influences promote the egress of water from the capillaries into the interstitial space. But other influences enhance lymphatic drainage. Therefore, the turnover rate may be quite large, but the total amount of water that accumulates in the lungs need not enlarge to abnormal levels, i.e., there is no pulmonary edema. As a corollary, the fact that the water space of the lung during

exercise may remain unchanged does not prove that capillary pressures
have remained unchanged. Capillary pressures can change considerably as long as lymphatic drainage is adequate to leave the water
content of the lung unchanged. It is commonly held that the
increased breathing movements during exercise promote lymphatic
flow.

Dempsey: We do have evidence that there is no accumulation of lung
water. Certainly there can be increased water turnover. Dr. Fishman what evidence do we have that there is increased lymphatic
drainage from increased water turnover in the lung or that capillary
pressures increase significantly during exercise? I'm impressed
by the fact that Wiltz has shown that at least the mechanisms
are there with recruitment for good protection of capillary
pressure during high flow conditions.

Fishman: I think that you have focused on an important question.
The evidence that I can give you is largely indirect and somewhat
incomplete. Drinker's experiments many years ago showed that
hyperventilation promoted lymphatic drainage. These experiments
have been utilized because of the abnormal conditions that had to
be created for successful cannulation of pulmonary lymphatic and
the difficulty in being sure that lymph is actually draining only
the lungs. More recent radiologic observations have, however,
supported Drinker's conclusion. Intuitively, I am drawn to this
notion, particularly because of its possible relation to Paintal's
concept of J-receptor. His idea is that interstitial edema
stretches juxta-capillary receptors in the interstitial space.
These J-receptors stimulate ventilation by way of the vagi.
If the increase in ventilation stimulates lympathic flow from the
lungs, it becomes possible to imagine an unchanged interstitial
water volume at the same time that interstitial water inflow and
outflow have increased.

Dempsey: Your points are excellent. I suppose the only resolution
is to actually measure lung water turnover in heavy exercise.

Gee: Are there data, using your inert gas methods, to remove the
$V_A:Q_c$ component and the shunt component and therefore see whether
diffusion is limiting O_2 transport during moderately severe exercise in hypoxia.

Gledhill: We measured $V_A:Q$ distribution in hypoxia at rest and I
don't believe that there was any significant diffusion limitation
down to as low as a 12% F_IO_2. There is a possibility that there
is incomplete alveolar-capillary equilibration in the very low
$V_A:Q$ units. That is, the compartments that had a $V_A:Q$ ratio of
around .5 for example, when the F_IO_2 is around 12%. I have to
speculate as far as exercise is concerned, but I think that very
probably during exercise in hypoxic conditions and especially
in the low $V_A:Q_c$ compartments, alveolar-capillary diffusion would
be incomplete.

Dempsey: I'd like to comment quickly on Dr. Gee's question. Bert
Forster, Bill Reddan and I have studied the A-a DO_2 and diffusion
at high altitudes (Resp. Physiol., 3:62-89, 1971). It seems to me
that the hyperventilation, especially in the chronically hypoxic
normal person after 3 weeks or more at high altitude, is so severe
(where arterial P_{CO_2} is in the low 20's during maximum exercise)
and the alveolar PO_2 is so high that there is a substantial
diffusion gradient and PaO_2 remains at resting levels. However,
once one gets up past 4000 m altitude and exercises, you can no
longer keep arterial PO_2 constant. John West showed this many
years ago as well. The PaO_2 falls and the A-a DO_2 is widening
because of a rise in alveolar and a drop in arterial PO_2. That
perhaps might be evidence of a diffusion limitation but you have
to perform very hard exercise and have pretty severe hypoxia,
in my opinion, for that to occur.

Rankin: I'd like to ask P. Wagner what we mean by diffusion
limitation. I teach my students that diffusion may be affected
by thickening the membrane, increasing the length of the diffusion
pathway or with a loss of surface area in the membrane. And yet
as I look at the scheme that you present, only one type of
diffusion defect would appear. I look at your patients with
emphysema and see no diffusion defect and yet I know instinctively
that there must be a tremendous loss of surface area for diffusion.
Therefore, it is difficult to say that diffusion in general is not
reduced if one is only measuring diffusion in terms of an end-
capillary gradient.

P. Wagner: I agree with your concepts. For example, in the COPD
where we appear to have areas of very high $VA:Q$, the most likely
mechanism is due to a loss of surface area in that there is
destruction of capillaries and of the alveolar walls, but with
some ventilation remaining. What gas does get in there probably
exchanges fairly well with what little blood flow is in there and,
therefore, doesn't give rise to an alveolar end-capillary difference.
No doubt, the mass of gas that is getting across is much less than
would be if the capillary bed were normal. But as you point out,
our particular viewpoint is in terms of the net effect on the
arterial PO_2.

Dempsey: How confident do you feel in using what you call your
indirect technique of just sampling arterial blood (and mixed
expired gas) and then by Fick, calculating the mixed venous values
rather than the direct method of sampling the mixed venous blood?
Can you think of specific examples of where you would suspect the
data when you just had to use the indirect vs. the direct technique?

P. Wagner: I would feel confident about the indirect approach under
all the conditions that both we and Dr. Gledhill have studied. We
have obtained mixed venous blood because this is the first time
that this approach has been used in patients and in experimental
animals. Scientifically, we must justify the fact that the subject

is in a steady-state, for example, and be able to account for all
the numbers in the Fick equation. It is not a question of not
trusting indirect methods, but rather to obtain extra evidence.
The calculation of the mixed venous blood values from the indirect
procedure are a reasonably accurate procedure given cardiac
output, ventilation, arterial and expired values and the
solubilities, because inert gases have a linear dissociation
curve and a single solubility co-efficient. But the same
cannot really be said for oxygen, certainly with the same level of
accuracy, because of the alinear dissociation curve, the problems
with small a-v differences when you are at rest, etc. We would
have to have direct measurements of venous PO_2 and PCO_2, particularly if we are trying to explain a 4-5 mm difference in PaO_2,
with assurance, in the exercising interstitial disease patients.

Summary & Conclusions

Alfred P. Fishman

As the conference draws to a close, I stand before you to summarize the proceedings. At this point, I am tempted to endorse
John Rankin's augury and to acknowledge that "I came as a stranger
and you took me in." However, I am disinclined to dwell on the
burdens of my assignment since I must confess that I enjoyed it.
These were certainly three lively days that slipped by impercepti-
bly in a general stream of excitement. There were no distractions
and no inconveniences. For the smooth sailing of the meeting we
are all grateful to Drs. Dempsey and Reed and their associates.

The focus of the conference was on the regulation of breathing
during exercise and exercise asthma. At least four minor themes
permeated the conference.

The first was historical and began with the chairman who recalled that the physiological giants of yesteryear were concerned
with many of the same topics. Krogh and Lindhard were just as
concerned as the present generation of respiratory physiologists
with the adjustments of the respiration and circulation at the
start of exercise. Barcroft regarded exercise as the only test of
the design of the human body. He wondered if there are overlapping
nervous and chemical controls of the regulation of ventilation and
about the extent to which they might substitute for each other. A
succession of respiratory physiologists sought to unravel the various physiological mechanisms other than the increase in minute ventilation during exercise and how they interrelate so as to shape
the integrate response.

The second theme dealt with the question of modeling the respiratory system. Grodins reviewed the concepts underlying models
which were designed to deal with optimization of the work of
breathing. He depicted how simple models might account for the
ventilatory pattern at rest and during exercise but illustrated how
heavily they relied on simplifying assumptions. As an example,
most mathematical models do not even separate the lungs from the
chest. Moreover, the "chest" lumps the ribs and abdomen, disregarding
the separate properties of each. Nonetheless, these models are
clearly valuable as a point of departure for experimentation.
The tragedy is that all too often they are regarded as an end in
themselves rather than as a basis for fresh exploration. One use-

ful product of his own model was the distinction between unchanged
arterial P_{CO_2} during exercise in contrast to the increase in arterial P_{CO_2} during exercise. Why this difference? The answer is not
yet available but is fundamental to the understanding of the regulation of ventilation during exercise.

The third motif stemmed from Kao's extended experience with the
peripheral neurogenic drive. From his elaborate preparations, he
became convinced that the peripheral neurogenic drive alone could
account for the hyperpnea of exercise. However, his broad experience also led him to recognize that in different preparations and
under different experimental conditions, multiple factors would be
required to explain the ventilatory response to exercise.

The final theme was contributed by Yamamoto. He described his
studies on the control of breathing as a search for the message and
the medium. During exercise, he pictured the arterial P_{CO_2} as the
message; but what is the medium? How do the swings in alveolar P_{CO_2}
and arterial P_{CO_2} during exercise relate to the regulatory process?
Now, fifteen years after he began to examine the problem, this question of the major stimulus to breathing during exercise, and how it
is communicated to the control centers, remains unsettled. In dealing with the integrated response of the ventilation, Yamamoto reminded the audience of Sherrington's "Occlusion Phenomenon" to
account, in part, for different ventilatory responses under different circumstances. By analogy with spinal reflexes, he reiterated
the point that co-existing, maximal or near maximal stimuli may exert less of an effect than would be expected than if the two were
measured separately and summated. The notion that the ventilatory
response is preconditioned by the state of the organism served as
an admonition that what is demonstrable in one experiment may not
be evident, albeit present, in another. His reflections finally
led him to enunciate Yamamoto's thirteenth law, "In any complex system where the repertoire of responses is less than the variety of
inputs, occlusion must occur." When the occlusion phenomenon is
weighed with respect to other influences that may modify experimental results arising from surgery, blood loss, prolonged manipulation,
"open-loops", and a host of interventions, it is clear that many of
the experimental results can only reflect a potential for response
rather than a measure of a spontaneous, balanced adjustment that
would be apt to occur under more natural circumstances.

Within these broad perspectives, a succession of papers dealt
with the breathing apparatus, exercise hyperpnea, the caliber of
the airways, exercise asthma and gas exchange during exercise.

The first session was concerned with the respiratory muscles
and the mechanics of breathing. Goldman considered the neuromuscular coordination of breathing of upright man at rest and during
exercise. His approach involved correlations between length-tension
and pressure-flow curves of the respiratory muscles and the EMG.
He described the remarkable interplay among these muscles.

At rest the diaphragm does all of the active work of breathing. During moderate exercise, the rib cage and abdominal muscles are recruited so that the diaphragm can devote more and more of its attention to the lung. He showed clearly how the pattern of coordination
during exercise differs from that during voluntary hyperpnea. These
are exciting observations. Although they represent only the first
phases of analysis of an elaborate mechanism, they already point new
directions for the understanding of the complicated interplay that
allows the ventilatory pump to function so efficiently.

Grimby carried the analysis further by considering the load on
the respiratory muscles in patients with obstructive disease of the
airways. By applying the approach of Konno and Mead for partitioning
the changes in lung volume and the work done by the respiratory muscles during breathing, he was able to contrast the load handled by
the respiratory muscles in normal subjects with that in the patients.
He demonstrated that in the normal subjects, the ventilation remains
efficient at the highest levels of exercise. In contrast, some patients with obstructive disease demonstrated inefficient ventilation, i.e. the maximum pleural pressure at a given lung volume became abnormally high without effecting an increase in air flow. The
studies by Grimby posed a provocative question with respect to conventional ways for determining the work of breathing done by the
respiratory muscles. His observations suggested that the method of
Campbell may underestimate the work of breathing not only in normal
subjects but particularly in patients with obstructive disease of the
airways where elastic inspiratory work is increased and the elastic
work of deforming the chest apparatus is appreciable. This challenging suggestion relies heavily on the validity of the Konno-Mead
method used to partition lung volume. Although simple in concept,
the accuracy and reproducibility of the method, particularly in patients with lung disease, remains to be shown.

Remmers turned from the mechanics of breathing to the motor
control of breathing. He used supine human subjects which complicated comparisons with those in Goldman's study who were upright.
From a careful analysis, he was able to show how both respiratory
center control and sensory-motor coordination interplay to effect
the regulation of breathing. The degree to which either type of
control predominates depends on the circumstance. During sleep,
the diaphragm is the predominant inspiratory muscle; presumably
the intercostal motor neurons or the gamma loop system is depressed.
While awake, the larynx contributes importantly. During exercise,
the rib cage is engaged. And, in contrast to CO_2 breathing, which
relies heavily on abdominal muscles, exercise relies more heavily
on the ribs.

Remmers' presentation stressed heavily the reflex pathways.
In the context of the length-tension relationship of muscle, he
singled out the muscle spindle as the ideal end organ by which demand could be automatically compared with execution. The identified
output of the muscle spindle is an error signal, indicating the

degree of matching between the actual and the desired position. He
offered these considerations as support for Campbell's concept of
length-tension inappropriateness which considers the perception of
mechanically-loaded or burden breath as the basis for dyspnea. This
remains an attractive hypothesis for some types of dyspnea. But, it
does seem unlikely that it will stand as a convincing explanation
for all. For example, quadriplegic human subjects, although de-
prived of sensory input from the periphery, are still capable of
experiencing the sensation of dyspnea.

The next session dealt with exercise hyperpnea. Levine examined the possible relevance of drug-induced hypermetabolism to
exercise hyperpnea. He showed that drugs which induced hypermetabolism do so along the VO_2-VE relationship that obtains during exercise. In a series of elaborate experiments designed to exclude nervous impulses, he has adduced evidence for a humoral substance.
Moreover, he was able to show that this substance acts by way of
extracranial chemoreceptors "in the thoracic region." His evidence
for the elusive "exercise factor" is rather convincing despite the
intricacies of the experimental arrangements. The idea that the
chemoreceptors for this stimulus are located within the thorax is
also consistent with Wasserman's observations on CO_2 flow and ventilatory control in unanesthetized man and dog. How to reconcile
Levine's conclusions with those of Kao, who also relied heavily on
cross-perfusion experiments, remains to be settled.

Wasserman's studies began some years ago as a result of his
mounting suspicion that the neurohumoral hypothesis, that he had
adopted for so long in explaining the abrupt increase in ventilation
at the start of exercise, was probably in error. Suspicion was
converted to certainty by the demonstration that the increase in
ventilation at the start of exercise is not associated with an increase in respiratory exchange ratio or a decrease in end-tidal P_{CO_2}.
If this is so, alveolar ventilation and pulmonary capillary blood
flow must be matched and a disproportionate neurogenic drive to ventilation does not exist.

In searching for the primary stimulus, he and his associates
examined the CO_2 delivery to the lungs (cardiac output X CO_2 content
in mixed venous blood). They manipulated flow and CO_2 content separately, using a variety of strategies, including drugs and came to
the conclusion that the CO_2 delivery to the lungs somehow elicits
the ventilatory drive. This mechanism suffices to maintain isocapnia in the arterial blood until other stimuli, such as metabolic
acidosis, supervene. At present, they are searching for the chemoreceptor which mediates this response; they believe that it lies
somewhere distal to the pulmonary capillaries.

It is important to view the CO_2 flow to the lungs as part of
an integrated mechanism for the control of breathing. In this sche-
ma, during exercise the conventional peripheral arterial chemorecep-

tors contribute attenuation and modulation to the predominant stimulus, CO_2 delivery to special post-pulmonary capillary receptors.
Thus, conventional chemical stimuli, particularly CO_2, pH, and PO_2,
continue to be pictured as essential elements in the regulation of
breathing during exercise. Primacy of any particular chemical
stimulus depends on the circumstance. But where the nervous stimuli fit into the picture is unclear.

Eldridge provided a fresh approach. He was concerned with
neural drive mechanisms of central origin. He pointed out that in
many situations chemical stimuli do not provide a complete answer
for the control of respiration during exercise. Nor have conventional neural stimuli filled in the gap. He envisages a superimposed mechanism that involves the central brain stem; this mechanism,
when fully engaged, sustains respiration after the primary stimulus has stopped. A good deal of his evidence for the existence of
this central mechanism is based on his experience as well as that
of others, with active and passive hyperventilation.

This central brain stem neural process is attractive as an
additive process. Depending on the circumstance, it can account
for up to 50% of the increase in ventilation that would be expected
from a primary stimulus acting alone. Thus, it is an amplifying
mechanism, an integral part of the respiratory control mechanism.
Eldridge sees a role for this mechanism in the increment in ventilation at the start and stop of exercise. It may also contribute
importantly to the ventilatory response to low PO_2 and high P_{CO_2}.
This attractive hypothesis has to be reconciled with the prevalent
notion of a fast component and a slow component in the ventilatory
response to exercise.

The first three papers of the next session were concerned with
the control of airway caliber. Coon, using an isolated lung preparation to achieve proper experimental control, somewhat in the
fashion of Nisel working in Liljestrand's laboratory many years ago,
found that CO_2 and O_2 tensions are less effective than pH in regulating airway caliber. His experiments underscored the primacy of
the hydrogen ion as the mediator of bronchomotor tone. Adkinson
provided a comprehensive overview of the endogenous chemical mediators that might be involved in the regulation of airway caliber.
He focused on histamine, slow-reacting substance of anaphylaxis
and prostanoic acid derivatives. He dealt with the implications of
the cholinergic innervation of the mast cell and indicated how much
had yet to be learned about these receptors. His presentation
underscored the vast intrapulmonary pharmacopeia that is available
in the lung and illustrated some of their potential relationships
to the control of the airways.

Sampson considered vagal receptors in the intrapulmonary
airways, particularly the rapidly-adapting receptors ("irritant
receptors", or "deflation receptors" or "expiration receptors").

These have always been somewhat of an enigma and a painstaking
attempt to elucidate their function is most welcome. At present,
too little is known about their stimulus-response patterns to define a role for them in the control of ventilation during exercise.

In closing this session, Bake turned from receptors to the
distribution of ventilation during exercise. In particular, he explored the effect of increased tidal volume, the effect of breathing
patterns and the effect of the pattern of inspiratory flow. His experiments, based on lung scanning, led to the conclusion that of the
three mechanisms that he explored, only the change in the breathing
pattern promotes uniformity of ventilation and the matching of alveolar ventilation to blood flow during exercise. His observations
led him to suggest that the asthmatic derangements in alveolar ven-
tilation-blood flow relationships probably represent inhomogeneities
within the different regions of the lung rather than variations from
region to region.

The session on exercise-induced bronchospasm (post-exercise
asthma) began with McFadden's presentation which identified exercise as one of many non-antigenic stimuli to bronchospasm. He advanced the concept of "bronchial lability" which is converted in
childhood to bronchoconstriction, possibly by infection. He called
attention to the poor correlation between exercise-induced asthma
and "clinical asthma" and deplored the use of non-standardized exercise which complicates comparisons among different studies.
Cropp, as part of an exhaustive analysis of the cardiopulmonary responses to exercise in severely asthmatic children, confirmed the
lack of correlation between exercise-induced asthma and pre-exercise
pulmonary performance. McFadden then returned to present preliminary observations on the role of lactic acid in mediating exercise-
induced asthma. Although he was inclined to favor the hydrogen ion
as the common denominator, a conclusion consistent with Coon's observations on the isolated lung, he left unsettled the role of the
lactate ion. Godfrey underscored the different asthmagenic potential
of different types of exercise and raised the provocative question
of why asthmatics tolerated swimming better than arm or leg exercise.
Bierman examined the effects of various agents in preventing exercise-induced asthma and outlined a systematic approach to therapy.
These last two papers were too detailed to be encompassed in this
brief summary. However, they did help to define some current un-
certainties in the understanding of exercise-induced asthma and
in suggesting possible approaches. For example, they made clear
that exercise testing should be standardized, even to the extent
of common equipment, such as the ergometer. Not only the equipment,
but also the work rate and oxygen consumption should be determined
in a standard way for the sake of comparison. Their presentations
prompted other questions: which pulmonary function tests might be
adopted for comparison among different laboratories? Is it possible
to categorize individuals on the basis of standardized equipment,
calibrated work rate and oxygen uptake, and standard pulmonary

function tests done in comparable ways?

The final session was a reminder of the important role of the
circulation in the adaptation to exercise. The opening remarks by
Peter Wagner described the problems in matching alveolar ventilation
and pulmonary circulation with respect to gas exchange in the lungs.
He emphasized the widening alveolar-arterial difference in oxygen
tension at certain levels of exercise despite an improved topographic
distribution of blood flow. He wondered about the question of capillary recruitment versus distention during exercise. In effect,
he underscored that many aspects of gas exchange during exercise
are uncertain.

Gledhill analyzed the alveolar ventilation-perfusion distribution during upright exercise in normal subjects using the approach
of Wagner and West. This approach focuses on the determinants of
blood gas tensions in arterial blood on the basis of the distribution of six inert gases. He found wide inhomogeneity of alveolar
ventilation-perfusion relationships. But the type of inhomogeneity
that was postulated was a bit unconventional. In order to reconcile these observations using inert gases with others that involved
the use of radioactive tracers and scanning, he had to postulate an
exaggeration in intra-regional inhomogeneity during exercise.

The theme was carried further by Peter Wagner who used the
same technique to examine distribution of exercise in patients with
diffuse pulmonary disease. The results were provocative. In the
patients with obstructive disease of the airways, ventilation was
much more deranged than blood flow. Most impressive was the failure
to provide evidence of difficulty in diffusion so that abnormalities
in arterial blood could be attributed, almost entirely, to disturbances in alveolar ventilation-perfusion supplemented by some shunting. The lack of diffusion limitation in obstructive disease of the
airways is difficult, but not impossible, to conceive. Much stranger
was the postulate of no diffusion impairment in patients with diffuse
interstitial disease. Clearly, the analysis of alveolar ventilation-
perfusion relationships by the Wagner-West approach are not easy to
relate to the traditional concepts involved in the Riley-Lilienthal
approach which includes diffusion limitation as a fundamental assumption. Also, to discount diffusion limitation as an important mechanism of arterial hypoxemia in patients with diffuse granulomatous or
fibrotic disease flies in the face of all anatomical experience.
Wagner and West have begun to rationalize their observations with
respect to the more conventional concepts of ventilation-perfusion
and diffusion abnormalities in normal subjects and in patients with
lung disease. During the next few years, the Wagner-West approach
will undoubtedly be subjected to critical appraisal from several
different points of view. Theoretical as well as practical limitations and implications will be examined. But, the novelty of the
approach has rekindled interest in alveolar-capillary gas exchange
and the reconciliation of old and new concepts will undoubtedly be

rewarding.

The other Wagner, W. Wagner, dealt with the regulation of pulmonary capillary blood flow using direct visualization techniques to distinguish between "lateral recruitment" and "longitudinal recruitment" (increase in velocity of blood flow). Of necessity, his observations were confined to the surface of the lung. They were quite dramatic. Unfortunately, small muscular arteries are out of sight in this preparation. Nonetheless, it was interesting to compare the automatic adjustments of the pulmonary capillary circulation to different stimuli. Gurtner completed the session by wondering if there is carrier-mediated transport of oxygen in the lung. Drawing upon previous experiments on the placenta, and relying heavily on the use of carbon monoxide as the test gas, he examined the liklihood that cytochrome P-450 may serve as a carrier for oxygen and carbon monoxide in the lung. In extreme physiologic conditions, he could not discount the possibility of facilitated diffusion. However, the extent to which this mechanism operates under more physiologic conditions was left unsettled.

If I have succeeded in transmitting the sense of excitement, query, scholarship and ingenuity that permeated the meeting, I will have satisfied my obligation as summarizer. Lively exchange and animated spirits characterized the proceedings. Dr. Kao may have captured its vital essence in a few lines of poetry that he credited to an anonymous Persian poet:

He who knows not and knows not that he knows not:

a fool, shun him

He who knows not and knows that he knows not:

a student, teach him

He who knows and knows not that he knows:

a poet, watch him

He who knows and knows that he knows:

a master, follow him.

This was a meeting of students, poets and masters.

Contributors & Participants
Index

Contributors & Participants

N. Franklin Adkinson, Jr.   Good Samaritan Hospital, Baltimore, MD
Bjorn Bake   University of Goteborg, Goteborg, Sweden
D. Bartlett, Jr.   Dartmouth Medical School, Hanover, NH
William L. Beaver   Stanford University, Stanford, CA
C. Warren Bierman   University of Washington, Seattle, WA
Harvey V. Brown   Sepulveda VA Hospital, UCLA School of Medicine
   Sepulveda, CA
Barry Burns   Johns Hopkins University, Baltimore, MD
Richard Casaburi   Harbor General Hospital, Torrance, CA
Robert L. Coon   Allen Bradley Medical Sciences Laboratories,
   Milwaukee, WI
Gerd J. A. Cropp   The Children's Hospital of Buffalo, Buffalo, NY
Frederic L. Eldridge   University of North Carolina School of
   Medicine, Chapel Hill, NC
Alfred P. Fishman   University of Pennsylvania School of Medicine,
   Philadelphia, PA
Allison B. Foese   Hospital for Sick Children, Toronto, Ontario,
   Canada
Norman Gledhill   York University and Hospital for Sick Children,
   Toronto, Ontario, Canada
Simon Godfrey   University of London and Hammersmith Hospital,
   London, England
Michael Goldman   Harvard University School of Public Health,
   Boston, MA
Gunnar Grimby   University of Goteborg, Goteborg, Sweden
Fred S. Grodins   University of Southern California, Los Angeles, CA
Gail H. Gurtner   Johns Hopkins University, Baltimore, MD
Hans L. Hahn   University of Poliklinik, Wurzburg, W. Germany
R. L. Haynes   Memorial Hospital, Atlanta, GA
R. H. Ingram   Peter Bent Brigham Hospital, Boston, MA
John Kampine   Allen Bradley Medical Sciences Laboratories,
   Milwaukee, WI
Frederick F. Kao   State University of New York, Brooklyn, NY
Leonard P. Latham   University of Colorado Medical Center, Denver, CO
Sanford Levine   Hospital of the University of Pennsylvania,
   Philadelphia, PA
E. R. McFadden, Jr.   Peter Bent Brigham Hospital, Boston, MA
Carlos J. Mendoza   Johns Hopkins University, Baltimore, MD

Hannah H. Peavy   National Institutes of Health, Bethesda, MD
W. E. Pierson   University of Washington, Seattle, WA
John E. Remmers   University of Texas Medical Branch, Galveston, TX
Sanford R. Sampson   University of California, San Francisco, CA
Gail G. Shapiro   University of Washington, Seattle, WA
Nobuo Tanakawa   Jefferson Davis Hospital, Houston, TX
E. H. Vidruk   University of California, San Francisco, CA
Peter D. Wagner   University of California, La Jolla, CA
Wiltz Wagner   University of Colorado Medical Center, Denver, CO
Karlman Wasserman   Harbor General Hospital, Torrance, CA
Brian J. Whipp   Harbor General Hospital, Torrance, CA
William S. Yamamoto   George Washington University Medical Center,
    Washington, DC
S. M. Yamashiro   University of Southern California, Los Angeles, CA

PARTICIPANTS

Deep Aggarwal   University of Wisconsin, Madison, WI
Murray D. Altose   Hospital of the University of Pennsylvania,
    Philadelphia, PA
James W. Bates   University of Wisconsin, Madison, WI
Jean Behrens-Tepper   University of Wisconsin, Madison, WI
Anne Berssenbrugge   Madison General Hospital, Madison, WI
P. V. Bhansali   University of Wisconsin, Madison, WI
Flemming Bonde-Petersen   Southwestern Medical School, Dallas, TX
Sheldon R. Braun   University of Wisconsin, Madison, WI
Eugene N. Bruce   Harvard University School of Public Health,
    Boston, MA
Robert K. Bush   University of Wisconsin, Madison, WI
William Busse   University of Wisconsin, Madison, WI
James I. Carlin   University of Wisconsin, Madison, WI
Frank J. Cerny   University of Windsor, Windsor, Ontario, Canada
Louis W. Chosy   University of Wisconsin, Madison, WI
Chryssanthos Chryssanthopoulos   Milwaukee Children's Hospital,
    Milwaukee, WI
Alan Claremont   University of Wisconsin, Madison, WI
Seymour B. Crepea   Syntex Corporation, Palo Alto, CA
David Cunningham   University of Western Ontario, London, Ontario,
    Canada
Ivan Daskalovic   University of Wisconsin, Madison, WI
Christopher A. Dawson   Medical College of Wisconsin, Milwaukee, WI
Warren Dennis   University of Wisconsin, Madison, WI
G. A. doPico   University of Wisconsin, Madison, WI
Harry P. DuVal   Indiana University, Bloomington, IN
Norman H. Edelman   Rutgers Medical School, Piscataway, NJ
Peyton A. Eggleston   University of Virginia Hospital, Charlottes-
    ville, VA
Geoff Elder   MacMaster University, Hamilton, Ontario, Canada
Jay Paul Farber   University of Iowa, Iowa City, IA
Giles Filley   University of Colorado Medical Center, Denver, CO
Hubert Forster   Allen Bradley Medical Sciences Laboratories,
    Milwaukee, WI

J. Bernard L. Gee   Yale University School of Medicine, New Haven, CT
R. C. Goode   University of Toronto, Toronto, Ontario, Canada
Michael H. Grieco   983 Park Avenue, New York, NY
Peter G. Hanson   University of Wisconsin, Madison, WI
Ralph L. Haynes   2118 Allaire Lane, Atlanta, GA
Franz Igler   Allen Bradley Medical Sciences Laboratories,
    Milwaukee, WI ·
Charles Irvin   University of Wisconsin, Madison, WI
Louis W. Jankowski   Universite de Montreal, Montreal, P.Q., Canada
Anthony Kiorpes   University of Wisconsin, Madison, WI
Howard G. Knuttgen   Boston University and Sargent College, Boston, MA
Shunsaku Koga   University of Wisconsin, Madison, WI
J. Brent Kooistra   University of Wisconsin, Madison, WI
Robert Kriz   University of Wisconsin, Madison, WI
E. H. Lanphier   University of Wisconsin, Madison, WI
Tee-Ping Lee   University of Wisconsin, Madison, WI
Peter Lemon   University of Wisconsin, Madison, WI
S. Martin Mastenbrook, Jr.   University of Wisconsin, Madison, WI
David A. Mathison   Scripps Clinic and Research Foundation,
    La Jolla, CA
Kathleen McCormick   University of Wisconsin, Madison, WI
Howard T. Milhorn, Jr.   University of Mississippi Medical Center,
    Jackson, MS
John P. Mullin   University of Wisconsin, Madison, WI
Timothy Musch   University of Wisconsin, Madison, WI
Francis Nagle   University of Wisconsin, Madison, WI
Gary Niehaus   University of Wisconsin, Madison, WI
E. B. Olson, Jr.   University of Wisconsin, Madison, WI
Dale Pelligrino   University of Wisconsin, Madison, WI
Robert Purvis   University of Wisconsin, Madison, WI
John Rankin   University of Wisconsin, Madison, WI
John H. G. Rankin   Madison General Hospital, Madison, WI
William G. Reddan   University of Wisconsin, Madison, WI
Lawrence C. Rohner   New Mexico State University, Los Cruces, NM
Michael T. Sharratt   University of Waterloo, Waterloo, Canada
James Skatrud   University of Wisconsin, Madison, WI
R. Michael Sly   Louisiana State University Medical Center, New
    Orleans, LA
Laurie Smith   National Institutes of Health, Bethesda, MD
Thomas J. Smith   University of Wisconsin, Madison, WI
Richard Stremel   Harbor General Hospital, Torrance, CA
John Sutton   MacMaster University, Hamilton, Ontario, Canada
George D. Swanson   University of Colorado Medical Center, Denver, CO
Benton C. Taylor   VA Hospital, Madison, WI
Charles M. Tipton   University of Iowa, Iowa City, IA
Monique Wanner   University of Wisconsin, Madison, WI
Phillip Weiser   The National Asthma Center, Denver, CO
James E. Wilkerson   Indiana University, Bloomington, IN
James Will   University of Wisconsin, Madison, WI
Brian A. Wilson   University of Guelph, Ontario, Canada
Edward J. Zuperku   Medical College of Wisconsin and Wood VA Hospital,
    Milwaukee, WI

Index

Abdominal muscles 5, 8-9, 44-46
Acetylcholine
    and cyclic CMP 291
    and irritant receptors 204
    and mast cells 214
Acidosis
    and bronchoconstriction 182,
    187-188, 192-193
    and EIA 282
Adrenergic receptors
    in airways 181, 290
Airway closure 225
    and distribution of ventila-
    tion 229
Alveolar-capillary diffusion
    A-a D_{CO_2} 362
    capillary transit time 321
    charged membrane hypothesis
    364
    cytochrome P-450 357
    DL_{CO} 317, 352, 358
    DL_{CO} and inspired CO 359
    DL_{CO} vs. DL_{O_2} 374
    facilitated diffusion 321, 357
    limitation to pulmonary O_2 trans-
    port 319, 345, 351, 354, 363
    O_2 vs. inert gas diffusion 321,
    357
    vs. placental diffusion 358
Airway resistance
    and distribution of ventila-
    tion 227
    and P_{CO_2} 190
    and sympathetic stimulations
    193
    and vagal stimulation 190
Anaerobic threshold 269
    normal vs. asthmatic children
    271
Anaphylaxis
    and mediator release 215
    and rapidly adapting irritant
    receptors 198
Anaphylatoxins 215
Anesthetics
    effect on smooth muscle 183
Aortic bodies 106
Aspirin
    and bradykinins 213
    and prostaglandin 213, 220

    effect on EIA 296
Asthamtic vs. normal children
    adaptation to exercise 272
    pulmonary function changes
    after exercise 269
Atropine
    as a bronchodilator 294
    effect on EIA 294

Baroreceptors
    and bronchoconstriction 181
Bradykinin 213-214
    and prostaglandin 218
Bronchial lability 249, 252
Bronchial smooth muscle
    and atropine 294
    and bradykinin 214
    and cyclic nucleotides 290
    and ether 183
    and histamine 182, 216
    and morphine 183
    and P_{CO_2} 180, 182, 187-189, 275
    and pH 182, 187-188, 192
    and P_{O_2} 180, 182, 187-188, 190
    and slow reacting substance of
    anaphylaxis and prostaglandins
    182, 219, 291, 296
    and sympathomimetic innervation
    179, 181, 212, 214, 253, 290, 292
    and theophylline 182
Bronchiolar responses 186, 192-193
    to CO_2 192-193
    to histamine 192
    to pH 192-193
    to sympathetic stimulation 193
    to vagal stimulation 192-193
Bronchitis and EIA 249, 251
Bronchoconstriction (see also bronchial
    smooth muscle and EIA)
    and pulmonary artery occlusion
    187-188, 192-193
    and rapidly adapting irritant
    receptors 198
    and vagal reflexes 198
Bronchomotor tone 190

Carbamazine
    effect on EIA 296
Carbon dioxide
    flow and ventilatory drive 68,

MANUFACTURED BY INTER-COLLEGIATE PRESS, INC.
SHAWNEE MISSION, KANSAS

Library of Congress Cataloging in Publication Data
Main entry under title:
Muscular exercise and the lung.
Includes bibliographical references and index.
1. Pulmonary function tests--Congresses. 2. Lungs--
Congresses. 3. Exercise--Physiological effect--
Congresses. 4. Bronchial spasm--Etiology--Congresses.
5. Respiration--Regulation--Congresses. 6. Ventilation
--perfusion ratio--Congresses. I. Dempsey, Jerome A.,
        1938-   II. Reed, Charles E., 1922-
[DNLM: 1. Respiratory system--Physiology--Congresses.
            WF102 M985 1976]
    RC733.M87   612'.2   76-16666
            ISBN 0-299-07220-7